Contemporary Cardiology

Series Editor

Peter P. Toth, Ciccarone Center for the Prevention of Cardiovascular Disease
Johns Hopkins University School of Medicine, Baltimore, MD, USA

For more than a decade, cardiologists have relied on the Contemporary Cardiology series to provide them with forefront medical references on all aspects of cardiology. Each title is carefully crafted by world-renown cardiologists who comprehensively cover the most important topics in this rapidly advancing field. With more than 75 titles in print covering everything from diabetes and cardiovascular disease to the management of acute coronary syndromes, the Contemporary Cardiology series has become the leading reference source for the practice of cardiac care.

Nicolas W. Shammas
Editor

Peripheral Arterial Interventions

Evolving Therapeutic Strategies

Springer

Editor
Nicolas W. Shammas
Midwest Cardiovascular Research Foundation
Davenport, IA, USA

ISSN 2196-8969 ISSN 2196-8977 (electronic)
Contemporary Cardiology
ISBN 978-3-031-09743-0 ISBN 978-3-031-09741-6 (eBook)
https://doi.org/10.1007/978-3-031-09741-6

This Springer imprint is published by the registered company Springer Nature Switzerland AG
The registered company address is: Gewerbestrasse 11, 6330 Cham, Switzerland

I dedicate this book to:

To my wife Gail Shammas for her relentless support and endless love and dedication to her family, to my late father Wahib Shammas who instilled in me discipline and hard work, to my mom Vera Shammas for all her continued sacrifices and love to her family, to my daughter Anna Shammas who makes me laugh and for her pure sweetness, to my sons W John Shammas and Andrew Shammas for their kindness, wonderful hearts, and love to their family, to my siblings Robert, Claudette, and Diana for being there for me when I needed them, and to my patients for being the source of my passion to research, education, and clinical cardiology.

Preface

Peripheral arterial disease (PAD) is a universal problem affecting 10–15% of the general population and is particularly prevalent with age. PAD is a marker for higher cardiovascular events and mortality. A broader approach to treat these patients is of paramount importance to reduce the morbidity and mortality of patients with this disease. There has been a shift in the PAD treatment from a focus on revascularization to implementing aggressive preventative therapies and improving the quality of life of these patients. Pharmacologic and structured exercise interventions are now first steps to improve the symptoms of patients with claudication. Revascularization is typically reserved for claudicants that fail medical therapy, and for patients with advanced limb ischemia with rest pain or ulcerations. Chronic limb-threatening ischemia (CLTI) needs to be addressed aggressively with simultaneous preventative, pharmacologic, and revascularization strategies to reduce its burden of amputation and mortality. Smoking, diabetes, and chronic kidney disease are major risk factors that need to be addressed and controlled. Several pharmacologic interventions including antiplatelets, statins or PCSK-9 inhibitors, low dose rivaroxaban, SGLT2 inhibitors, and others are now available for the endovascular specialist to treat the PAD patient.

The endovascular treatment of peripheral arterial disease has gained momentum and surpassed surgical therapies. Since early endovascular treatment of PAD with balloon angioplasty, multiple newer therapies have emerged including second-generation self-expanding stents, atherectomy devices, specialty balloons and wires, drug-coated balloons and drug-eluting stents, and crossing catheters and devices. The strategy to leave the least metal behind has gained momentum particularly in traditional no-stent zones such as the common femoral and popliteal arteries, younger patients, in-stent restenosis, long and complex disease, and vessels below the knee. An optimal strategy to treat infrainguinal arterial disease with the least metal behind focuses on vessel prepping to gain the maximum minimal luminal area without disruption of the deeper layers of the vessel, protecting the distal vascular bed, and applying antiproliferative therapy to reduce restenosis. Although stenting is endorsed by the guidelines, and in the short- and intermediate term provides good outcomes, loss of patency is evident in the long term along with stent fractures and thrombosis. Carpet stenting becomes a real problem in the long term with a progressive disease that requires multiple recurrent treatments. The least stent approach allows overall excellent results with the combination of vessel prepping and drug-eluting balloons while keeping the doors opened for future therapies, a particularly important strategy in younger patients. Randomized trials have not compared best-stent strategy to a no-stent strategy of vessel prepping and antiproliferative therapy.

In this book, we review peripheral arterial atherogenesis with a focus on risk factors and the global nature of atherosclerotic disease. Exercise and pharmacologic therapies are then discussed followed by a review of strategies and devices and how to approach different plaque morphologies in various vascular beds. Well-powered randomized trials are unfortunately scarce in the field of PAD treatment. However, world experts have been assembled in this book to fill in some of the gaps on how to approach various PAD treatments. The last chapter puts it all together to provide operators an optimal strategy for peripheral arterial interventions.

I am grateful to the many people who have contributed to this book and to the excellent team at Springer for agreeing to publish it. This book is the culmination of efforts by many experts dedicated to improve and prolong the lives of PAD patients. A special thanks to our patients who voluntarily and willingly participated in the many clinical trials that led to advancing this field. For them, we are forever indebted. Furthermore, I could have not done this book without my wonderful wife, Gail Shammas, for her relentless dedication to our research program, and her overwhelming unconditional love and support to me and my family. Finally, I am also grateful to our children W John, Andrew Nicolas, and Anna Elizabeth for appreciating and understanding the need to be away from them for long hours and days, and to the entire Midwest Cardiovascular Research Foundation staff for being there for me when I needed them. I do hope you will enjoy and make good use of this book. This book is not intended to give medical advice or be a substitute to the medical advice or a substitute to the medical judgment and decisions of endovascular specialists and other providers.

Davenport, IA, USA Nicolas W. Shammas

Contents

About the Editor

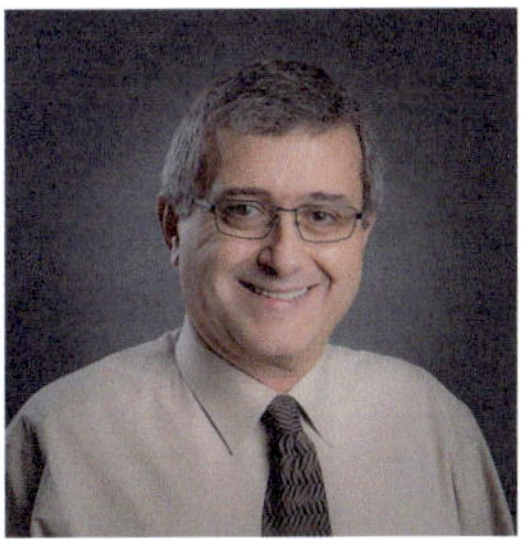

Nicolas Shammas, MD, EJD, MS, FACC, FSCAI, FSVM is the Founder and Research Director of the Midwest Cardiovascular Research Foundation, Iowa, USA. He is also the Medical Director of Cardiology Services at Trinity Bettendorf Hospital and an Adjunct Clinical Associate Professor of Medicine at the University of Iowa Hospitals. Dr. Shammas is also an Interventional Cardiologist at Cardiovascular Medicine, LLC in Davenport, Iowa. He attended the American University of Beirut in Beirut, Lebanon, for his MD and MS in cardiac physiology combined program. Dr. Shammas completed both a residency program and postgraduate training in Interventional Cardiology at the University of Iowa Hospitals and General Cardiology training at the University of Rochester Medical Center in Rochester, New York. Dr. Shammas is board certified in Internal Medicine, Cardiology, Endovascular Medicine, and Interventional Cardiology. Dr. Shammas has published over 425 manuscripts, abstracts, book chapters, and books and participated in over 220 national clinical trials. He was the immediate past Governor of the American College of Cardiology, Iowa Chapter.

Chapter 1
Peripheral Arterial Atherogenesis

Joseph M. Meyer, Thorsten M. Leucker, Steven R. Jones, Seth S. Martin, and Peter P. Toth

Peripheral Artery Disease

The terms describing the diseases of peripheral arteries are not uniformly used [1–3]. In general, *peripheral arterial disease* is atherosclerosis of the vertebral, carotid, mesenteric, and renal arteries and arteries of the upper and lower extremities. *Peripheral artery disease* (PAD) technically refers to atherosclerosis in the upper and lower extremities [4]. However, atherosclerosis of the lower extremities is more common and more often symptomatic and thus will be the focus of this chapter [5]. Atherosclerosis of the upper extremities most commonly involves the brachiocephalic trunk and subclavian and axillary arteries [1]. The clinical spectrum of PAD ranges from asymptomatic to critical limb ischemia (CLI) with limb loss (Table 1.1). CLI is due to chronic ischemia with ankle pressures usually ≤50 mmHg and is defined by rest pain or gangrene [6]. Chronic PAD severity is staged by the Fontaine or Rutherford classifications (Table 1.2). Non-atherosclerotic processes, such as external compression, vasculitis, or embolism, may mimic the signs and symptoms of PAD, but are separate entities of peripheral *arterial* disease and will not be addressed in this chapter.

J. M. Meyer · T. M. Leucker · S. R. Jones · S. S. Martin
Ciccarone Center for the Prevention of Cardiovascular Disease, Johns Hopkins University School of Medicine, Baltimore, MD, USA
e-mail: jmeyer52@jhmi.edu; tleucke1@jhmi.edu; sjones64@jhmi.edu; smart100@jhmi.edu

P. P. Toth (✉)
Ciccarone Center for the Prevention of Cardiovascular Disease, Johns Hopkins University School of Medicine, Baltimore, MD, USA

CGH Medical Center, Sterling, IL, USA
e-mail: Peter.toth@cghmc.com

N. W. Shammas (ed.), *Peripheral Arterial Interventions*, Contemporary Cardiology, https://doi.org/10.1007/978-3-031-09741-6_1

Table 1.1 Common terms to describe the symptoms of peripheral artery disease

	Hemodynamics	Limb symptoms	Function
Asymptomatic PAD	Abnormal ABI at rest or after exercise[a] or other objective evidence of PAD (duplex ultrasound, computed tomographic angiography, magnetic resonance angiography)	None recognized	Limited date available, but reduced walking endurance and slower walking velocity have been documented; rate of decline in walking performance is at least as great as for patients with intermittent claudication
Atypical claudication	Abnormal ABI at rest or after exercise	Leg pain on exertion that is not consistent with classic "claudication"; may include calf, thigh, or buttock	Limited walking distance and exercise performance due to PAD may be present; symptoms may or may not be reproducible on a daily basics as for classic claudication
Claudication	Abnormal ABI at rest or after exercise	Reproducible lower-extremity muscle fatigue or discomfort on exertion, relieved by rest within 10 min	Limited walking distance, exercise performance due to PAD
Critical limb ischemia	Hemodynamics evidence of severe PAD	Distal leg pain at rest, with or without ischemic ulcers or gangrene	Very limited, usually ambulatory only for short distance
Acute limb ischemia	Hemodynamics evidence of severe PAD	Acute limb pain, neurological dysfunction	Very limited as above
Additional terms			
Nonvascular claudication	Normal leg hemodynamics at rest and with exercise	Typical or atypical limb discomfort with effort	May be caused by rheumatologic or neuromuscular disease

ABI ankle–brachial index

Table from Hiatt [4]

[a] An abnormal ABI has previously been defined as <0.90, but recent evidence suggests that an ABI <1.00 is indicative of PAD and an increased risk of systemic atherosclerotic events. In the presence of diabetes mellitus, pressure measurements may be unreliable in some patients

PAD is traditionally defined by the resting ankle brachial pressure index (ABI) <0.9, which is the ratio of ankle blood pressure to brachial artery blood pressure. If abnormal, segmental blood pressure measurements of the lower extremity may be performed to localize the stenosis. On physical exam, PAD may manifest as diminished or absent distal pulses, a femoral bruit, or discoloration of the lower extremity, particularly pallor with elevation or dependent rubor. Other means to diagnose PAD include the toe-brachial index (TBI), tissue oxygen pressure (TcPO2), and skin perfusion pressure, which may be particularly useful when clinical suspicion is high despite a normal ABI, or when ABI >1.4, which suggests the artery is noncompressible secondary to extensive calcification.

Table 1.2 Peripheral artery disease severity described by the Fontaine and Rutherford classifications

Stages of peripheral artery disease		
Fontaine classification		
	Stage I	Asymptomatic
	Stage II	Intermittent claudication without rest pain
	IIa	Claudication walking >200 m
	IIb	Claudication walking <200 m
	Stage III	Nocturnal pain or pain at rest
	Stage IV	Tissue loss (ulcers or gangrene)
Rutherford classification		
Grade 0	Category 0	Asymptomatic
Grade I	Category 1	Mild claudication
	Category 2	Moderate claudication
	Category 3	Severe claudication
Grade II	Category 4	Ischemic rest pain
Grade III	Category 5	Minor tissue loss
	Category 6	Major tissue loss

Adapted from Aboyans [1]

Epidemiology and Risk Factors

PAD is a common disease with growing worldwide prevalence, particularly in low- and middle-income countries (LMIC). Globally, an estimated 236.6 million people, or 5.6% of the population aged 25 or older, are living with PAD as of 2015, an increase from 202 million in 2010 [7, 8]. Between 2010 and 2015, the rise in PAD was mostly observed in LMIC, where the prevalence rose over 22% compared to a 4.5% rise in high-income countries (HIC) [7].

The prevalence of PAD increases with age, particularly in HIC where the odds of PAD increased 65% for each decade of life over age 25 years [7]. PAD steadily rises after age 50, with a prevalence of 5.7% in patients aged 50–54, 9.1% in patients aged 60–64, 14.1% in patients aged 70–74, 21.2% in patients aged 80–84, and 31.3% in patients aged 90 and older (Fig. 1.1). As the share of the US population above age 65 is expected to continue to rise, the total burden of PAD is also expected to rise [9]. In LMIC, factors such as rising pollution, sedentary lifestyle, psychological stressors, and adoption of the Western diet may explain the recent rise of PAD in these countries, which is expected to continue increasing [3]. In the USA, it is estimated that approximately 30% of African American men and 27.6% of African American women will develop PAD by the age of 80, compared to an estimated 19% of white men and women and 22% of Hispanic men and women [10]. This racial difference remains even after adjusting for traditional risk factors [10], and socioeconomic factors that limit access to healthcare and risk factor modification likely account for some of this disparity [11].

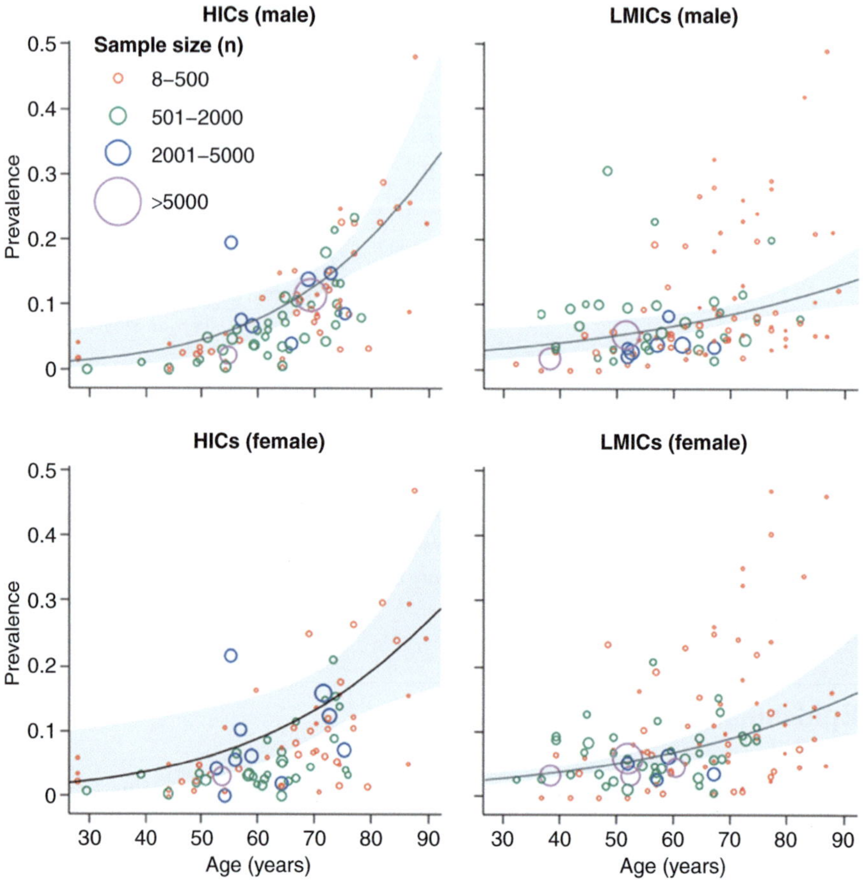

Fig. 1.1 Prevalence of peripheral artery disease in high-income countries (HIC) and low- to medium-income countries (LMIC) by sex. Prevalence rises with age for men and women. (Figure from Song [7]. This is an open-access article distributed under the terms of the Creative Commons CC-BY license, which permits unrestricted use, distribution, and reproduction in any medium, provided the original work is properly cited. You are not required to obtain permission to reuse this article)

Other significant risk factors for PAD include a history of cigarette smoking and diabetes [12]. Hypertension, dyslipidemia, concomitant cardiovascular disease (CVD), and renal dysfunction are also associated with PAD (Table 1.3) [7, 10]. While early studies recognized male sex as a risk factor, a more contemporary sample suggests that women <65 years of age are 24% more likely to have PAD (ABI <0.9) compared to men, a finding that was attenuated but remained even in older age [10]. A meta-analysis of worldwide population data showed men were 26% less likely to have PAD than women after adjustment for risk factors, including age by decade, driven primarily by women in LMIC despite these women having lower prevalence of current smoking, hypertension, and diabetes [7]. In the Reduction of

Table 1.3 Risk of peripheral artery disease for common risk factors, expressed as odds ratios (OR)

Risk factor	OR (95% CI)
Age (per 10-year increase)	1.55 (1.38–1.75)
Male sex	0.74 (0.61–0.91)
Current smoker	2.82 (2.0–3.98)
Former smoker	1.70 (1.39–2.09)
Hypertension	1.67 (1.50–1.86)
Diabetes	1.89 (1.68–2.13)
Hypercholesterolemia	1.34 (1.17–1.53)
Cardiovascular disease	2.31 (1.89–2.83)
Obesity	0.96 (0.82–1.13)
Renal impairment[a]	1.79 (1.03–3.12)

Data are from pooled observational studies of worldwide populations
Adapted from Song [7]
[a] High-income countries only

Atherothrombosis for Continued Health (REACH) registry, a large, diverse sample of outpatients with established CVD (coronary, cerebrovascular, or peripheral) showed these atherosclerotic diseases have a broad overlap of risk factors, yet only one in six patients had symptomatic polyvascular disease (disease of two or more vascular territories). [13] This finding suggests that while atherosclerosis is a systemic disease, risk factor exposure affects individual patients differently. While there is significant overlap in risk factors in ASCVD, cigarette smoking and diabetes are strongly linked to PAD [14]. Observational data suggest that current smokers have a two- to threefold increase in risk of developing PAD [3, 7]. Patients with diabetes are particularly at risk for severe complications of PAD, namely, due to reduced recognition of wounds due to diabetic neuropathy and poor wound healing [15].

The clinical phenotype of PAD also varies depending on the presence of risk factors. Among consecutive patients undergoing endovascular therapy for PAD (Fontaine Stages II–IV), the distribution of PAD was classified as iliac (proximal), femoropopliteal, or crural (distal) [14]. As depicted in Fig. 1.2 with the reference comparator of femoropopliteal disease, current smoking and hypercholesterolemia are associated with proximal disease, whereas age and diabetes are more highly associated with distal disease. Hypertension has a relatively uniform impact on all vascular territories, and male sex is more prevalent in proximal and distal disease. Similar results were found in a large sample of outpatients referred for PAD evaluation, which re-demonstrated proximal and distal phenotypes of PAD linked to specific risk factors: smoking, hypertension, and dyslipidemia associated with proximal disease and older age, male sex, and diabetes associated with distal disease [16]. However, it is not currently possible to accurately prognosticate outcomes based on disease location, likely due to the heterogeneous nature of PAD and differing clinical status of selected patients [16, 17].

The presence and severity of PAD are associated with increased morbidity and mortality [18–27]. Regardless of the presence of symptoms, patients with PAD are

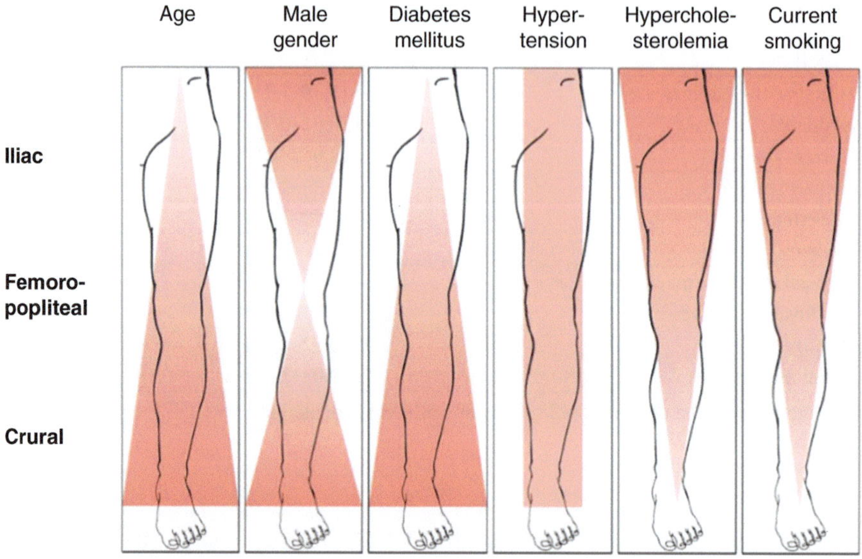

Fig. 1.2 Association of risk factors to the distribution of target lesions in a group of patients with endovascular intervention for peripheral artery disease. Disease was classified as iliac (proximal), femoropopliteal, or crural (distal), and wider and darker shading represents increase prevalence for a given risk factor. (Figure from Diehm [14])

less active, have reduced functional capacity, and have reduced quality of life [18, 19]. The incidence of all-cause mortality was 19% after 5 years in patients with asymptomatic PAD, which was nearly 50% higher than healthy controls. Furthermore, the risk of disease progression from asymptomatic PAD to intermittent claudication (IC) was 7% and IC to critical limb ischemia was 21% after 5 years [20, 21]. Perhaps predictably, all-cause mortality in symptomatic patients was even higher, occurring in 27% of patients after 5 years with a 2.8-fold higher rate of CV mortality compared to healthy controls [20]. The risk of CV and all-cause mortality increases as the ABI becomes progressively more abnormal (either <0.9 or >1.4) [22], and the addition of ABI improves risk prediction when combined with the Framingham risk score [23]. Among symptomatic patients with PAD in the Examining Use of Ticagrelor in Peripheral Artery Disease (EUCLID) trial, 10.7% of patients experienced CV death, myocardial infarction, or ischemic stroke; 1.7% of patients were hospitalized for acute limb ischemia; and 12.5% underwent lower extremity revascularization over a 30-month follow-up period [24]. The French COhorte de Patients ARTériopathes (COPART) registry followed 940 hospitalized patients with PAD. The risk of mortality and amputation increased with severity of symptoms, ranging from IC to rest pain, and ultimately tissue loss. In patients with tissue loss, mortality was highest at 28.7%, and the rate of amputation was 24.2% at 1 year [25]. More than half of amputees require contralateral amputation within 3 years, and mortality was as high as 50% at 5 years after first amputation [26]. In a population study in Germany, the risk of CV events, amputation, or mortality increased significantly with Rutherford category (Fig. 1.3). Even among patients

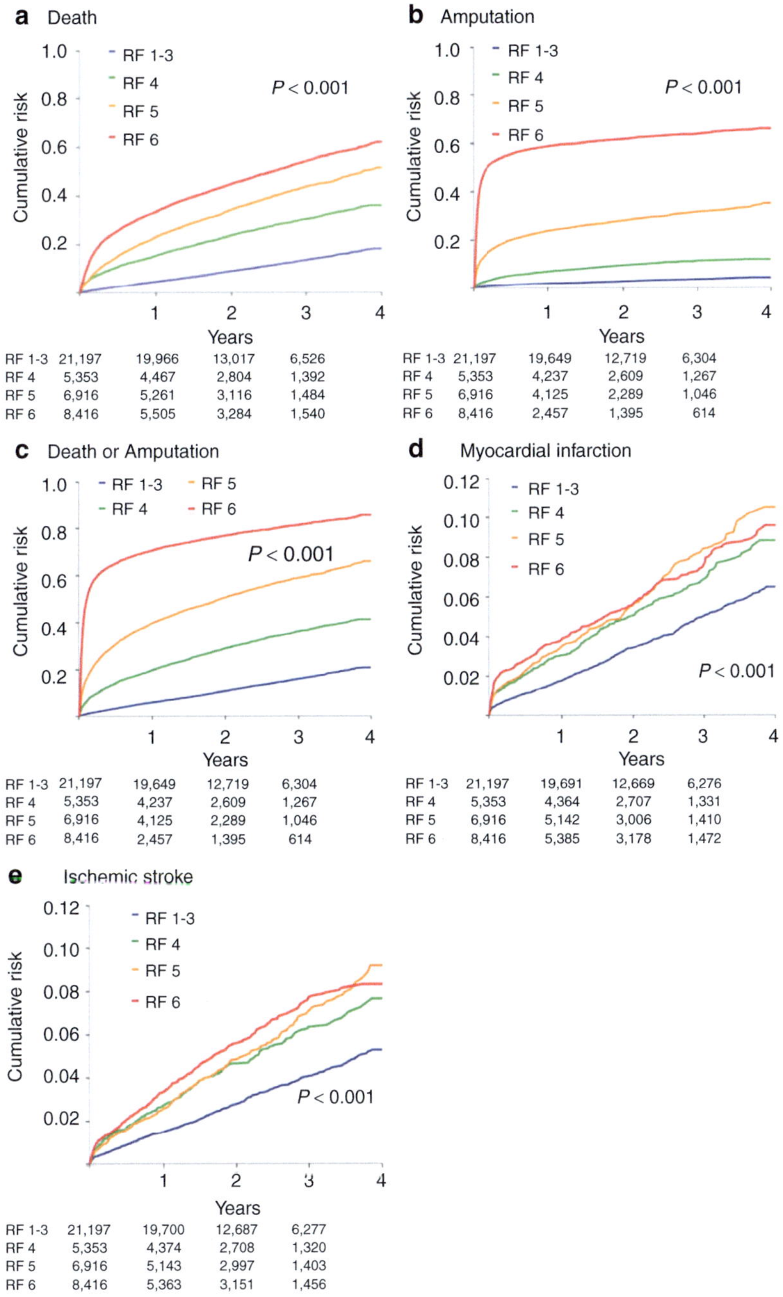

Fig. 1.3 Kaplan-Meier curves in a population with peripheral artery disease. The rate of death (**a**), amputation (**b**), myocardial infarction (**c**), death or amputation (**d**), and ischemic stroke (**e**) generally increased with increasing Rutherford category, a measure of disease severity. The p value is a log-rank test to determine differences between subgroups. (Figure from Reinecke [27])

with less severe PAD (Rutherford categories 1–3), the risk of amputation and mortality was 4.6 and 18.9% at 4-year follow-up, respectively, and the incidence of myocardial infarction and ischemic stroke after 4 years was 6.6% and 5.4%, respectively [27].

In summary, while risk factors associated with PAD overlap with other CVD, there is significant heterogeneity in the location and severity of atherosclerosis. However, once PAD is clinically apparent, the risk of death, limb amputation, myocardial infarction, and stroke rises, and this risk further increases as PAD becomes more severe and symptomatic.

Detection of PAD

Clinical Findings and Imaging

PAD may be diagnosed after a complete history and physical, but is often detected by non-invasive imaging techniques in asymptomatic patients [1]. The classic symptom of PAD is IC, which is muscle discomfort, cramping, or pain distal to an arterial stenosis that is consistently induced with exercise and relieved with rest [2]. As the superficial femoral artery (SFA) most commonly develops obstructive disease, calf pain is most commonly reported as the presenting symptom [28]. Atypical leg symptoms, defined as pain that does not involve the calves or does not resolve with 10 min of rest, are also common [2, 29]. In patients who do not report IC, 39% of patients developed leg pain during a 6-min walk test, suggesting patient inactivity may mask inducible leg ischemia [30]. Patients may also develop non-healing wounds or gangrene, which should trigger an evaluation for PAD [2].

In clinical practice, PAD screening is recommended for patients aged 65 years or older; patients aged 50–64 with risk factors for atherosclerosis (e.g., diabetes, cigarette smoking history, hyperlipidemia, hypertension, or family history of PAD); patients <50 years with type 1 diabetes mellitus and one additional risk factor for atherosclerosis; or those with known atherosclerotic disease in another vascular bed [2, 31]. It is estimated that only 20–33% of patients with PAD will have IC, making it important for clinicians to screen patients at high risk of the disease and explain why PAD is under-detected in routine clinical practice [1]. In the Progression of Early Subclinical Atherosclerosis (PESA) study, 4184 bank employees ranging from 40 to 54 years of age without CVD were screened with ABI, vascular ultrasound, and computed tomography (CT) scan. This evaluation revealed that 71% of men and 48% of women had subclinical atherosclerosis, of which ilio-femoral disease was the most common (53% of men and 29% of women) [32]. Disease progression by 3 years correlated significantly with baseline ASCVD risk [33]. In the MESA (Multi-Ethnic Study of Atherosclerosis) study, 16.8% of the population had an abnormal ABI (defined in the study as <1.0 or >1.3) despite not having traditional ASCVD risk factors [34]. Furthermore, while the ABI is the standard for diagnosing PAD, 21% of patients undergoing revascularization for CLI had normal preoperative ABIs (0.91–1.4), 11% had non-compressible ABI (>1.4), and only 16% had ABI ≤0.4 [35]. The IN.PACT DEEP (Randomized IN.PACT Amphirion Drug-Coated Balloon vs. Standard Percutaneous Transluminal Angioplasty for the Treatment of Below-the-Knee Critical Limb Ischemia) trial found similar results with a normal (0.91–1.4) and severely abnormal ABI (<0.4) in 19% and 6% of patients, respectively [36].

Consequently, vascular imaging is useful to obtain additional anatomic information. Duplex ultrasound, CT and magnetic resonance (MR) angiography, or invasive angiography can all localize and characterize PAD [2]. Functional imaging, such as flow-mediated dilation (FMD) of the brachial artery, may offer additional prognostic information, as FMD is predictive of events in symptomatic patients with PAD and an ABI <0.9 (particularly with an ABI <0.65) [37].

Biomarkers

As PAD is often underrecognized, there is increasing interest in biomarkers to detect and assess the severity of disease. General categories of biomarkers for PAD with some common examples are listed in Table 1.4 [40]. Levels of circulating oxidized phospholipids (OxPLs) and lipoprotein (a) (Lp(a)), the latter the major carrier of OxPL in plasma, are both correlated with an increased risk of PAD with nearly a twofold increased risk in the highest tertile [41]. A recent meta-analysis evaluated a number of biomarkers, including inflammatory markers (high-sensitivity C-reactive protein (hs-CRP), growth differentiation factor 15 (GDF-15), myeloperoxidase, the neutrophil-lymphocyte ratio (NLR)), coagulation markers (fibrinogen, D-dimer), cardiac markers (high-sensitivity cardiac troponin T (hs-cTnT) and N-terminal pro-brain natriuretic peptide (NT-proBNP)), and markers of arterial damage (asymmetric dimethylarginine (ADMA), adiponectin, and homocysteine) [42]. Each of these parameters is associated with a relatively modest increase in mortality, major acute coronary events (MACE) or major adverse limb events (MALE), ranging from a 1.2- to 4.6-fold increase in patients with PAD. P-selectin is marginally associated with prevalence and incidence of PAD (OR 1.17 [1.11–1.53] and OR 1.30 [1.11–1.53], respectively) [43].

Other novel biomarkers have also been assessed, including noncoding RNA, proprotein convertase subtilisin/kexin type 9 (PCSK9), endothelial progenitor cells (EPCs), thrombospondin-1 (TSP-1), and trimethylamine N-oxide (TMAO), as well as genetic factors. Noncoding RNAs, including microRNAs (miRNA) and long noncoding RNAs (lncRNA), are important regulators of mRNA expression and are linked to PAD. A number of circulating miRNA were identified to discriminate patients with PAD from normal, matched controls, including miRNA involved in vascular endothelial growth factor-A (VEGF-A) and transforming growth factor β (TGF-β) signaling and vascular adhesion [40, 44]. Of these, miR-15b, miR-16, and

Table 1.4 General categories of biomarkers for peripheral artery disease by pathophysiologic pathway with some representative examples

Pathophysiologic pathway	Biomarkers
Inflammatory cytokines and acute-phase reactant proteins	• CRP • IL-6 • β_2-microglobulin • TNF-α[a] • SAA
Markers of endothelial cells/ leukocyte activation and chemokines	• VCAM-1 • ICAM-1 • P-selectin • MCP-1 • CD40 ligand • MPO
Markers of thrombosis cascade	• VWF • tPA • D-dimer • tPA antigen • PAI antigen • VWF:ADAMTS13 ratio • Fibrinogen
Lipids, apolipoproteins, and phospholipids	• Lp-PLA_2 • Lipoprotein(a)
Modulators of angiogenesis	• VEGF-A • Soluble tunica intima endothelial kinase 2 (TIE-2) • Angiopoietin-2
Oxidative stress and other biomarkers	• Homocysteine • ADMA • Glutathione peroxidase 1 activity • 8-isoprostaglandin $F_{2\alpha}$ • Heme oxygenase-1 • Matrix metalloproteinases [38, 39]
Circulating microRNAs	microRNAs let 7e, miR-15b, -16, -20b, -25, -26b, -27b, -28-5p, -126, -195, -335, -363, -130a, -210, and -27b

ADMA asymmetric dimethylarginine, *CRP* C-reactive protein, *ICAM-1* intercellular adhesion molecule-1, *La PLA2* lipoprotein associated phospholipid A2, *MCP-1* monocyte chemoattractant protein-1, *MPO* myeloperoxidase, *PAI* plasminogen activator inhibitor, *SAA* serum amyloid apolipoprotein, *TNF-α* tumor necrosis factor-α, *tPA* tissue plasminogen activator, *VCAM-1* vascular cell adhesion molecule-1, *VEGF-A* vascular endothelial growth factor A, *VWF* von Willebrand factor
Table from Hazarika [40]

miR-363 were most predictive (receiver operating characteristic AUC >0.92) [44]. Most of the identified miRNA are downregulated, resulting in increased expression of downstream genes. Only miRNA-210 was found to have significantly higher expression in atherosclerotic plaque [45], suggesting that depletion of circulating miRNA is not related to translocation into plaques. miRNA-26b, which is downregulated in PAD [44] and acute ischemia [46], enhances angiogenesis, as well as endothelial cell (EC) survival and proliferation [46]. A number of miRNA are linked to angiogenesis, EC health and permeability, cholesterol regulation, and macrophage phenotype switching, to name a few key regulatory mechanisms (fully reviewed elsewhere [47]). Several lncRNA are linked to angiogenesis, particularly in hypoxic conditions, but are less conserved between mice and humans making them more difficult to study [47]. Noncoding RNAs offer potential diagnostic and therapeutic utility, but will require further investigation prior to routine clinical use.

PCSK9 regulates low-density lipoprotein receptor (LDLR) degradation in the liver (reviewed elsewhere [48]). Commercially available PCSK9 inhibitors have demonstrated significant reductions in low-density lipoprotein (LDL) cholesterol and CV events, as well as a modest reduction in Lp(a) [49, 50]. PCSK9 inhibition also significantly reduced the risk of MALE by 42% in patients with PAD enrolled in the FOURIER (Further Cardiovascular Outcomes Research with PCSK9 Inhibition in Subjects With Elevated Risk) trial [51]. Additionally, administration of a PCSK9 inhibitor improved coronary endothelial function at 6-week follow-up as measured by coronary MR imaging [52]. Comparing patients with intermittent claudication with matched controls, plasma PCSK9 and Lp(a) were both significantly higher in patients after controlling for multiple ASCVD risk factors, including smoking and diabetes [53]. PCSK9 was significantly higher in a population with asymptomatic PAD (ABI <0.9) compared to patients at risk without atherosclerotic disease, and PCSK9 was significantly higher as the extent of PAD worsened as assessed by CT angiography [54].

Tissue ischemia increases circulating EPCs, suggesting a possible role to augment neovascularization [55]. In patients with PAD, while circulating EPCs were significantly higher than controls, the proangiogenic capacity of these circulating EPCs was reduced [54]. Additionally, levels of apoptotic circulating ECs were also higher. Interestingly, the higher levels of circulating EPCs were previously shown to associate with a lower risk of CV mortality and ASCVD events in patients with CAD, but these EPCs were also dysfunctional [56]. Understanding how EPC level and function are regulated in PAD requires further investigation, particularly relative to other atherosclerotic diseases.

TSP-1 is significantly elevated in patients with PAD relative to normal controls [57]. TSP-1 is increased in response to ischemia and is released by activated platelets, whereas other angiogenic growth factors including VEGF and placental growth factor (PlGF) were not significantly different. TSP-1 has both pro- and anti-angiogenic properties and remains a possible diagnostic and therapeutic target for PAD [57].

TMAO levels may help assess PAD severity and predict CV and all-cause mortality. TMAO is a gut-derived metabolite of dietary choline that modulates platelet reactivity and increases thrombotic risk in a dose-dependent manner and is, in part, believed responsible for the increased risk of CV events in Western diets [58]. In symptomatic patients with IC or CLI, TMAO levels were associated with PAD severity and CV mortality (particularly when levels exceeded 2.26 μmol/L) [59].

Specific genetic factors correlate with PAD risk. Using genetic data from the Million Veteran Program, a large sample identified 19 loci associated with PAD

[60]. Of these, 11 were also associated with atherosclerosis of coronary and carotid arteries, including lipid-related genes (*LDLR*, *LPL*, and *LPA*, corresponding to LDL receptor, lipoprotein lipase, and Lp(a)), hypertension (*PTPN11)*, and diabetes (*TCF7L2)*. However, four were unique to PAD, most notably *F5* variant responsible for Factor V Leiden, supporting the observation that thrombus formation may be particularly important in the pathogenesis of PAD.

Given the heterogeneity of PAD, it remains possible that a marked abnormality of a specific biomarker could help individualize treatment (e.g., as a hypothetical example, if a pro-coagulation marker was high, a patient may derive greater benefit from anticoagulation). However, further investigation of biomarkers and response to therapies is required.

Vascular Anatomy and Rheology

The primitive embryonic vascular plexus is generated by angioblasts derived from mesodermal cells during vasculogenesis [61]. We learned from animal studies that vascular cords are established starting on embryologic day 6.5–7 through a complex process of cell proliferation, migration, and aggregation that creates the primitive vascular network required to support ensuing organ development [62]. Angiogenesis is the process of expanding the primitive network by forming new blood vessels from the existing vascular plexus, and this begins by embryologic day 9.5 [62]. ECs, derived from angioblasts, are activated to proliferate, secrete matrix metalloproteinases (MMPs), and migrate toward angiogenic factors, such as VEGF [63]. The subsequent primitive vessels are stabilized and form the expansive network of closed-circuit blood vessels, including arteries, arterioles, capillaries, veins, and lymphatic vessels [62, 63]. As will be further described below, angiogenesis can be triggered in the setting of lower extremity ischemia. The lower extremity artery anatomy and Doppler pulse waveforms are shown in Fig. 1.4.

Arterial blood flow in the lower extremities is dependent on upstream pressure and downstream resistance. At rest, the lower extremities receive approximately one-third of the blood volume passing through the thoracic aorta and have a relatively high vascular resistance in the low metabolic state. The remaining two-thirds of blood perfuse the low-resistance renal arteries and celiac artery [66]. With activity, lower extremity arteries vasodilate in response to hypoxia and sympathetic stimulation [67, 68]. The resulting reduction in vascular resistance coupled with the rise in cardiac output increases blood flow to the lower extremities to try to match metabolic demand. This normal response involves a complex interaction of local and systemic signaling (biochemical and neurological) to affect arteries and their constituent wall components [67].

Even in the apparently healthy population, the lower extremity (particularly iliofemoral region) is commonly the first anatomic location to develop atherosclerosis [32]. It has been recognized that atherosclerotic lesions tend to occur at atheroprone regions where blood flow is non-laminar, which occurs primarily at vessel

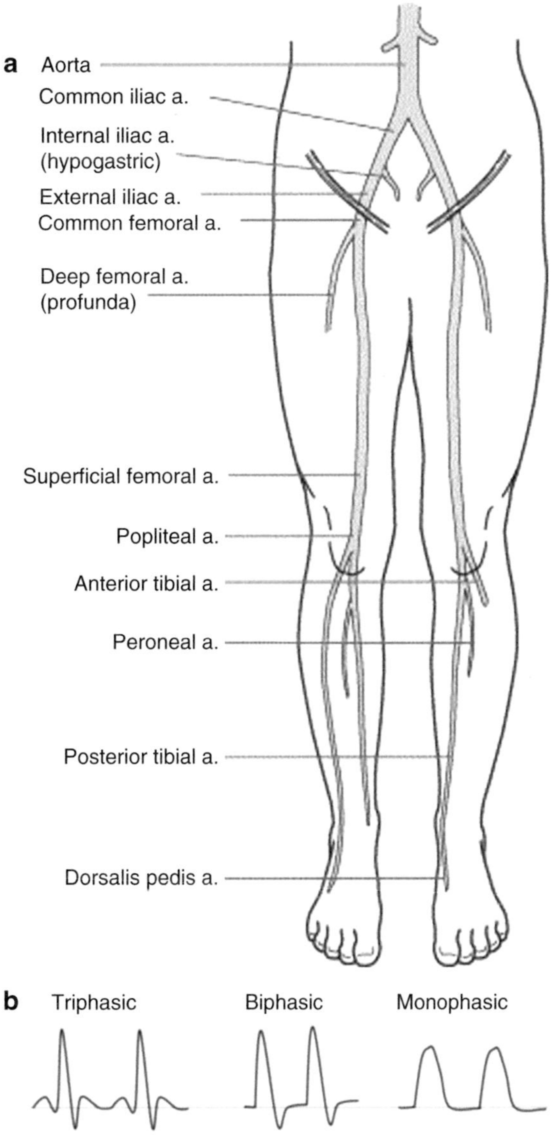

Fig. 1.4 (**a**) Arteries of the lower extremity. (**b**) Schematic tracings of arterial Doppler signals of the lower extremities. Normal Doppler signals are triphasic with a sharp systolic upstroke, short retrograde wave, and diastolic runoff. With proximal stenosis, the waveform is initially biphasic, but eventually becomes monophasic with severe arterial obstruction. (Figures from Sieggreen [64] and Del Conde [65])

arborization or curvature where there is low shear stress, high oscillatory flow, or turbulent flow [69, 70]. The SFA is a common site for atherosclerosis particularly within the adductor canal, a region where the artery passes through muscle bodies with marked tortuosity. This region was noted to form early atherosclerosis in a spiral distribution, suggesting that blood flow disturbances play a role in atherosclerosis [71]. The hemodynamic pattern of flow in the SFA in young men and women was mapped with MR imaging, showing complex cross-sectional flow patterns with distinct longitudinal regions of low shear stress and oscillatory shear. These locations of disturbed flow are similar to the distribution of atherosclerosis seen in postmortem samples [71]. The pathophysiology of atherosclerosis in these athero-prone regions is further described below.

Arterial Structure

Arterial walls consist of three tunicae, the intima, media, and adventitia, each of which plays an essential role in normal blood flow and regulation (Fig. 1.5) [72, 73]. These layers are separated by two layers of elastin, the inner and outer elastic laminae, and the components of each vessel layer vary based on the size and function of

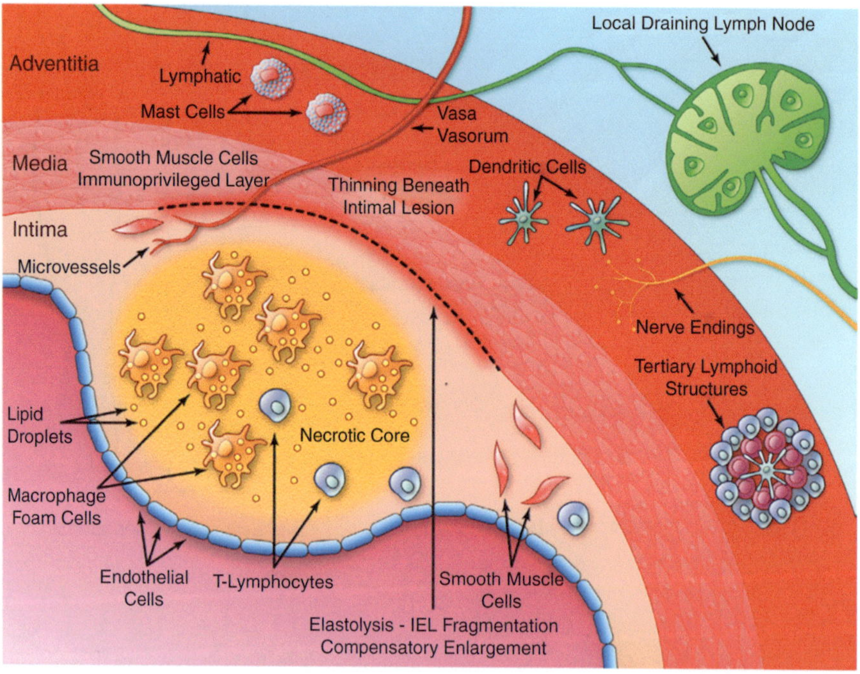

Fig. 1.5 Depiction of the arterial wall, consisting of the vascular lumen and three tunicae (or layers), the intima, media, and adventitia. The endothelium is a continuous layer of endothelial cells that lines the vascular lumen. Vascular smooth muscle cells are the predominant cell in the media in the normal artery. The adventitia contains resident immune cells that can be activated in response to inflammatory signals. In large arteries with a wall exceeding 0.5 mm, a small blood vessel network called the vasa vasorum supplies nutrients and a pathway for cellular migration. Arteries are also supported by a lymphatic system that removes cholesterol via the reverse cholesterol transport system, as well as other cellular debris and fluid. Inflammatory cells migrate and differentiate in attempt to clear the pro-inflammatory lipids that are retained in the subendothelial space. (Figure from Libby [72])

the artery. Three additional components support the normal function of arteries, including the vasa vasorum, autonomic nerves, and lymphatic vessels.

The most inner layer, the tunica intima, has a single, continuous layer of ECs attached to a basement membrane composed of a thin elastin layer called the internal elastic lamina. ECs are aligned parallel to the direction of blood flow, except at branch points, and any disruption of orientation (e.g., with vascular trauma) is rapidly corrected [74]. ECs in atheroprone areas are often disorganized and fail to align [75]. In a model allowing acute changes in blood flow direction, endothelial nitric oxide synthetase (eNOS) was maximally activated when flow was parallel to the orientation of ECs, whereas the inflammatory NF-κB (nuclear factor kappa-light-chain-enhancer of activated B cells) pathway was activated with perpendicular flow [76]. Furthermore, perpendicular flow results in higher levels of reactive oxygen species (ROS) and lower nitric oxide (NO) generation. These effects were suppressed if ECs were not aligned, suggesting EC alignment is important to maintain normal function [76]. ECs exhibit significant structural and biochemical variation across the vascular tree depending on the local tissue. Veins and arteries, responsible for the transfer of blood to and from the heart, have a continuous layer of ECs that limits extravasation, while capillaries, particularly those of filtering organs like the liver and kidney, have a fenestrated or even discontinuous endothelial layer that enables the tissue to function [77]. ECs vary in thickness, ranging from 0.1 μm in capillaries to 1 μm in the aorta, and have a total surface area of 4000–7000 m^2 in adults [74, 78, 79].

The middle layer is the tunica media and contains layers of vascular smooth muscle cells (VSMCs) intermixed with an extracellular matrix (ECM) composed of elastic and collagen fibers. Collagen fibers of the ECM are aligned predominately circumferentially to restrict pulsatile expansion under physiologic conditions. VSMCs are responsible for maintaining the ECM and inducing vascular constriction or relaxation; the latter is regulated by ECs and autonomic signaling.

The outer tunica adventitia is a complex milieu containing resident inflammatory cells, autonomic and nociceptive nerves, vasa vasorum, and lymphatics. While this layer was previously overlooked for its biological role, it is now clear the adventitia plays an essential role in normal vascular function, as well as in atherogenesis. The adventitia houses a number of resident cells types, including fibroblasts, pericytes, and immune cells, including macrophages, dendritic cells, T and B cells, and mast cells [80]. While the intima has EPCs and the media has vascular smooth muscle progenitor cells, the adventitia has multiple types of progenitors, including VSMC, EPCs, mesenchymal stem cells, and myeloid progenitor cells. These progenitor cells are particularly numerous in the stem cell niche (or vasculogenic zone) at the outer interface of the media and adventitia [80]. Fibroblasts are the most numerous cell type in healthy adventitia and are responsible for synthesizing type I and type III collagen. Collagen fibers in the adventitia are stiffer with a biaxial alignment (circumferential and axial) and are primarily responsible for limiting axial (longitudinal) expansion [81]. Under healthy conditions, the adventitia is thought to serve primarily in immunosurveillance and cell trafficking while providing structural and nutrient support to the artery [80–82].

The vasa vasorum are microvessels that penetrate from the adventitia to supply blood to the media. When the arterial wall exceeds 0.5 mm (>29 lamellar units), simple diffusion from the tunica intima or adventitia is inadequate to supply the metabolic requirements of the VSMCs [80, 83].

Autonomic innervation of the artery, acting through ECs or VSMC, is partly responsible for regulating vascular tone. Perivascular nerves are confined to the adventitia and are not known to penetrate into the media regardless of vessel size [80]. Both parasympathetic and sympathetic nerve endings release neurotransmitters intercellularly that bind ECs or VSMCs to induce constriction or relaxation [80, 84].

Finally, an extensive lymphatic plexus surrounds arteries to support the removal of extravasated fluid, solutes, and macromolecules, including lipids and immune cells. Cholesterol homeostasis in peripheral tissues is heavily dependent on the reverse cholesterol transport (RCT) pathway and high-density lipoprotein (HDL), and this will be described further below [85, 86]. Lymphatic vessels are also important for immunosurveillance and immunoregulation. Lymphocytes and antigen-presenting cells that return from the periphery via the lymphatic system can induce an immune response to pathogens. Additionally, the lymphatic system directly removes antigens and cytokines and thus influences the intensity and duration of the immune response [85].

Normal Function of the Endothelium

Given its location at the interface between blood and tissues, the endothelium is a key regulator of vascular hemostasis and responds to various physical and chemical signals. As ECs are directly exposed to blood, they play a crucial role in barrier function, trafficking nutrients and cells, regulating blood flow and thrombogenesis, as well as angiogenesis [39, 74].

In its most basic role, the endothelium serves as a physical semi-permeable barrier between the blood and the surrounding tissue. ECs are linked by two main types of intercellular junctions that are responsible for cell-to-cell adhesion: tight junctions and adherens junctions [74, 87]. A third type called gap junctions mediates cell-to-cell communication [87]. The spatial distribution of these junctions varies based on the primary function of the vessel, and tight junctions, in particular, control vessel permeability. For example, proximal arteries have a well-developed network of tight junctions to withstand the arterial pulsatility and pressure of conduit arteries. In conduit arteries with a continuous endothelial layer, only particles under 3 nm in molecular radius (M_r) cross paracellularly (between ECs), which includes water, glucose, and amino acids, and their migration is dictated by solute gradients and Starling forces [88]. More distally, this tight network becomes porous, which allows the transcellular transfer of cells and nutrients [74]. Consistent with this, ECs of specific organs express unique transcriptomes, further suggesting ECs serve their local environment [89]. Hemodynamic shear stress regulates EC alignment and intercellular junction expression [90, 91]. When bovine aortic ECs were cultured at increasing shear stress within physiologic ranges (up to 8 dynes/cm^2), ECs changed from polygonal to ellipsoidal shape and aligned with the direction of blood flow within 48 h [90]. Mechanical shear stress is a key factor in modifying the permeability of the endothelial layer [88, 91].

ECs mediate the transfer of biochemical signals, nutrients, and cells from blood to meet the specific metabolic requirements of local tissue [77]. While small molecules can cross paracellularly, larger molecules require transcellular transport. The glycocalyx, the negatively charged luminal proteins expressed on ECs, repels negatively charged macromolecules (e.g., red blood cells, albumin) and may allow charge-selective transcellular transport, particularly for positively charged molecules [88].

ECs also regulate blood flow through anti-thrombotic effects and by affecting VSMC tone via local NO signaling. NO limits platelet and neutrophil binding, making an anti-thrombotic surface on the endothelial wall [92, 93]. NO also induces vasorelaxation in healthy arteries, as seen directly with the administration of sublingual nitroglycerin or indirectly (i.e., endothelium-dependent) via the administration of acetylcholine [94]. NO is generated from L-arginine by eNOS, the isoform of NOS that regulates vascular tone. This enzyme is activated via multiple stimuli, through either the calcium-independent pathway as seen in shear stress or the calcium-dependent pathway involving calmodulin triggered by acetylcholine, bradykinin, or histamine [95]. NO generated from either pathway, which has a half-life of 3–5 s depending on oxygen tension, diffuses down its concentration gradient into the VSMC layer of the tunica media and regulates vascular tone in three ways (fully reviewed elsewhere [95]).

Briefly, the first occurs under normal conditions, where NO induces a powerful vasodilatory effect by stimulating soluble guanylyl cyclase (sGC). sGC catalyzes the production of cyclic guanosine monophosphate (cGMP), which activates protein kinase G (PKG). PKG induces intracellular calcium depletion by inhibiting extracellular calcium influx (via the voltage-dependent calcium channel), decreases calcium release from the sarcoplasmic reticulum (via binding to inositol 1,4,5-trisphosphate (IP_3) receptor), and increases reuptake of cytosolic calcium into the sarcoplasmic reticulum (via the sarco-/endoplasmic reticulum calcium ATPase [SERCA]). Calcium depletion activates myosin light chain phosphatase (MLCP) and inactivates calmodulin and subsequently myosin light chain kinase (MLCK), the net result of breaking actin-myosin cross-bridging and inducing vasorelaxation. The second mechanism is activated under hypoxic conditions, where sGC generates inosine-3′, 5′-cyclic monophosphate (cIMP), which activates Rho-associated protein kinase (ROCK) to inhibit MLCP and activate MLCK, inducing paradoxical vasoconstriction [96]. In the third pathway, NO produces S-nitrosylated proteins from cysteine thiols. These *S*-nitrosylated proteins induce a number of effects, such as increase the activity of SERCA to induce vasodilation and regulate G protein-coupled receptors (GPCR) signaling, particularly GPCR kinase 2, which is involved in β-adrenergic signaling in the myocardium and peripheral vessels. Notably, NO can also be generated by endothelium-independent pathways using nitrite or nitrate stores predominately under hypoxic conditions, including by deoxyhemoglobin, xanthine oxidoreductase, and mitochondrial cytochrome *c* oxidase [95]. Normal arteries adapt to maintain a basal level of wall stress, which is 15–20 dynes/cm^2 across a number of species [66]. In the short term, arteries dilated in response to increased shear stress (e.g., exercise). Over time, arteries remodel to maintain this baseline of shear stress [66].

The intact endothelium maintains hemostasis by inactivating pro-thrombotic pathways while secreting anti-thrombotic vasodilators [97]. First, tissue factor, which is the primary physiologic activator of the clotting cascade, is not expressed on the luminal surface of ECs, but is abundant in cells of the media and adventitia, including VSMCs and fibroblasts. In the event of vascular injury with disruption of the endothelial barrier, platelets are activated by the exposed tissue factor and collagen. Second, ECs express enzymes to hydrolyze ATP and ADP into adenosine, which has anti-inflammatory effects. Additionally, as ADP is a key mediator of platelet activation and aggregation, EC hydrolysis of ADP limits platelet activation and aggregation [97, 98]. Third, ECs release NO and prostacyclin I_2 that induce vasodilation, although both also have antiadhesive and antiaggregating effects. Fourth, ECs express a number of membrane-bound proteins, including heparin-like proteoglycans, thrombomodulin, tissue factor pathway inhibitor, and protein receptor C (PRC). PRC also stabilizes EC barrier function and induces the expression of anti-apoptotic and anti-inflammatory regulators. In the event of vascular injury, ECs rapidly promote hemostasis by releasing a number of agents, including von Willebrand factor (VWF), P-selectin, angiopoietin-2, and endothelin-1, which contribute to platelet activation and aggregation, as well as a cascade of other pro-thrombotic effects [79].

Finally, ECs rarely proliferate under normal circumstances, but have the potential to rapidly expand in the event of vascular injury or when triggered for angiogenesis [63]. When tissue is hypoxic or nutrient-deprived, angiogenic signals are released, such as VEGF. ECs are activated to secrete MMPs that enables tip ECs, followed by stalk ECs, to migrate and proliferate toward the angiogenic signal. Once tip ECs intersect, progenitor cells follow to build the normal arterial structure. With restoration of sufficient oxygen and nutrients, angiogenic signals decrease, and ECs return to a dormant state.

Development of Atherosclerosis

Pathogenesis of Atherosclerosis

As there is significant heterogeneity of vascular phenotype and function under healthy conditions, it is unsurprising that atherosclerosis itself manifests as a heterogeneous disease. The structure of the atherosclerotic plaque in peripheral arteries differs from coronary arteries [99]. There has been significant progress in the understanding of atherosclerosis in the last century. Much of this work has been on CAD, but there is now increased attention being paid to PAD. However, there remain significant gaps in our understanding of the pathogenesis and progression of atherosclerosis and even more uncertainty in atherogenesis in the lower extremities.

Historically, the response-to-injury hypothesis suggested that atherosclerosis resulted from an injury to the medium- and large-vessel ECs. This focal injury caused endothelial denudation and allowed abnormal binding of circulating plasma cells, namely, platelets which were thought to induce intimal VSMC proliferation and eventual formation of atherosclerotic plaque [100, 101]. After repeated injuries, it was hypothesized that the plaque would expand to cause significant flow obstruction. However, autopsies of young patients between 15 and 34 years of age demonstrated that an intact endothelial layer formed over most atherosclerotic lesions and that early atherosclerosis occurred in a somewhat predictable distribution [102]. At these locations, fluid mechanical forces were shown to induce a change in EC shape and orientation, surface protein expression, and alteration in the configuration of cytoskeletal and intercellular junctional proteins, and these changes were thought to allow increased lipid deposition [103].

But it was also clear that the increase in cholesterol influx alone could not explain the formation of atherosclerotic plaque; in fact, studies differed on whether athero-prone areas demonstrated increased or decreased cholesterol entry [101]. A model that relied only on cholesterol influx, particularly in response to endothelial shear stress, was too narrow to explain the pathogenesis of atherosclerosis.

This realization led to the response-to-retention hypothesis [101]. As LDL crossed the endothelial layer in healthy and diseased arteries (at that time through unknown pathways), Williams and Tabas postulated that retention of atherogenic cholesterol induced a series of alterations that propagated atherogenesis, including expansion of proteoglycans and glycosaminoglycans in the ECM (which binds LDL), cellular chemotaxis (including monocytes and VSMCs), and expression of endothelial adhesion molecules, all of which enhanced further cholesterol influx and retention. Retention also required insufficient cholesterol efflux, although it was believed cholesterol was only removed passively from the arterial wall at that time. Four years later, Ross expanded upon this hypothesis and emphatically acknowledged that atherosclerosis is better explained as an inflammatory disease [39]. While parts of the response-to-injury theory remain accepted today, atherosclerosis is now recognized as an inflammatory disease that occurs in response to lipid deposition and retention, called the inflammatory hypothesis of atherosclerosis [103]. Further investigation has uncovered significant heterogeneity in how ECs respond to shear stress, resulting in changes in morphology, metabolism, and immunoregulatory regulation, that yield either an atheroprotective or atheroprone responses in the local vascular territory [78, 103]. It has become increasingly apparent that atherogenesis is a highly complex and maladaptive process involving endothelial dysfunction of arteries and lymphatics, surrounding vasa vasorum, macrophages and other inflammatory cells, VSMCs, the adventitia, and numerous lipid receptors [104].

Even prior to lipid deposition, diffuse intimal thickening (DIT) is observed in atheroprone arterial segments and can develop in fetal life or in young infants. These regions contain VSMC and an expanded ECM including elastin and proteoglycans that are well-organized, but notably do not contain lipid deposits or neovessels, and are thought to arise secondary to mechanical stress on the vascular wall [105]. VSMCs in DIT serve a more synthetic role, as suggested by increased representation of synthetic organelles relative to contractile proteins, and are the thought to generate the majority of the expanded ECM in DIT [106].

It remains unclear what transforms DIT into pathologic intimal thickening (PIT), and not all DIT becomes pathologic. Historically, this transformation was thought secondary to lipid-laden macrophage apoptosis that allowed extracellular deposition [105]; however, as the mechanisms of lipid handling are being better elucidated, it appears increasingly likely that the rate of lipid influx and efflux contributes to this transformation. As such, it is important to consider how lipids enter and exit the arterial wall.

Entry of LDL into the Subendothelial Space

Circulating apolipoprotein B (apoB)-containing lipid particles, particularly LDL, are causal in the development of atherosclerotic plaque. For some time, macromolecule transfer across the endothelium was thought to be passive through paracellular pores down molecular gradients [107]. However, research has shown LDL is too large (up to 70 nm in diameter) to cross through the narrow gap junctions of intact endothelium to any significant degree and an intact endothelium is seen in early atherosclerotic lesions. Instead, LDL is transported through a process called transcytosis [104, 107, 108]. While LDL receptors (LDLR) are expressed on ECs, their role in the regulation of LDL transport in the vascular endothelium remains unclear, but they do not appear to be a major contributor to the extravascular transfer of lipids in atherosclerosis. This is particularly apparent as patients with *LDLR* mutations (as seen in familial hypercholesterolemia) are at heightened risk for atherosclerosis. Administration of PCSK9 results in almost complete loss of murine coronary endothelial LDLR in vitro, yet the transfer of LDL is unaffected [109]. LDL transcytosis is mediated by scavenger receptor-B1 (SR-B1) and activin receptor-like kinase 1 (ALK1) as shown in Fig. 1.6.

SR-B1 is involved in LDL transcytosis. Upregulation of *Scarb1*, the gene encoding SR-B1, in mouse ECs results in a 50% increase of LDL transcytosis, whereas knockout SR-B1 mice experienced a >40% reduction in aortic LDL accumulation over a 3-h period [109]. In early work, SR-B1 and apoE double knockout mice demonstrated rapid and extensive atherosclerosis, but this was attributed to loss of hepatic SR-B1 function responsible for HDL binding in hepatocytes in the RCT pathway [111, 112]. However, an elegant study showed that mice with selective silencing of endothelial-specific SR-B1 had marked reduction in transcytosis of LDL and oxidized (oxLDL), as well as intermediate- and very-low-density

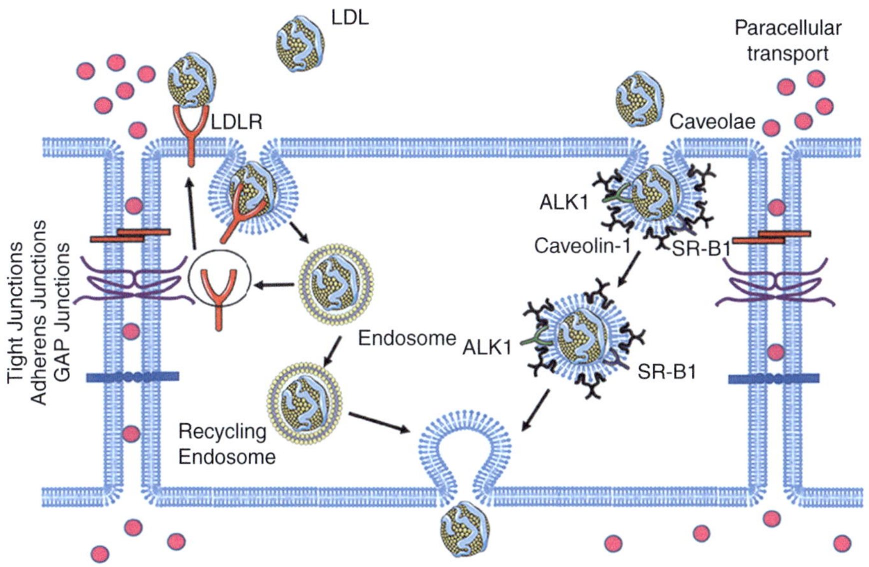

Fig. 1.6 Schematic of the endothelium and the mechanism of transcytosis of low-density lipoprotein (LDL) cholesterol. Endothelial cells (ECs) are connected by tight junctions and adherens junctions, which maintain cell-to-cell adhesion, and gap junctions, which mediate cell-to-cell communication. Small molecules (<3 nm in molecular radius) are able to cross paracellularly. LDL receptors (LDLR) are expressed on the apical aspect of ECs, but do not appear to be involved in LDL transcytosis. Scavenger receptor-B1 (SR-B1) and activin receptor-like kinase 1 (ALK1), which are expressed in caveolae (small plasma membrane rafts), are primarily responsible for LDL transcytosis and eventual entry into the subendothelial space. (Figure from Zhang [110]. This is an open-access article distributed under the terms of the **Creative Commons Attribution License (CC BY)**. The use, distribution, or reproduction in other forums is permitted, provided the original author(s) and the copyright owner(s) are credited and that the original publication in this journal is cited, in accordance with accepted academic practice)

lipoproteins (IDL and VLDL, respectively) [112]. This study further demonstrated that LDL binds to SR-B1 with colocalized dedicator of cytokinesis 4 (DOCK4) and suppression of *Dock4* resulted in reduced LDL transcytosis, confirming that both SR-B1 and DOCK4 are involved in LDL transcytosis. mRNA expression of both *SR-B1* and *Dock4* was increased in atherosclerotic-prone areas (i.e., lesser curvature of the aorta), and expression of both of these molecules was higher in atherosclerotic arteries compared to normal arteries.

Further investigation revealed a positive feedback loop between nuclear high mobility group box 1 (HMGB1) and SR-B1 expression [113]. HMGB1 is highly expressed in human atherosclerotic plaques, and local expression of HMGB1 is increased in the setting of inflammation. In the presence of HMGB1, monocytes release various cytokines, including TNF-α, IL-1, and IL-6 [114]. These cytokines stimulate ECs to increase expression of intercellular cell adhesion molecule-1 (ICAM-1), vascular cell adhesion molecule-1 (VCAM-1), and tissue plasminogen factor (tPA) [115], which in turn induce VSMC reorganization and migration into the intima [115]. Knockdown of nuclear HMGB1 results in reduced LDL transcytosis, and loss of HMGB1 results in reduced SR-B1 (but not ALK1) and sterol regulatory element-binding protein 2 (SREBP2), a critical transcriptional regulator of genes involved in cholesterol handling, such as *LDLR* and *Scarb1*. Importantly, when ECs are incubated with LDL, levels of HMGB1 increased, suggesting a positive feedback loop where LDL induces increased HMGB1 expression, which subsequently increases SR-B1 expression and further accelerates transcytosis of LDL [113]. SR-B1 is also linked to HDL transcytosis and has been extensively investigated in its role in hepatic HDL uptake. In the periphery, HDL and LDL competitively bind SR-B1, and excess LDL reduces HDL transcytosis [107, 109]. SR-B1 is also thought to be at least partially responsible for the atheroprotectiveness of estrogen. Previously, estrogen was shown to increase LDLR receptors on hepatocytes, resulting in a reduction in circulating LDL. In more recent studies, compared to cells from premenopausal women, ECs from men and a postmenopausal woman had increased LDL transcytosis. When these ECs were exposed to physiologic levels of estrogen, there was a dose-dependent reduction in coronary endothelial SR-B1 (but not ALK1) and LDLR with subsequent reduction in LDL transcytosis, but no effect on hepatocytes [116]. Neither HMGB1 nor estrogen appeared to affect endothelial barrier function, and their effects were specific for LDL transcytosis. Therefore, SR-B1 is a crucial regulator of LDL transcytosis and appears to be a pathway by which inflammation induces and accelerates atherosclerosis, as well as how estrogen is atheroprotective.

ALK1 also plays an independent role in vascular LDL transport. ALK1 was initially found by genome-wide RNAi screening (which also identified *Scrab1*, though not studied in the publication) and is a TGF-β-type receptor that is highly expressed by ECs [117]. ALK1 knockdown in mice resulted in a significant reduction in LDL transcytosis; however, ALK1 is required for embryologic vascular development. As such, long-term studies of ALK1 inhibition or silencing are prohibitively lethal [117].

Caveolae, the small plasma membrane rafts classically involved in endocytosis, have also recently been shown to mediate lipid transcytosis [118, 119]. In apoE knockout mice with deleted caveolin-1 (Cav1), the protein responsible for caveolae formation, atherosclerosis is significantly reduced despite hyperlipidemic conditions. Recently, Cav1 deletion was shown to significantly reduce LDL influx (approximately 80% reduction) in LDLR knockout mice [120]. Three key observations were generated from this work. First, the atheroprone lesser curvature of murine aorta showed increased expression of Cav1 and more abundant intracellular caveolae compared to the atheroresistant greater curvature. Intracellular caveolae and lipid influx were completely abolished in atheroprone regions in *CAV1* knockout mice, and reintroduction of Cav1 showed rapid accumulation of lipids in the vascular wall. These findings support the conclusion that mechanical signaling appears to control caveolae morphology and location. Second, Cav1 knockout mice had reduced surface expression of ICAM-1 and VCAM-1, as well as reduced fibronectin deposition and macrophage infiltration, a finding that persisted even in the presence of inflammatory cytokines. Third, ECs exposed to oscillatory shear stress, a model of disrupted blood flow, demonstrated a two- to threefold increase in

ICAM-1, VCAM-1, and p65 phosphorylation, and these increases were silenced in Cav1 knockout mice. Notably, these Cav1 knockout mice demonstrated cardiac hypertrophy, as seen in previous reports. In short, Cav1 appears to be a key mediator of lipid transcytosis, fibronectin deposition, and regulation of adhesion molecule expression in response to abnormal shear stress or inflammation.

Both SR-B1 and ALK1 are expressed on the EC apical surface within caveolae, and inhibition of each receptor individually results in an approximately 50% reduction in immediate LDL transcytosis, whereas combined inhibition reduces LDL transcytosis by 70% [112]. Consequently, other means of LDL transcytosis are likely undiscovered. Notably, LDLR, cluster of differentiation 36 (CD36), and oxidized LDL receptor-1 (LOX-1) bind LDL, but these receptors are not involved in LDL transcytosis in vascular ECs outside of the brain [112]. Additionally, the uptake of other lipoproteins or modified lipoproteins (e.g., oxLDL, modified non-oxidized lipoproteins) likely contributes to atherogenesis, although the contribution of these pathways is less clear. For example, LOX-1 is the primary receptor for oxLDL for ECs, and expression is significantly amplified by inflammatory cytokines, creating an additional positive feedback loop [121]. Binding of oxLDL to LOX-1 on ECs results in EC activation with increased expression of adhesion molecules, activation of the NF-κB pathway, and reduced EC vasorelaxation, among other effects [121].

Once lipids cross the luminal membrane of ECs, relatively little is known about the trafficking and modification of cholesterol within the EC. This transfer is believed to occur within minutes, and it is unclear if LDL undergoes any modification, such as oxidation, while still in the EC [107]. However, caveolae containing the LDL integrate into the basal membrane, likely mediated by soluble *N*-ethylmaleimide-sensitive factor (NSF) attachment protein receptor (SNARE) machinery, which allows exocytosis of LDL into the subendothelial space.

Transluminal influx of LDL appears to be the primary pathway of lipid accumulation in arterial walls. While there may be some component of cholesterol influx via the vasa vasorum, this appears to be relatively modest [107].

Clearance of LDL into the Subendothelial Space

Peripheral cells are unable to catabolize cholesterol, so accumulated and excess cholesterol in the vessel wall needs to be recycled and returned to the liver via the central circulation [122]. In the vessel wall, LDL is engulfed by macrophages and VSMCs, effluxed to extracellular HDL, and transported back to the liver for excretion in the bile in the RCT pathway. Alternatively, the liver can also either convert the cholesterol into bile salts via 7α-hydroxylase or simply package it back into apoB containing particles and re-secrete it into the circulation.

Once across the EC barrier, positively charged lipoproteins on native LDL, which is LDL that is not yet modified, bind with negatively charged proteoglycans and glycosaminoglycans deposited by VSMC to become aggregated LDL [123].

Aggregated LDL (agLDL) uptake by macrophages is primarily mediated by the LDL receptor-related protein 5 (LRP5), an enzyme that is part of the LDLR family [124]. In human macrophages, LRP5 is located in the cytoplasm, but is translocated to the cell membrane and upregulated in response to agLDL. PCSK9 expression, which is nearly undetectable in monocytes, increases significantly as macrophages differentiate in response to agLDL. Together, PCSK9 and LRP5 form a complex, and LRP5 appears involved in the release of PCSK9. Selective inhibition of either PCSK9 or LRP5 leads to a significant reduction in cholesterol ester (CE) accumulation in macrophages, and simultaneous silencing of both led to a nearly 70% drop in intracellular CE after 24 h. Furthermore, in the presence of agLDL, silencing RNA (siRNA) against PCSK9 reduced TNF-α and IL-1β expression to baseline levels and reduced NF-κB pathway signaling. In mice, PCSK9 is not expressed in normal aortas, but is increased in atherosclerotic plaques. Silencing of PCSK9 (with siRNA) reduces TNF-α, IL-1β, and monocyte chemoattractant protein-1 (MCP-1) expression by inhibiting the toll-like receptor 4 (TLR4)/NF-κB signaling pathway, despite no significant change in circulating lipids [125]. Recent data demonstrated that TNF-α reduced eNOS activation and NO production, but that administration of PCSK9 siRNA restored eNOS function and NO production even in the presence of TNF-α [126]. There is also evidence of cross-talk between LOX-1 and PCSK9 such that each can positively upregulate the expression of the other [127]. These studies support the conclusion that agLDL induces a pro-inflammatory state and that blocking PCSK9 reduces atherosclerosis by inhibiting inflammatory signaling, in addition to its known role in augmenting hepatic LDL uptake to reduce plasma LDL levels.

Aggregated LDL deposits may then undergo further modification (e.g., oxidization), which makes them more atherogenic by producing oxysterols, as well as OxPLs (including oxLDL) and fatty acids. A number of lipid receptors have a recognized role in atherosclerosis (reviewed elsewhere [104]), but key receptor will be reviewed.

Macrophages, the primary immune cell involved in atherosclerosis, identify and internalize oxLDL (by either phagocytosis or pinocytosis) via scavenger receptors (SRs) that are primed to detect oxidation-specific epitopes (OSE), which are moieties on oxidized lipids that are particularly pro-atherogenic. The functions of the macrophage with lipid handling are depicted in Fig. 1.7. A number of these scavenger receptors exist, although in vitro up to 90% of macrophage uptake of fully oxidized LDL is mediated by CD36, SR-A1, and SR-B1 [129, 130]. LOX-1 also binds oxLDL, though primarily delipidated oxLDL and partially oxidized LDL. Under normal conditions, LOX-1 expression is low, but expression can be significantly increased in response to inflammation and thus may be an additional minor pathway of macrophage uptake of oxLDL [121, 131]. The two primary OSEs, OxPL and malondialdehyde (MDA)-modified amine groups, bind to cellular pattern recognition receptors (PRRs) CD36 and SR-A, respectively, although other OSEs are known to bind these scavenger receptors as well. Toll-like receptors (TLRs) appear to work in concert with SRs to mediate a sterile inflammatory response. For example, CD36 was shown to recognize oxLDL and trigger the formation of a

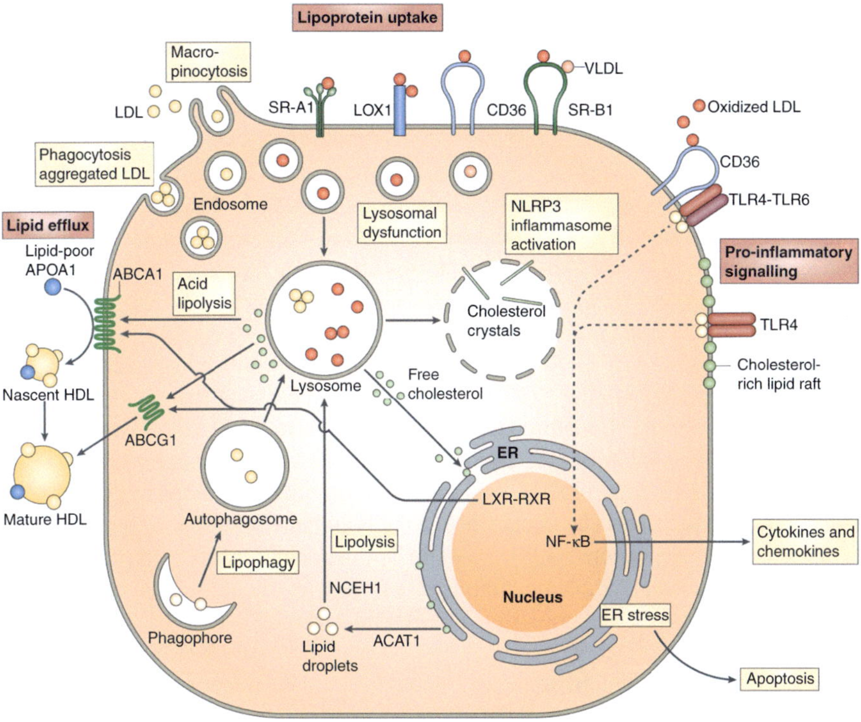

Fig. 1.7 Lipoprotein uptake and efflux by macrophages from the extracellular matrix. **Normal state:** Macrophages uptake lipoproteins, including native low-density lipoprotein (LDL), aggregated LDL, and oxidized LDL (oxLDL), via phagocytosis or pinocytosis, or by receptor-mediated uptake via scavenger receptor-A1 (SR-A1), oxidized LDL receptor-1 (LOX-1), cluster of differentiation 36 (CD36), and SR-B1. Upon entry, lipids are degraded in lysosomes into free cholesterol, which may be effluxed to lipid-poor apolipoprotein-A1 (apo-A1) or high density lipoprotein (HDL) via ATP-binding membrane cassette transport protein A1 (ABCA1) or ABCG1, destined for the reverse cholesterol transport pathway. Free or oxidized cholesterol may also be stored by converting them into cholesterol esters via acetyl-CoA acetyltransferase-1 (ACAT1) to form lipid droplets. Accumulated cholesterol activates nuclear liver X receptor-retinoid X receptor (LXR-RXR), which enhances expression of ABCA1 and ABCG1. Lipid droplets are mobilized by either lipolysis by neutral cholesterol ester hydrolase 1 (NCEH1) or lipophagy to return to lysosomes. **Pathologic state:** oxLDL is recognized by toll-like receptors (e.g., TLR4) or scavenger receptors, such as the CD36-TLR4/TLR6 heterotrimer, which activate NF-κB signaling and the production of cytokines. Excess free cholesterol can also precipitate to form cholesterol crystals, which are potent activators of the NLRP3 (NOD−, LRR−, and pyrin domain-containing 3) inflammasome. With significant oxidative stress, macrophages may be triggered to undergo apoptosis or secondary necrosis. (Figure from Moore [128])

CD36-TLR4/TLR6 heterotrimer, a complex that activates the NF-κB pathway and increased expression of cytokines, such as IL-1β [132]. CD36 also forms a heterotrimer with TLR2/TLR6 and can induce macrophage apoptosis and plaque necrosis in the setting of endoplasmic reticulum stress [133]. Soluble PRRs, such as CRP, are known to bind OSEs of apoptotic cells and inhibit the cellular PRR response, triggering the alternative complement pathway to clear OSE-expressing cellular debis [134]. Given the variety of OSE generated by lipid peroxidation combined with the various PRRs, there are likely numerous undiscovered signaling pathways involved in oxidized lipid handling.

Engulfed OxPLs in macrophages are converted into CEs via acetyl-CoA acetyltransferase-1 (ACAT1) on the endoplasmic reticulum to prevent free cholesterol toxicity. Under normal conditions, a balance of phospholipids and CE is maintained without significant accumulation of lipids in the vascular wall, but macrophages can become foam cells, the prototypical cell of atherosclerotic plaque, as more lipid is retained [108]. To clear lipids, CEs are converted back to free cholesterol via neutral cholesterol ester hydrolase (nCEH) and effluxed by macrophages to lipid-poor apoA-1 or HDL [131, 135]. This is accomplished either by direct efflux to free apoA-1 via the ATP-binding membrane cassette transport protein A1 (ABCA1) or by efflux to mature HDL particles via ABCG1 [122]. Mature HDL is generated by conversion of free cholesterol into CE via lecithin/cholesterol acyltransferase (LCAT). Mature HDL then travels predominately via the lymphatic system to return to the liver. The importance of the lymphatic system was demonstrated in a series of observations [136]. First, in apoE knockout mice, hyperlipidemia resulted in impaired lymphatic drainage, as well as accumulation of fluid (as edema), macrophages, and cholesterol. When treated with ezetimibe, which inhibits dietary and biliary cholesterol absorption and increases VEGF-C, lymphatic drainage improved. Lymphatic vessels dilated with a subsequent improvement in edema and a reduction in accumulated lipids. Second, labelled cholesterol-loaded macrophages injected into a mouse were first detected in the lymph and then later in the plasma, liver, and eventually feces. When lymph drainage was surgically disrupted, labeled HDL was poorly cleared from peripheral tissue, and labeled HDL concentrations in the lymphatic fluid and plasma of were reduced 90% and 80%, respectively. Finally, downregulation of lymphatic SR-B1 impaired HDL uptake by 80%, suggesting that HDL primarily binds to SR-B1 on lymphatic ECs to be removed from the periphery. These findings demonstrated that the lymphatic system is a key player in lipid homeostasis and that venous efflux of cholesterol was insufficient to support physiologic requirements [136]. Hyperlipidemia and inflammation impair clearance of lipids via obstructing lymphatic flow. Furthermore, expression of ABAC1 and ABCG1 is downregulated in response to inflammation of atherosclerosis, further reducing cholesterol transfer from macrophages to HDL [131].

Additionally, VSMC are also important in lipid clearance. With lipid accumulation, VSMC undergo phenotypic switching to become macrophage-like cells via the Krüpple-like factor 4 (KLF4) pathway [137]. KLF4 is a transcription factor that regulates VSMC differentiation and proliferation that is stimulated by platelet-derived growth factor (PDGF) released by macrophages [137]. AgLDL uptake by VSMC appears to be mediated by LRP1 [138]. The SRs responsible for oxLDL uptake in VSMC are similar to those in macrophages, including SR-A1, SR-A2, CD36, and LOX-1 (Fig. 1.8) [139]. An estimated 30–40% of foam cells are derived

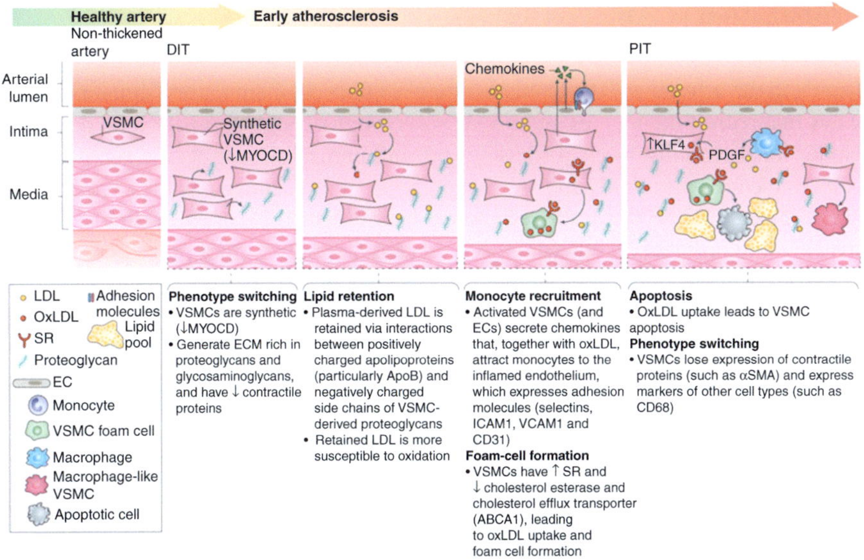

Fig. 1.8 Roles of vascular smooth muscle cells (VSMCs) in atherosclerosis. In early atherosclerosis, VSMC migrate from the media to the intima and deposit proteoglycans and glycosaminoglycans in the extracellular matrix (ECM) to induce diffuse intimal thickening (DIT). Myocardin (MYOCD) family proteins increase the expression of contractile genes of VSMCs, and expression of MYOCD decreases as VSMC phenotype switch from a contractile to synthetic function. Low-density lipoprotein (LDL) trancytoses through the endothelial cell (EC) wall where positively charged lipid moieties bind negatively charged proteoglycans resulting in lipid retention. Retained LDL undergoes modification, including oxidation, which is pro-inflammatory and promotes monocyte recruitment, secretion of cytokines and chemokines, and expression of adhesion molecules that leads to pathologic intimal thickening (PIT). Macrophages release platelet-derived growth factor (PDGF) that induces the Krüpple-like factor 4 (KLF4) pathway, a transcription factor that upregulates VSMC differentiation and proliferation. VSMC phenotype switches into a macrophage-like state, marked by reduced contractile proteins (e.g., α-smooth muscle actin, αSMA) and increased expression of cluster of differentiation 68 (CD68), a protein that is typically expressed on macrophages. Macrophage-like VSMCs and macrophages use scavenger receptors (SR) to uptake oxidized LDL (oxLDL) and offload it to the reverse cholesterol transport pathway (not shown) via ATP-binding membrane cassette transport protein A1 (ABCA1) or ABCG1, but can become foam cells with significant cholesterol uptake that are at risk for apoptosis if inflammation is sustained. *ICAM-1* intercellular adhesion molecule-1, *VCAM-1* vascular cell adhesion molecule-1. (Figure from Basatemur [106])

from VSMCs, suggesting they play a significant role in lipid uptake and clearance. VSMC may be particularly susceptible to form cell formation in response to enzyme-modified non-oxidative LDL [140].

After the lymph fluid is returned to the circulation via the thoracic duct, CEs in HDL undergo uptake to the liver either directly via HDL binding to hepatic SR-B1 or indirectly whereby cholesteryl ester transfer protein (CETP) offloads cholesterol from HDL to apoB-containing lipids and binds to hepatic LDLR for hepatic uptake [122].

Propagation of Atherosclerosis

Lipids in the arterial wall upregulate a number of pro-inflammatory signaling pathways that recruit monocytes and VSMCs to recognize and eliminate lipid deposits. Under ideal circumstances, a transient pro-inflammatory state would recruit these cells to clear excess lipids and subsequently be downregulated as the excess lipids are eliminated. However, if the response is insufficient to clear excess lipids, a positive, pro-inflammatory feedback loop is created that only further propagates atherogenesis, particularly in pro-atherogenic states, such as hyperlipidemia, diabetes, or chronic systemic inflammation [39, 101].

Macrophages exist throughout most tissues and act to maintain tissue homeostasis through antimicrobial defense, clearance of cellular debris, and regulation of the inflammatory response via inflammatory signaling [141]. Various phenotypes of macrophages exist in tissues, and their phenotype is likely controlled via the inflammatory signaling of the microenvironment, which enables macrophages to dynamically mediate either a pro- or anti-atherosclerotic response [142].

Retained lipoproteins in the subendothelial space continue to undergo oxidation through various enzymatic and nonenzymatic pathways that further induce inflammation [143]. Oxidative reactions are essential for the survival of eukaryotes, including for the generation of energy and cellular signaling [129]. However, these vital reactions also induce oxidative stress, and the balance of essential versus excessive ROS generation skews toward harm in pathologic states [134, 144]. Lipids, particularly phospholipids, are major targets for peroxidation that produces OSE that are recognized by PRRs of the innate immune system [134, 145]. Membrane phospholipids in apoptotic macrophages and VSMCs are also a source of OSE, and the generation and clearance of OSE-expressing cells is an important signaling mechanism for clearance of cellular debris in normal or pathologic cell turnover [146].

OxPLs induce a number of pro-inflammatory signaling pathways, including activating macrophages to release various cytokines (e.g., IL-6, IL-8, MCP-1) [147] and chemokines (e.g., CCL2 (C-C motif chemokine ligand 2) and CX_3CL1), resulting in further monocyte recruitment and differentiation into macrophages at the site of injury [128]. VSMCs also are responsible for secreting some of these chemoattractants [106]. OxPLs also activate monocytes via the NLRP3 (NOD-, LRR-, and pyrin domain-containing 3) inflammasome, which is also involved in responding to danger signals and exogenous threats (e.g., bacterial lipopolysaccharides (LPS)). However, distinctly different than the immune response to exogenous ligands, OxPLs trigger the binding of only monocytes to luminal surface of ECs instead of both monocytes and neutrophils. This allows enhanced migration and homing of monocytes in response to OxPL deposition in the subendothelial vascular space. OxPL activates ECs that results in the increased expression of IL-8, CXCL2 (C-X-C motif ligand 2), and CXCL3 and the activation of NF-κB pathway; surface adhesion molecules E-selectin, P-selectin, VCAM-1, and ICAM-1; MCP-1; and CD40/CD40L pathway [121]. oxLDL also decreases NO production, increases ROS formation, and induces EC apoptosis [121]. With accumulation and continued retention of lipids in the subendothelial space, apoB-containing lipoproteins, particularly those that are oxidized, initiate a complex positive feedback loop of inflammation and cellular recruitment that propagates the formation of atherosclerotic plaque as depicted in Fig. 1.9.

OxPLs also stimulate angiogenesis via upregulating expression of VEGF [148]. As the vascular wall expands due to lipid accumulation, inflammatory cell recruitment, and ECM expansion, neovessels form to support the increased metabolic requirements. In particular, VEGF stimulates proliferation and migration of ECs, increases EC production of ROS via the NOX family of NADPH oxidases, and promotes monocyte migration via VEGF receptor 1 (VEGFR-1) [148, 149]. While the density of vasa vasorum correlates with the quantity of monocytes in atherosclerotic plaques, it remains uncertain to what extent these neovessels allow further plaque expansion, such as by increasing delivery of lipids and inflammatory cells.

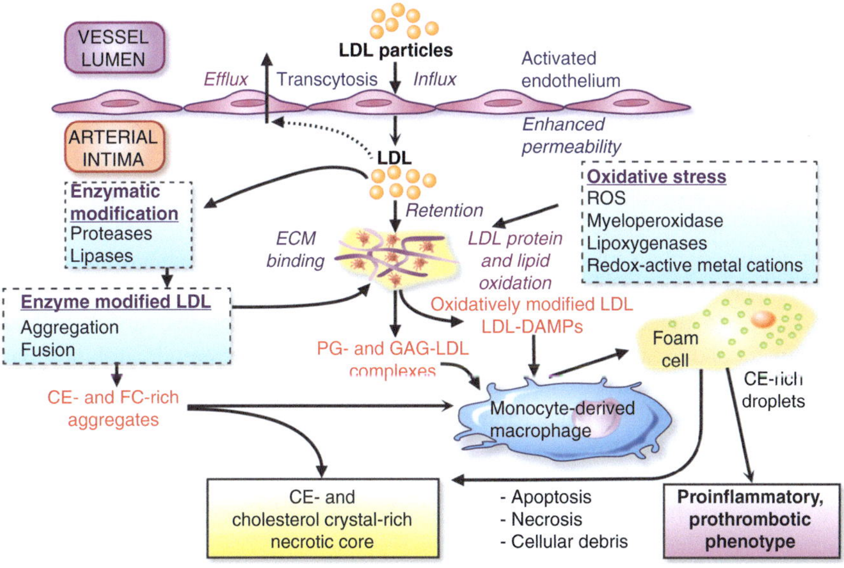

Fig. 1.9 The response-to-retention hypothesis of atherogenesis. Low-density lipoprotein (LDL) enters the arterial wall via transcytosis and binds proteoglycans (PG) and glycosaminoglycans (GAG) and in the extracellular matrix (ECM). Retained LDL undergoes enzymatic modification (e.g., oxidation) to enzyme-modified oxidized LDL and non-oxidized LDL, which creates cholesterol esters (CE) and free cholesterol (FC) aggregates. These modified lipids are particularly pro-inflammatory and express oxidation-specific epitopes (recognized as damage-associated molecular patterns, DAMPs) that are recognized by macrophages and macrophage-like vascular smooth muscle cells (latter not shown) that try to contain and remove inflammatory lipids via the reverse cholesterol transport pathway. As lipids accumulate in these cells, they become foam cells rich in CE and may undergo apoptosis or necrosis. Increased oxidative stress and DAMPs expressed by dead immune cells results in a positive feedback loop that further stimulates the inflammatory cascade. ROS, reactive oxygen species. (Figure from Borén [108])

Additionally, up to 20–30% of IgM in serum of healthy mice bind OSEs, particularly to MDA epitopes, suggesting involvement of the adaptive immune system [129]. These antibodies bind OxPL and activate T and B cells. Initially, the adaptive immune system appears to favor atheroprotective effects, but as atherosclerosis progresses, the adaptive immune system becomes pro-atherogenic, and adaptive immune cells release pro-inflammatory mediators, including interferon-γ (INF-γ), IL-2, IL-3, TNF, and lymphotoxin, which further activate macrophages and T cells [150].

These inflammatory signaling pathways recruit macrophages and VSMCs to clear the pro-inflammatory lipids. However, if excess intracellular CEs accumulate, macrophages and VSMCs phenotypically become foam cells. Foam cells secrete an abundance of inflammatory mediators, which further propagates atherogenesis [150]. Additionally, cholesterol can precipitate as extracellular crystals, which are also potent stimulators of the immune system, including the NLRP3-depdent inflammasome (Fig. 1.7). While most crystals are thought to arise from macrophages, a recent study demonstrated apoE knockout mice showed rapid accumulation of cholesterol crystals in the aortic arch, even prior to significant macrophage recruitment with significant compromise of the EC barrier [151]. This may represent an additional pathway of cholesterol crystal deposition mediated by ECs, particularly in early atherosclerosis formation, but further investigation is required. With enhancement of the response with foam cell and cholesterol crystal formation, sustained inflammation induces significant oxidative stress, which can trigger macrophage and VSMC apoptosis. VSMCs are also susceptible to apoptosis particularly in response to oxLDL [152].

In advanced atherosclerotic plaque, PIT can progress to fibroatheromas, which notably have a characteristic necrotic core and fibrous cap. Non-resolving inflammation due to defective lipid and cellular clearance propagates further cellular recruitment and escalation of the inflammatory response. Increased cytokines, particularly IL-8 and IL-1β, reduce efferocytosis, the process of removing apoptotic cells, including lipid-laden macrophages that underwent cell death due to excessive oxidative stress [108]. Efferocytosis pertaining to cholesterol handling involves the adhesion G protein-coupled receptor B1 (ADGRB1), which allows direct contact with the macrophage (acting as an efferocyte), or indirection via the MER proto-oncogene tyrosine kinase (MERTK) with a bridging molecule growth arrest-specific protein 6 (GAS6) or LDL-related protein 1 (LRP1) receptors, shown in Fig. 1.10 [153]. ADGRB1 promotes the assembly of engulfment and cell motility protein 1 (ELMO1) with downstream activation of RAC1 to facilitate phagocytosis of the apoptotic cell. With indirect binding of MERTK or LRP1, free cholesterol is internalized and converted to CEs by ACAT. Both direct and indirect pathways (the latter through LXR) induce ABCA1 expression, which effluxes cholesterol to the ECM to prevent excess intracellular cholesterol accumulation. Atherosclerosis can induce defective efferocytosis. Several possible mechanisms exist to explain this, such as proteolytic destruction of MERTK or downregulation of LRP1 in response to oxLDL, although apoptotic cells may have inappropriate expression of CD47, a

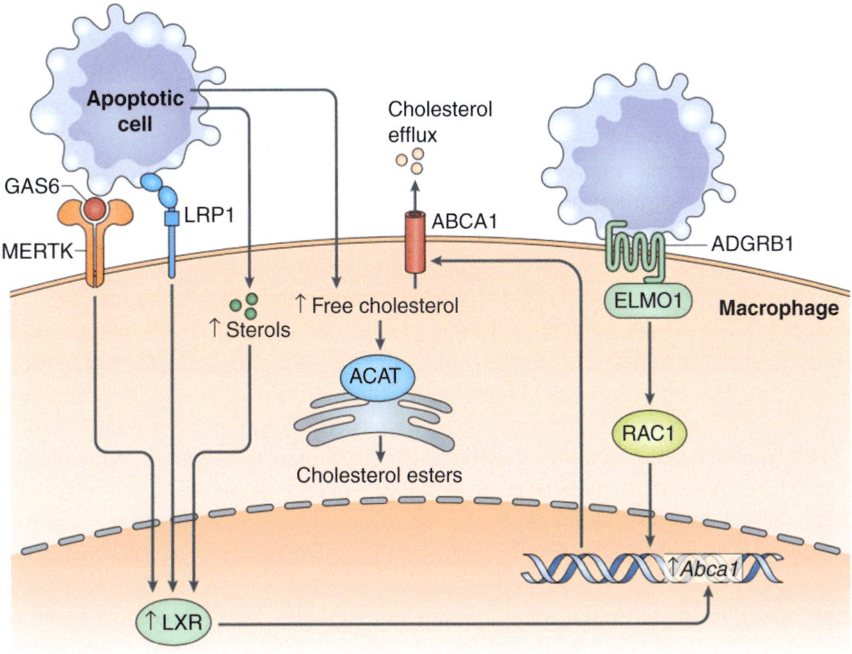

Fig. 1.10 Clearance of cholesterol of apoptotic cells by efferocytosis. Apoptotic, lipid-laden macrophages are recognized by other macrophages serving as efferocytes. Direct adhesion to the macrophage surface via adhesion G protein-coupled receptor B1 (ADGRB1) promotes the assembly of engulfment and cell motility protein 1 (ELMO1) with downstream activation of RAC1 to facilitate phagocytosis of the apoptotic cell for further intracellular processing. Indirect adhesion via either MER proto-oncogene tyrosine kinase (MERTK) with a bridging molecule growth arrest-specific protein 6 (GAS6) or LDL-related protein 1 (LRP1) receptors facilitates offloading of cholesterol to be processed into cholesterol esters by acetyl-CoA acetyltransferase-1 (ACAT1). Both the direct and indirect pathway (latter via upregulation of nuclear liver X receptor (LXR)) induce expression of ATP-binding membrane cassette transport protein A1 (ABCA1), which effluxes cholesterol extracellularly. (Figure from Doran [153])

signal that makes apoptotic cells resistant to efferocytosis [153]. Additionally, VSMC are relatively poor at efferocytosis [154].

Uncleared apoptotic cells eventually undergo secondary necrosis. In this relatively uncontrolled pathway, membrane dissolution releases the cellular contents, which further exacerbates inflammation by the release of damage-associated molecular patterns (DAMPs) molecules. A necrotic core results within the plaque, which is covered and contained by a fibrous cap. There is increasing evidence to support that both intimal and medial VSMCs are responsible for synthesizing the ECM and collagen of the fibrous cap in response to pro-inflammatory cytokines, including TGF-β, IL-1, PDGF, and others [106]. Depending on the local milieu of cell signaling, activated inflammatory cells, and MMP activity, VSMCs may develop a thick protective fibrous cap or release enzymes that promote plaque erosion and rupture

[140]. What controls the fate of advanced atherosclerotic plaques and the stability of the fibrous cap remains uncertain, but appears dependent on the balance of specialized pro-resolving mediators (SPMs) and pro-inflammatory signaling (e.g., prostaglandins and leukotrienes). There are at least four distinct SPM families, including lipoxins, resolvins, protectins, and maresins, and a higher ratio of SPM to inflammatory signals is correlated with a smaller necrotic core and thicker fibrous cap [155]. Administration of resolvin E1, an SPM generated by endogenous oxidation of eicosapentaenoic acid (EPA), to atherosclerotic-prone mice attenuated atherosclerotic lesion area, appeared to slow the progression of atherosclerotic lesions, and reduced INF-γ and TNF-α [156]. SPMs were also shown to enhance efferocytosis [153]. As advanced atherosclerotic plaques have lower SPMs compared to earlier lesions, this likely contributes to a thinner fibrous cap and reduced efferocytosis [153]. The fibrous cap is vulnerable to rupture if it is thin, and it is estimated that 95% of plaque ruptures in coronary arteries occur when the cap is <65 μm [108].

Lastly, arterial calcification is associated with all-cause mortality and is prominent in PAD, particularly in patients with diabetes or end-stage renal disease (ESRD) [157]. While bulkier calcification (≥3 mm) appears relatively stable, "spotty" microcalcifications (0.2–3 mm) are unstable and susceptible to rupture [108]. Atherosclerotic debris allows hydroxyapatite deposition to form microcalcifications, which further stimulates the inflammatory cascade [157]. The mechanism of arterial calcification is not well understood, although VSMCs appear to be the primary cell mediator. Enzyme-modified non-oxLDL, another modified LDL component of atherosclerotic plaque produced by hydrolytic enzymes, appears to be particularly important in transforming VSMCs into an osteoblast-like phenotype to promote arterial calcification [140]. Further, oxidized lipoproteins inhibit osteoclastic differentiation of macrophages [157]. Additional investigation is required to understand what controls plaque calcification, as well as what lipoproteins are implicated in this (e.g., Lp(a) may have significant causal role in calcification) [108].

This pro-inflammatory feedback loop can be disrupted to improve CV outcomes, as demonstrated by the use of canakinumab [158] or colchicine [159] in patients following a myocardial infarction. Additionally, reduction in LDL also improves CV outcomes [49, 160, 161]. In LDLR knockout mice fed a high-cholesterol diet to develop atherosclerosis, subsequent treatment with an anti-apoB antisense oligonucleotide to reduce plasma cholesterol showed that LDL permeability of ECs fell within 1 week, followed by a substantial reduction in foam cells and increased plaque collagen content by 4 weeks [162]. There was no change in the size of the necrotic core by 4 weeks, but the duration of follow-up was likely insufficient to see this effect [162]. These studies suggest that even advanced plaques can be rescued with anti-inflammatory or lipid-reducing therapies.

In summary, the presence of sustained lipid transcytosis in excess of clearance results in a chronic inflammatory milieu that supports plaque expansion. Aggregated phospholipids are modified, and OxPLs induce the expression of inflammatory cytokines and chemokines to recruit inflammatory cells, stimulate pro-adhesion molecules on ECs, and enhance neovascularization. Monocytes respond to inflammatory signals, differentiate predominately into macrophages, and, with VSMCs, attempt to clear OxPLs. If these mechanisms fail to clear excess lipids, chronic inflammation induces plaque expansion, cellular death with necrotic core formation, and vascular calcification, all of which increase the risk of plaque rupture.

Atherosclerosis in Peripheral Artery Disease

The pathogenesis and progression of PAD are assumed to be similar to CAD. However, while similar risk factors and biological pathways are likely involved, there is growing evidence that the pathogenesis and phenotype of atherosclerosis vary widely depending on the vascular bed. Recent analysis of gene expression in atherosclerotic plaques of aortic, carotid, and femoral arteries demonstrated that 156 pathways were altered compared to controls, but only approximately 50% of genetic pathways overlap across all three arterial beds [163]. Additionally, the hallmark of coronary atherosclerosis is PIT and formation of a fibrous cap with abundance of lipid deposition and inflammatory cells. Acute coronary syndrome occurs in the setting of plaque rupture with formation of overlying thrombus and sudden onset myocardial ischemia in approximately two-thirds of cases and plaque erosion, where the endothelial layer is denuded resulting in an exposed subendothelial layer, in one-third of cases [164]. However, these findings are less common in PAD [165]. Several studies investigated the distribution and histopathology of atherosclerosis in PAD. Among patients with CLI undergoing amputation, multiple studies demonstrate several distinguishing phenotypical features of PAD compared to CAD [165–168].

First, there is significant intimal thickening (>90% of samples, mostly in a concentric distribution) with a relative paucity of lipid deposition and absence of macrophages, found in only one-quarter (39% in Soor [167]) and one-third of patients, respectively [166]. Intimal thickening and macrophage presence did not differ among patients with diabetes, smoking, or ESRD. These results were similar in a more recent study evaluating the location of maximum stenosis of amputations from patients predominately with CLI. Despite stenosis ≥70%, insignificant atherosclerosis was found in 29 and 59% of patients with above-the-knee (AK) and below-the-knee (BK) amputations, respectively [165]. In those patients with atherosclerosis, the majority of plaques were fibrocalcific (57% in AK and 60% in BK) instead of fibroatheromas (39% in AK and 30% in BK). A more recent MR-based study of the SFA in patients with PAD found that only 24% had lipid-rich necrotic cores and 59% had arterial calcification; interestingly, only the presence of a lipid-rich core was predictive of future PAD events [169]. Whether non-atherosclerotic intimal thickening is similar to DIT observed in CAD or is instead an end-stage form of atherosclerosis in PAD remains unclear.

Second, calcification is significantly more prevalent in PAD and occurs most commonly in the tunica media adjacent to the internal elastic lamina (IEL). Prevalence of medial calcification increases with age [170] and is higher in patients with cigarette smoking history [166], ESRD [167], and diabetes [167]. The severity (defined by percent circumference) of medial calcification was higher in arteries below the knee, and there was a trend for higher prevalence (59% in AK, 73% in BK) [165]. Intimal calcification was noted in 43% of patients and was typically continuous with a calcified IEL and medial calcification. Interestingly, in amputation samples in patients without PAD, the prevalence of intimal thickening, lipid accumulation, and calcification were all similar, but less severe [166]. Vascular calcification in PAD is thought to be deposited by VSMCs similar to atherosclerosis in CAD, but why it is more common in PAD remains unclear [170]. Vascular calcification, particularly in the tunica media, causes arterial stiffening that limits vasomotor reactivity and increases systolic blood pressure due to reduced arterial elasticity [99].

Finally, there appear to be significant differences in the etiology of stenosis in AK versus BK lesions. In amputated limbs with ≥70% stenosis, 73% had acute or chronic thrombi, and, of those, 68% did not have significant underlying atherosclerosis, suggestive that plaque rupture is less common in PAD compared to CAD [165]. Further, the presence of chronic thrombi without atherosclerosis was significantly higher in BK, whereas acute thrombi were more common in AK compared to BK. Similar results were noted in a small study that compared CT findings to arterial histopathology extending from proximal SFA to distal leg vessels in patients with risk factors for PAD (but notably not clinically diagnosed) [168]. In this study, acute thrombosis was exclusively found AK and usually associated with calcified nodules, whereas BK stenoses were mostly chronic total occlusions, of which half appeared to be related to embolization from a proximal source. Layered chronic thrombus in distal vessels suggests repeat embolization leading to progressive stenosis [168]. In CLI, these findings suggest de novo thrombus formation is more likely AK, whereas distal embolization is more likely BK.

Taken together, these studies demonstrate that PAD differs substantially from CAD in the nature of intimal thickening, prevalence and severity of calcification, and characteristics of thrombus formation. These studies are limited by relatively small sample sizes, differing clinical status and accompanying comorbidities, observation at an advanced stage of disease (often using amputations), and lack of standardization as to the extent of lower extremity arteries assessed.

Despite having an extensive investigation into the pathogenesis of atherosclerosis in other vascular territories, particularly CAD, these histologic differences should prompt further investigation specifically into the pathogenesis of PAD. There are likely overlapping, but differing, mechanisms for lipid handling, cellular dysfunction, and propagation of inflammation. Recent studies combining imaging and histology offer a promising strategy to better study PAD phenotypes.

Ischemia-Induced Changes

Limb ischemia occurs when there is inadequate tissue perfusion and is a major cause of reduced quality of life and morbidity in PAD. Depending on the time of onset, limb ischemia is termed acute limb ischemia (ALI) if the onset of hypoperfusion is less than 2 weeks' duration or CLI if ischemia results in rest pain lasting longer than 2 weeks' duration [21].

Acute limb ischemia is recognized by the "6 Ps" pneumonic, including paresthesia, pain at rest, pallor, pulselessness, poikilothermia (impaired temperature regulation of the limb), and paralysis (or noted limb weakness) [171]. The acute loss of adequate blood flow, typically with a measured ankle blood pressure <50 mmHg, results in cellular ischemia and death. The outcome of ALI depends on the rapid recognition and treatment to restore blood flow [171, 172]. The estimated annual incidence is 1.5 cases per 10,000 people [171]. While a number of mechanisms can result in ALI, such as trauma, dissection, external compression (e.g., compartment syndrome), or use of vasoactive medications, thromboembolic causes are most common. In the large population-based Oxford Vascular (OXVASC) study in the UK, ALI was most commonly embolic (46% of cases), followed by thrombotic with accompanying atherosclerosis (24% of cases) [173]. Of those with ALI, age was significantly associated with incidence, and the incidence of ALI rose drastically after 75 years of age. CV risk factors were present in 99% of ALI cases, with ever smoking (69% of cases, RR 2.07 [CI 1.22–3.50]), hypertension (61% of cases, RR 2.04 [CI 1.18–3.53]), and atrial fibrillation (39%, RR not calculated) the most prevalent. Only 42% of patients with ALI carried a diagnosis of PAD. Notably, of the ALI patients who were independent prior to the event (defined by the modified Rankin score of ≤2), only 52% were able to remain independent at 6 months. In patients with symptomatic PAD enrolled in the TRA2°P-TIMI 50 (Thrombin Receptor Antagonist in Secondary Prevention of Atherothrombotic Ischemic Events—Thrombolysis in Myocardial Infarction) study, the incidence of ALI was 1.3% per year and was more common in patients with an ABI that was very low or high (≤0.5 or ≥1.3) or those who were actively smoking or had prior peripheral revascularization [174]. The majority of ALI cases were due to thrombosis of a surgical graft (62%) or peripheral stent (9%); the remainder were due to native vessel thrombosis (25%) or thromboembolic disease (4%), suggesting that the pre-event diagnosis of PAD changes the etiology of ALI events compared to a general population, which in part may be related to significant baseline differences in medication use [174].

The hallmark signs and symptoms of CLI are rest pain, non-healing wounds, or tissue loss in the setting of proven ischemia lasting over 2 weeks [21]. It is estimated that the annual incidence of CLI is 2.2–35 cases per 10,000 people and as many as 11% of patients with PAD may have CLI [21]. In the OXVASC study, the majority of patients with CLI had underlying PAD (71%), and the most prevalent risk factors were ever smoking (71% of cases, RR 2.22 [CI 1.31–3.76]), hypertension (71% of cases, RR 3.28 [CI 2.12–5.09]), hyperlipidemia (55%, RR not calculated), and diabetes (44% of cases, RR 5.96 [CI 3.15–11.26]) [173]. CLI was similarly debilitating compared to ALI, where only 46% of CLI patients who were previously independent remained so at 6 months after a CLI event.

In response to chronic hypoperfusion, the arterioles dilate and are less sensitive to vasodilator stimuli [175]. Additionally, distal ischemic tissue responds to promote collateral circulation through angiogenesis. ECs and VSMCs migrate and proliferate to form neovasculature in response to growth factors, namely, VEGF, hepatocyte growth factor (HGF), and fibroblast growth factor (FGF) [176]. The resulting angiogenesis may be adequate in the early stages of PAD, but is generally inadequate as PAD progresses, leading to persistent tissue ischemia [175]. VEGF is the most studied of these growth factors. Acute hypoxia creates ROS that stimulate hypoxia-inducible factor 1-α (HIF 1-α), which increases the expression of VEGF. Results differ in amputated samples regarding the expression of pro-angiogenic growth factors and capillary density [177], again suggesting significant heterogeneity in the PAD phenotype. In skeletal muscle samples analyzed from amputated extremities with acute-on-chronic ischemia, gene expression of HIF 1-α and VEGF, as well as TNF-α, was upregulated; interestingly, in amputation samples from patients with CLI, HIF 1-α and VEGF were downregulated, whereas anabolic factors insulin growth factor-1 (IGF-1) and IGF-2 were upregulated [178]. IGF promotes VEGF expression and is thought to play an important role in skeletal muscle survival and regeneration in ischemia [178]. Another study noted significant heterogeneity of the expression of pro-angiogenic growth factors, with 38% of samples demonstrating upregulation of *VEGF-A* and *HIF1A*, the genes corresponding to VEGF-A and HIF 1-α [179]. Further research showed increased VEGF expression in the skin and muscle of the foot compared to more proximal samples from the calf and thigh, and VEGF mRNA was increased in skin bordering ischemic ulcers and gangrene [180]. While surgical or endovascular revascularization remains the preferred treatment in CLI, there are an increasing number of studies investigating the use of pro-angiogenic growth factors, progenitor cells (e.g., EPCs), and scaffolds for CLI that have so far produced mixed results [181, 182].

Chronic ischemia results in downstream effects on ECs and skeletal muscle cells. As noted above, FMD of the brachial artery is reduced in patients with PAD, suggesting systemic endothelial dysfunction [37]. More recently, ECs from amputated samples showed increased albumin extravasation, suggesting increased EC permeability, as well as increased evidence of inflammation, cellular adhesion marker expression, and macrophage infiltration [183]. These changes were linked to Dhh (desert hedgehog), which is downstream of KLF2 and downregulated by inflammatory cytokines. An agonist of Dhh (Smo agonist—SAG) resulted in improved endothelial function with reduced permeability, capillary perfusion, and skeletal muscle organization [183]. As for skeletal muscle, chronic ischemia results in reduced muscle area and increased fat infiltration, decreased mitochondrial activity, and increased mitochondrial damage [177]. Changes in myofiber typing are heterogeneous in PAD with studies reporting disparate findings regarding the composition of type I and type II myofibers in ischemic tissue (see McDermott) [177]. Samples from amputations of severe PAD patients revealed immature muscle fibers with increased areas of fibrosis [183]. Mitochondrial cell DNA (mtDNA), which accumulates mutations faster than nuclear DNA due to its proximity to ROS, accumulates mutations with ischemia. In patients with PAD, the mixture of mutated mtDNA, called heteroplasmy, in the gastrocnemius was significantly increased compared to controls, suggesting increased oxidative stress [184]. Furthermore, among those patients with PAD, those with a lower level of mitochondrial damage had better walking performance [184].

In addition to atherosclerosis of the large arteries in PAD, microvascular dysfunction (MVD) is also recognized as an independent risk factor for adverse limb events. MVD is considered a systemic process similar to atherosclerosis that clinically manifests as retinopathy, nephropathy, and peripheral neuropathy [26]. Patients with MVD involvement in one territory often have evidence of MVD in all other territories [26]. Diabetes is a common cause of MVD, and patients with diabetes have a 1.7-fold and 2.9-fold higher risk of ischemic rest pain and ischemic ulcers compared to non-diabetic patients after controlling for ABI [185, 186]. As noted above in patients undergoing revascularization for CLI, between 19 and 21% of patients had a normal ABI [35, 36]. The presence of MVD may explain why some patients with a normal ABI can still have limb symptoms or CLI [26, 36]. MVD is defined as disease of the arterioles and capillaries <100 μm [26]. Biopsy samples from the lower extremity (gastrocnemius or vastus lateralis) of patients with IC demonstrated reduced capillary density [187–189], although a study in patients with PAD largely without IC showed increased capillary density [190]. It remains unclear whether symptoms develop secondary to capillary atrophy or from inadequate angiogenesis, but capillary density increased significantly in patients with IC after exercise training which preceded subsequent improvements in peak VO_2 [191]. Exercise therapy was shown to significantly improve walking distance and pain-free walking distance [189]. In a large observational study of veterans, patients with MVD defined by the presence of peripheral neuropathy, retinopathy, or proteinuria had a 3.7-fold increase in the risk of amputation [192]. Moreover, the presence of PAD or PAD with MVD resulted in a 13.9- and 22.7-fold higher risk of amputation, respectively. In patients with MVD alone, accounting for 18% of all amputations, 73% of amputations were below the ankle, whereas 53% of amputations in patients with PAD alone were above the ankle, suggesting MVD more commonly affects the distal lower extremity. Patients with PVD with MVD represented only 4% of the population, but accounted for 40% of all amputations. The use of the toe-brachial index may help diagnose MVD in patients with symptoms concerning for CLI with a normal ABI [2].

Conclusion

PAD is a common and underrecognized atherosclerotic disease that can result in progressive loss of function from claudication, gangrene, or limb amputation. Patients with PAD have a significant risk of ASCVD events and an even higher risk of all-cause mortality compared to patients with CAD or prior stroke. Our understanding of atherosclerosis has significantly advanced especially over the last few decades, highlighting the complexity of lipid influx, modification, and clearance in the subendothelial space. However, numerous areas of uncertainty remain within atherogenesis, particularly pertaining to PAD and its unique phenotype.

References

1. Aboyans V, Ricco JB, Bartelink MLEL, et al. 2017 ESC guidelines on the diagnosis and treatment of peripheral arterial diseases, in collaboration with the European Society for Vascular Surgery (ESVS). Eur Heart J. 2018;39(9):763–816. https://doi.org/10.1093/eurheartj/ehx095.
2. Gerhard-Herman MD, Gornik HL, Barrett C, et al. 2016 AHA/ACC guideline on the management of patients with lower extremity peripheral artery disease: executive summary: a report of the American College of Cardiology/American Heart Association task force on clinical practice guidelines. Circulation. 2017;135 https://doi.org/10.1161/CIR.0000000000000470.
3. Fowkes FGR, Aboyans V, Fowkes FJI, McDermott MM, Sampson UKA, Criqui MH. Peripheral artery disease: epidemiology and global perspectives. Nat Rev Cardiol. 2017;14(3):156–70. https://doi.org/10.1038/nrcardio.2016.179.
4. Hiatt WR, Goldstone J, Smith SC, et al. Atherosclerotic peripheral vascular disease symposium II: nomenclature for vascular diseases. Circulation. 2008;118(25):2826–9. https://doi.org/10.1161/CIRCULATIONAHA.108.191171.
5. Touyz RM, Delles C. Textbook of vascular medicine. Cham: Springer; 2019. https://doi.org/10.1007/978-3-030-16481-2.
6. Gallino A, Aboyans V, Diehm C, et al. Non-coronary atherosclerosis. Eur Heart J. 2014;35(17):1112–9. https://doi.org/10.1093/eurheartj/ehu071.
7. Song P, Rudan D, Zhu Y, et al. Global, regional, and national prevalence and risk factors for peripheral artery disease in 2015: an updated systematic review and analysis. Lancet Glob Health. 2019;7(8):e1020–30. https://doi.org/10.1016/S2214-109X(19)30255-4.
8. Fowkes FGR, Rudan D, Rudan I, et al. Comparison of global estimates of prevalence and risk factors for peripheral artery disease in 2000 and 2010: a systematic review and analysis. Lancet. 2013;382(9901):1329–40. https://doi.org/10.1016/S0140-6736(13)61249-0.
9. Vespa J, Medina L, Armstrong D. Demographic turning points for the United States: population projections for 2020 to 2060. Curr Popul Rep. 2020;P25–1144:1–13. https://census.gov/programs-surveys/popproj.html
10. Matsushita K, Sang Y, Ning H, et al. Lifetime risk of lower-extremity peripheral artery disease defined by ankle-brachial index in the United States. J Am Heart Assoc. 2019;8(18):e012177. https://doi.org/10.1161/JAHA.119.012177.
11. Vart P, Coresh J, Kwak L, Ballew SH, Heiss G, Matsushita K. Socioeconomic status and incidence of hospitalization with lower-extremity peripheral artery disease: atherosclerosis risk in communities study. J Am Heart Assoc. 2017;6(8):e004995. https://doi.org/10.1161/JAHA.116.004995.
12. Hiatt WR, Armstrong EJ, Larson CJ, Brass EP. Pathogenesis of the limb manifestations and exercise limitations in peripheral artery disease. Circ Res. 2015;116(9):1527–39. https://doi.org/10.1161/CIRCRESAHA.116.303566.
13. Bhatt DL, Ohman EM, Hirsch AT, Richard AJ, Wilson PWF. International prevalence, recognition, and treatment of cardiovascular risk factors in outpatients with atherothrombosis. JAMA. 2006;295(2):180–9. http://www.ncbi.nlm.nih.gov/pubmed/16403930
14. Diehm N, Shang A, Silvestro A, et al. Association of cardiovascular risk factors with pattern of lower limb atherosclerosis in 2659 patients undergoing angioplasty. Eur J Vasc Endovasc Surg. 2006;31(1):59–63. https://doi.org/10.1016/j.ejvs.2005.09.006.
15. Singer AJ, Tassiopoulos A, Kirsner RS. Evaluation and management of lower-extremity ulcers. N Engl J Med. 2017;377(16):1559–67. https://doi.org/10.1056/nejmra1615243.
16. Chen Q, Smith CY, Bailey KR, Wennberg PW, Kullo IJ. Disease location is associated with survival in patients with peripheral arterial disease. J Am Heart Assoc. 2013;2(5):12–4. https://doi.org/10.1161/JAHA.113.000304.
17. Aboyans V, Desormais I, Lacroix P, Salazar J, Criqui MH, Laskar M. The general prognosis of patients with peripheral arterial disease differs according to the disease localization. J Am Coll Cardiol. 2010;55(9):898–903. https://doi.org/10.1016/j.jacc.2009.09.055.

18. McDermott MM, Guralnik JM, Ferrucci L, et al. Asymptomatic peripheral arterial disease is associated with more adverse lower extremity characteristics than intermittent claudication. Circulation. 2008;117(19):2484–91. https://doi.org/10.1161/CIRCULATIONAHA.107.736108.
19. Regensteiner JG, Hiatt WR, Coll JR, et al. The impact of peripheral arterial disease on health-related quality of life in the peripheral arterial disease awareness, risk, and treatment: new resources for survival (PARTNERS) program. Vasc Med. 2008;13(1):15–24. https://doi.org/10.1177/1358863X07084911.
20. Sigvant B, Lundin F, Wahlberg E. The risk of disease progression in peripheral arterial disease is higher than expected: a meta-analysis of mortality and disease progression in peripheral arterial disease. Eur J Vasc Endovasc Surg. 2016;51(3):395–403. https://doi.org/10.1016/j.ejvs.2015.10.022.
21. Farber A. Chronic limb-threatening ischemia. N Engl J Med. 2018;379(2):171–80. https://doi.org/10.1056/nejmcp1709326.
22. Resnick HE, Lindsay RS, McDermott MMG, et al. Relationship of high and low ankle brachial index to all-cause and cardiovascular disease mortality: the strong heart study. Circulation. 2004;109(6):733–9. https://doi.org/10.1161/01.CIR.0000112642.63927.54.
23. Fowkes G, Fowkes FGR, Murray GD, et al. Ankle brachial index combined with Framingham risk score to predict cardiovascular events and mortality: a meta-analysis. J Am Med Assoc. 2008;300(2):197–208. https://doi.org/10.1001/jama.300.2.197.
24. Hiatt WR, Fowkes FG, Heizer G, Berger JS, Baumgartner I, Held P, et al. Ticagrelor versus Clopidogrel in symptomatic peripheral artery disease. N Engl J Med. 2017;376:32–40. https://doi.org/10.1056/NEJMoa1611688.
25. Cambou JP, Aboyans V, Constans J, Lacroix P, Dentans C, Bura A. Characteristics and outcome of patients hospitalised for lower extremity peripheral artery disease in France: the COPART registry. Eur J Vasc Endovasc Surg. 2010;39(5):577–85. https://doi.org/10.1016/j.ejvs.2010.02.009.
26. Behroozian A, Beckman JA. Microvascular disease increases amputation in patients with peripheral artery disease. Arterioscler Thromb Vasc Biol. 2020;40:534–40. https://doi.org/10.1161/ATVBAHA.119.312859.
27. Reinecke H, Unrath M, Freisinger E, et al. Peripheral arterial disease and critical limb ischaemia: still poor outcomes and lack of guideline adherence. Eur Heart J. 2015;36(15):932–8. https://doi.org/10.1093/eurheartj/ehv006.
28. Norgren L, Hiatt WR, Dormandy JA, Nehler MR, Harris KA, Fowkes FGR. Inter-society consensus for the management of peripheral arterial disease (TASC II). J Vasc Surg. 2007;45(1 Suppl):5–67. https://doi.org/10.1016/j.jvs.2006.12.037.
29. McDermott MMG, Mehta S, Greenland P. Exertional leg symptoms other than intermittent claudication are common in peripheral arterial disease. Arch Intern Med. 1999;159(4):387–92. https://doi.org/10.1001/archinte.159.4.387.
30. McDermott MMG, Greenland P, Liu K, et al. Leg symptoms in peripheral arterial disease associated clinical characteristics and functional impairment. J Am Med Assoc. 2001;286(13):1599–606. https://doi.org/10.1001/jama.286.13.1599.
31. Conte MS, Pomposelli FB, Clair DG, et al. Society for Vascular Surgery practice guidelines for atherosclerotic occlusive disease of the lower extremities: management of asymptomatic disease and claudication. J Vasc Surg. 2015;61(3):2S–41S.e1. https://doi.org/10.1016/j.jvs.2014.12.009.
32. Fernández-Friera L, Peñalvo JL, Fernández-Ortiz A, et al. Prevalence, vascular distribution, and multiterritorial extent of subclinical atherosclerosis in a middle-aged cohort the PESA (progression of early subclinical atherosclerosis) study. Circulation. 2015;131(24):2104–13. https://doi.org/10.1161/CIRCULATIONAHA.114.014310.
33. López-Melgar B, Fernández-Friera L, Oliva B, et al. Short-term progression of multiterritorial subclinical atherosclerosis. J Am Coll Cardiol. 2020;75(14):1617–27. https://doi.org/10.1016/j.jacc.2020.02.026.

34. Aboyans V, McClelland RL, Allison MA, et al. Lower extremity peripheral artery disease in the absence of traditional risk factors. The multi-ethnic study of atherosclerosis. Atherosclerosis. 2011;214(1):169–73. https://doi.org/10.1016/j.atherosclerosis.2010.10.011.
35. Sukul D, Grey SF, Henke PK, Gurm HS, Grossman PM. Heterogeneity of ankle-brachial indices in patients undergoing revascularization for critical limb Ischemia. JACC Cardiovasc Interv. 2017;10(22):2307–16. https://doi.org/10.1016/j.jcin.2017.08.026.Heterogeneity.
36. Shishehbor MH, Hammad TA, Zeller T, Baumgartner I, Scheinert D, Rocha-Singh KJ. An analysis of IN.PACT DEEP randomized trial on the limitations of the societal guidelines-recommended hemodynamic parameters to diagnose critical limb ischemia. J Vasc Surg. 2016;63(5):1311–7. https://doi.org/10.1016/j.jvs.2015.11.042.
37. Brevetti G, Silvestro A, Schiano V, Chiariello M. Endothelial dysfunction and cardiovascular risk prediction in peripheral arterial disease: additive value of flow-mediated dilation to ankle-brachial pressure index. Circulation. 2003;108(17):2093–8. https://doi.org/10.1161/01.CIR.0000095273.92468.D9.
38. The top 10 causes of death. Geneva: World Health Organization; 2020. https://www.who.int/es/news-room/fact-sheets/detail/the-top-10-causes-of-death
39. Ross R. Atherosclerosis—an inflammatory disease. Epstein FH, ed. N Engl J Med. 1999;340(2):115–26. https://doi.org/10.1056/NEJM199901143400207.
40. Hazarika S, Annex BH. Biomarkers and genetics in peripheral artery disease. Clin Chem. 2017;63(1):236–44. https://doi.org/10.1373/clinchem.2016.263798.
41. Bertoia ML, Pai JK, Lee J-H, et al. Oxidation-specific biomarkers and risk of peripheral artery disease. J Am Coll Cardiol. 2013;61(21):2169–79. https://doi.org/10.1016/j.jacc.2013.02.047.
42. Kremers B, Wübbeke L, Mees B, Ten Cate H, Spronk H, Ten Cate-Hoek A. Plasma biomarkers to predict cardiovascular outcome in patients with peripheral artery disease: a systematic review and meta-analysis. Arterioscler Thromb Vasc Biol. 2020;40:2018–32. https://doi.org/10.1161/ATVBAHA.120.314774.
43. Wassel CL, Berardi C, Pankow JS, et al. Soluble P-selectin predicts lower extremity peripheral artery disease incidence and change in the ankle brachial index: the multi-ethnic study of atherosclerosis (MESA). Atherosclerosis. 2015;239(2):405–11. https://doi.org/10.1016/j.atherosclerosis.2015.01.022.
44. Stather PW, Sylvius N, Wild JB, Choke E, Sayers RD, Bown MJ. Differential microRNA expression profiles in peripheral arterial disease. Circ Cardiovasc Genet. 2013;6(5):490–7. https://doi.org/10.1161/CIRCGENETICS.111.000053.
45. Raitoharju E, Lyytikäinen LP, Levula M, et al. miR-21, miR-210, miR-34a, and miR-146a/b are up-regulated in human atherosclerotic plaques in the Tampere vascular study. Atherosclerosis. 2011;219(1):211–7. https://doi.org/10.1016/j.atherosclerosis.2011.07.020.
46. Martello A, Mellis D, Meloni M, et al. Phenotypic miRNA screen identifies miR-26b to promote the growth and survival of endothelial cells. Mol Ther Nucleic Acids. 2018;13:29–43. https://doi.org/10.1016/j.omtn.2018.08.006.
47. Pérez-Cremades D, Cheng HS, Feinberg MW. Noncoding RNAs in critical limb ischemia. Arterioscler Thromb Vasc Biol. 2019;40:523–33. https://doi.org/10.1161/ATVBAHA.119.312860.
48. Shapiro MD, Tavori H, Fazio S. PCSK9 from basic science discoveries to clinical trials. Circ Res. 2018;122(10):1420–38. https://doi.org/10.1161/CIRCRESAHA.118.311227.
49. Sabatine MS, Giugliano RP, Keech AC, et al. Evolocumab and clinical outcomes in patients with cardiovascular disease. N Engl J Med. 2017;376(18):1713–22. https://doi.org/10.1056/nejmoa1615664.
50. Schwartz GG, Steg PG, Szarek M, et al. Alirocumab and cardiovascular outcomes after acute coronary syndrome. N Engl J Med. 2018;379(22):2097–107. https://doi.org/10.1056/nejmoa1801174.
51. Bonaca MP, Nault P, Giugliano RP, et al. Low-density lipoprotein cholesterol lowering with Evolocumab and outcomes in patients with peripheral artery disease: insights from

the FOURIER trial (further cardiovascular outcomes research with PCSK9 inhibition in subjects with elevated risk). Circulation. 2018;137(4):338–50. https://doi.org/10.1161/CIRCULATIONAHA.117.032235.
52. Leucker TM, Gerstenblith G, Schär M, et al. Evolocumab, a PCSK9-monoclonal antibody, rapidly reverses coronary artery endothelial dysfunction in people living with HIV and people with dyslipidemia. J Am Heart Assoc. 2020;9(14):e016263. https://doi.org/10.1161/JAHA.120.016263.
53. Kheirkhah A, Lamina C, Rantner B, et al. Elevated levels of serum PCSK9 in male patients with symptomatic peripheral artery disease: the CAVASIC study. Atherosclerosis. 2021;316:41–7. https://doi.org/10.1016/j.atherosclerosis.2020.11.025.
54. Chao TH, Chen IC, Li YH, Lee PT, Tseng SY. Plasma levels of proprotein convertase Subtilisin/Kexin type 9 are elevated in patients with peripheral artery disease and associated with metabolic disorders and dysfunction in circulating progenitor cells. J Am Heart Assoc. 2016;5(5):1–12. https://doi.org/10.1161/JAHA.116.003497.
55. Takahashi T, Kalka C, Masuda H, et al. Ischemia- and cytokine-induced mobilization of bone marrow-derived endothelial progenitor cells for neovascularization. Nat Med. 1999;5(4):434–8. https://doi.org/10.1038/7434.
56. Werner N, Kosiol S, Schiegl T, et al. Circulating endothelial progenitor cells and cardiovascular outcomes. N Engl J Med. 2005;353(10):999–1007. https://doi.org/10.1056/nejmoa043814.
57. Smadja DM, D'Audigier C, Bièche I, et al. Thrombospondin-1 is a plasmatic marker of peripheral arterial disease that modulates endothelial progenitor cell angiogenic properties. Arterioscler Thromb Vasc Biol. 2011;31(3):551–9. https://doi.org/10.1161/ATVBAHA.110.220624.
58. Zhu W, Gregory JC, Org E, et al. Gut microbial metabolite TMAO enhances platelet hyperreactivity and thrombosis risk. Cell. 2017;165(1):111–24. https://doi.org/10.1016/j.cell.2016.02.011.Gut.
59. Roncal C, Martínez-Aguilar E, Orbe J, et al. Trimethylamine-N-oxide (TMAO) predicts cardiovascular mortality in peripheral artery disease. Sci Rep. 2019;9(1):1–8. https://doi.org/10.1038/s41598-019-52082-z.
60. Klarin D, Lynch J, Aragam K, et al. Genome-wide association study of peripheral artery disease in the million veteran program. Nat Med. 2019;25(8):1274–9. https://doi.org/10.1038/s41591-019-0492-5.
61. Risau W. Mechanisms of angiogenesis. Nature. 1997;386(6626):671–4. https://doi.org/10.1038/386671a0.
62. Patel-Hett S, D'Amore PA. Signal transduction in vasculogenesis and developmental angiogenesis. Int J Dev Biol. 2011;55(4–5):353–69. https://doi.org/10.1387/ijdb.103213sp.
63. Eelen G, Treps L, Li X, Carmeliet P. Basic and therapeutic aspects of angiogenesis updated. Circ Res. 2020;127:310–29. https://doi.org/10.1161/CIRCRESAHA.120.316851.
64. Sieggreen M. Lower extremity arterial and venous ulcers. Nurs Clin North Am. 2005;40(2):391–410. https://doi.org/10.1016/j.cnur.2004.09.016.
65. Del Conde I, Benenati JF. Noninvasive testing in peripheral arterial disease. Interv Cardiol Clin. 2014;3(4):469–78. https://doi.org/10.1016/j.iccl.2014.06.006.
66. Ku DN. Blood flow in arteries. Annu Rev Fluid Mech. 1997;29:399–434. https://doi.org/10.1146/annurev.fluid.29.1.399.
67. Dinenno FA. Skeletal muscle vasodilation during systemic hypoxia in humans. J Appl Physiol. 2016;120(2):216–25. https://doi.org/10.1152/japplphysiol.00256.2015.
68. Bruno RM, Ghiadoni L, Seravalle G, Dell'Oro R, Taddei S, Grassi G. Sympathetic regulation of vascular function in health and disease. Front Physiol. 2012;3:1–15. https://doi.org/10.3389/fphys.2012.00284.
69. VanderLaan PA, Reardon CA, Getz GS. Site specificity of atherosclerosis: site-selective responses to atherosclerotic modulators. Arterioscler Thromb Vasc Biol. 2004;24(1):12–22. https://doi.org/10.1161/01.ATV.0000105054.43931.f0.

70. Chatzizisis YS, Coskun AU, Jonas M, Edelman ER, Feldman CL, Stone PH. Role of endothelial shear stress in the natural history of coronary atherosclerosis and vascular remodeling—molecular, cellular, and vascular behavior. J Am Coll Cardiol. 2007;49(25):2379–93. https://doi.org/10.1016/j.jacc.2007.02.059.
71. Wensing PJW, Meiss L, Mali WPTM, Hillen B. Early atherosclerotic lesions spiraling through the femoral artery. Arterioscler Thromb Vasc Biol. 1998;18(10):1554–8. https://doi.org/10.1161/01.ATV.18.10.1554.
72. Libby P, Hansson GK. Inflammation and immunity in diseases of the arterial tree: players and layers. Circ Res. 2015;116(2):307–11. https://doi.org/10.1161/CIRCRESAHA.116.301313.
73. Chandran KB, Rittgers SE, Yoganathan AP. Rheology of blood and vascular mechanics. In: Biofluid mechanics the human circulation. Boca Raton: CRC Press; 2012. p. 109–54.
74. Aird WC. Phenotypic heterogeneity of the endothelium: I. Structure, function, and mechanisms. Circ Res. 2007;100(2):158–73. https://doi.org/10.1161/01.RES.0000255691.76142.4a.
75. Davies PF. Flow-mediated endothelial mechanotransduction. Physiol Rev. 1995;75(3):519–60. https://doi.org/10.1152/physrev.1995.75.3.519.
76. Wang C, Baker BM, Chen CS, Schwartz MA. Endothelial cell sensing of flow direction. Arterioscler Thromb Vasc Biol. 2013;33(9):2130–6. https://doi.org/10.1161/ATVBAHA.113.301826.
77. Potente M, Mäkinen T. Vascular heterogeneity and specialization in development and disease. Nat Rev Mol Cell Biol. 2017;18(8):477–94. https://doi.org/10.1038/nrm.2017.36.
78. Bierhansl L, Conradi LC, Treps L, Dewerchin M, Carmeliet P. Central role of metabolism in endothelial cell function and vascular disease. Physiology. 2017;32(2):126–40. https://doi.org/10.1152/physiol.00031.2016.
79. Yau JW, Teoh H, Verma S. Endothelial cell control of thrombosis. BMC Cardiovasc Disord. 2015;15(1):1–11. https://doi.org/10.1186/s12872-015-0124-z.
80. Tinajero MG, Gotlieb AI. Recent developments in vascular adventitial pathobiology: the dynamic adventitia as a complex regulator of vascular disease. Am J Pathol. 2020;190(3):520–34. https://doi.org/10.1016/j.ajpath.2019.10.021.
81. Chen H, Slipchenko MN, Liu Y, et al. Biaxial deformation of collagen and elastin fibers in coronary adventitia. J Appl Physiol. 2013;115(11):1683–93. https://doi.org/10.1152/japplphysiol.00601.2013.
82. Stenmark KR, Yeager ME, El Kasmi KC, et al. The adventitia: essential regulator of vascular wall structure and function. Annu Rev Physiol. 2013;75:23–47. https://doi.org/10.1146/annurev-physiol-030212-183802.
83. Boyle EC, Sedding DG, Haverich A. Targeting vasa vasorum dysfunction to prevent atherosclerosis. Vasc Pharmacol. 2017;96–98(June):5–10. https://doi.org/10.1016/j.vph.2017.08.003.
84. Chistiakov DA, Ashwell KW, Orekhov AN, Bobryshev YV. Innervation of the arterial wall and its modification in atherosclerosis. Auton Neurosci. 2015;193:7–11. https://doi.org/10.1016/j.autneu.2015.06.005.
85. Brakenhielm E, Alitalo K. Cardiac lymphatics in health and disease. Nat Rev Cardiol. 2019;16(1):56–68. https://doi.org/10.1038/s41569-018-0087-8.
86. Oliver G, Kipnis J, Randolph GJ, Harvey NL. The lymphatic vasculature in the 21st century: novel functional roles in homeostasis and disease. Cell. 2020;182(2):270–96. https://doi.org/10.1016/j.cell.2020.06.039.
87. Bazzoni G, Dejana E. Endothelial cell-to-cell junctions: molecular organization and role in vascular homeostasis. Physiol Rev. 2004;84(3):869–901. https://doi.org/10.1152/physrev.00035.2003.
88. Mehta D, Malik AB. Signaling mechanisms regulating endothelial permeability. Physiol Rev. 2006;86(1):279–367. https://doi.org/10.1152/physrev.00012.2005.
89. Paik DT, Tian L, Williams IM, et al. Single-cell RNA sequencing unveils unique transcriptomic signatures of organ-specific endothelial cells. Circulation. 2020;142(19):1848–62. https://doi.org/10.1161/CIRCULATIONAHA.119.041433.

90. Dewey CF, Bussolari SR, Gimbrone MA, Davies PF. The dynamic response of vascular endothelial cells to fluid shear stress. J Biomech Eng. 1981;103(3):177–85. https://doi.org/10.1115/1.3138276.
91. Stanicek L, Lozano-Vidal N, Bink DI, et al. Long non-coding RNA LASSIE regulates shear stress sensing and endothelial barrier function. Commun Biol. 2020;3(1):1–13. https://doi.org/10.1038/s42003-020-0987-0.
92. Provost P, Lam JYT, Lacoste L, Merhi Y, Waters D. Endothelium-derived nitric oxide attenuates neutrophil adhesion to endothelium under arterial flow conditions. Arterioscler Thromb. 1994;14(3):331–5. https://doi.org/10.1161/01.atv.14.3.331.
93. Radomski MW, Palmer RMJ, Moncada S. Endogenous nitric oxide inhibits human platelet adhesion to vascular endothelium. Lancet. 1987;330(8567):1057–8. https://doi.org/10.1016/S0140-6736(87)91481-4.
94. Furchgott R, Zawadski JV. The obligatory role of endothelial cells in the relaxation of atrial smooth muscle. Nature. 1980;288(November):373–6.
95. Zhao Y, Vanhoutte PM, Leung SWS. Vascular nitric oxide: beyond eNOS. J Pharmacol Sci. 2015;129(2):83–94. https://doi.org/10.1016/j.jphs.2015.09.002.
96. Gao Y, Chen Z, Leung SWS, Vanhoutte PM. Hypoxic vasospasm mediated by cIMP: when soluble guanylyl cyclase turns bad. J Cardiovasc Pharmacol. 2015;65(6):545–8. https://doi.org/10.1097/FJC.0000000000000167.
97. Borissoff JI, Spronk HMH, ten Cate H. The hemostatic system as a modulator of atherosclerosis. Schwartz RS, ed. N Engl J Med. 2011;364(18):1746–60. https://doi.org/10.1056/NEJMra1011670.
98. Stafford NP, Pink AE, White AE, Glenn JR, Heptinstall S. Mechanisms involved in adenosine triphosphate-induced platelet aggregation in whole blood. Arterioscler Thromb Vasc Biol. 2003;23(10):1928–33. https://doi.org/10.1161/01.ATV.0000089330.88461.D6.
99. Narula N, Olin JW, Narula N. Pathologic disparities between peripheral artery disease and coronary artery disease. Arterioscler Thromb Vasc Biol. 2020;40:1982–9. https://doi.org/10.1161/ATVBAHA.119.312864.
100. Ross R, Glomset J, Harker L. Response to injury and atherogenesis. Am J Pathol. 1977;86(3):675–84.
101. Williams KJ, Tabas I. The response-to-retention hypothesis of early atherogenesis. Arterioscler Thromb Vasc Biol. 1995;15(5):551–62. https://doi.org/10.1161/01.atv.15.5.551.
102. Katsuda S, Boyd HC, Fligner C, Ross R, Gown AM. Human atherosclerosis: III. Immunocytochemical analysis of the cell composition of lesions of young adults. Am J Pathol. 1992;140(4):907–14.
103. Gimbrone MA, García-Cardeña G. Endothelial cell dysfunction and the pathobiology of atherosclerosis. Circ Res. 2016;118(4):620–36. https://doi.org/10.1161/CIRCRESAHA.115.306301.
104. Mineo C. Lipoprotein receptor signalling in atherosclerosis. Cardiovasc Res. 2020;116(7):1254–74. https://doi.org/10.1093/cvr/cvz338.
105. Nakashima Y, Wight TN, Sueishi K. Early atherosclerosis in humans: role of diffuse intimal thickening and extracellular matrix proteoglycans. Cardiovasc Res. 2008;79(1):14–23. https://doi.org/10.1093/cvr/cvn099.
106. Basatemur GL, Jørgensen HF, Clarke MCH, Bennett MR, Mallat Z. Vascular smooth muscle cells in atherosclerosis. Nat Rev Cardiol. 2019;16(12):727–44. https://doi.org/10.1038/s41569-019-0227-9.
107. Jang E, Robert J, Rohrer L, von Eckardstein A, Lee WL. Transendothelial transport of lipoproteins. Atherosclerosis. 2020;315(July):111–25. https://doi.org/10.1016/j.atherosclerosis.2020.09.020.
108. Borén J, John Chapman M, Krauss RM, et al. Low-density lipoproteins cause atherosclerotic cardiovascular disease: pathophysiological, genetic, and therapeutic insights: a consensus statement from the European Atherosclerosis Society Consensus Panel. Eur Heart J. 2020;41(24):2313–30. https://doi.org/10.1093/eurheartj/ehz962.

109. Armstrong SM, Sugiyama MG, Fung KYY, et al. A novel assay uncovers an unexpected role for SR-BI in LDL transcytosis. Cardiovasc Res. 2015;108(2):268–77. https://doi.org/10.1093/cvr/cvv218.
110. Zhang X, Sessa WC, Fernández-Hernando C. Endothelial transcytosis of lipoproteins in atherosclerosis. Front Cardiovasc Med. 2018;5(September):1–6. https://doi.org/10.3389/fcvm.2018.00130.
111. Braun A, Trigatti BL, Post MJ, et al. Loss of SR-BI expression leads to the early onset of occlusive atherosclerotic coronary artery disease, spontaneous myocardial infarctions, severe cardiac dysfunction, and premature death in apolipoprotein E-deficient mice. Circ Res. 2002;90(3):270–6. https://doi.org/10.1161/hh0302.104462.
112. Huang L, Chambliss KL, Gao X, et al. SR-B1 drives endothelial cell LDL transcytosis via DOCK4 to promote atherosclerosis. Nature. 2019;569(7757):565–9. https://doi.org/10.1038/s41586-019-1140-4.
113. Ghaffari S, Jang E, Nabi FN, et al. Endothelial HMGB1 is a critical regulator of LDL transcytosis via an SREBP2–SR-BI axis. Arterioscler Thromb Vasc Biol. 2021;41:200–16. https://doi.org/10.1161/atvbaha.120.314557.
114. Andersson U, Wang H, Palmblad K, et al. High mobility group 1 protein (HMG-1) stimulates proinflammatory cytokine synthesis in human monocytes. J Exp Med. 2000;192(4):565–70. https://doi.org/10.1084/jem.192.4.565.
115. Fiuza C, Bustin M, Talwar S, et al. Inflammation-promoting activity of HMGB1 on human microvascular endothelial cells. Blood. 2003;101(7):2652–60. https://doi.org/10.1182/blood-2002-05-1300.
116. Ghaffari S, Nabi FN, Sugiyama MG, Lee WL. Estrogen inhibits LDL (low-density lipoprotein) transcytosis by human coronary artery endothelial cells via GPER (G-protein-coupled estrogen receptor) and SR-BI (scavenger receptor class B type 1). Arterioscler Thromb Vasc Biol. 2018;38(10):2283–94. https://doi.org/10.1161/ATVBAHA.118.310792.
117. Kraehling JR, Chidlow JH, Rajagopal C, et al. Genome-wide RNAi screen reveals ALK1 mediates LDL uptake and transcytosis in endothelial cells. Nat Commun. 2016;7:13516. https://doi.org/10.1038/ncomms13516.
118. Frank PG, Pavlides S, Cheung MWC, Daumer K, Lisanti MP. Role of caveolin-1 in the regulation of lipoprotein metabolism. Am J Physiol Cell Physiol. 2008;295(1):242–8. https://doi.org/10.1152/ajpcell.00185.2008.
119. Fernández-Hernando C, Yu J, Dávalos A, Prendergast J, Sessa WC. Endothelial-specific overexpression of caveolin-1 accelerates atherosclerosis in apolipoprotein E-deficient mice. Am J Pathol. 2010;177(2):998–1003. https://doi.org/10.2353/ajpath.2010.091287.
120. Ramírez CM, Zhang X, Bandyopadhyay C, et al. Caveolin-1 regulates atherogenesis by attenuating low-density lipoprotein transcytosis and vascular inflammation independently of endothelial nitric oxide synthase activation. Circulation. 2019;140(3):225–39. https://doi.org/10.1161/CIRCULATIONAHA.118.038571.
121. Pirillo A. LOX-1, OxLDL, and atherosclerosis. Mediat Inflamm. 2013;2013(March):12.
122. Rader DJ, Alexander ET, Weibel GL, Billheimer J, Rothblat GH. The role of reverse cholesterol transport in animals and humans and relationship to atherosclerosis. J Lipid Res. 2009;50(Suppl):189–94. https://doi.org/10.1194/jlr.R800088-JLR200.
123. Hurt-Camejo E, Olsson U, Wiklund O, Bondjers G, Camejo G. Cellular consequences of the association of ApoB lipoproteins with proteoglycans. Arterioscler Thromb Vasc Biol. 1997;17(6):1011–7. https://doi.org/10.1161/01.ATV.17.6.1011.
124. Badimon L, Luquero A, Crespo J, Peña E, Borrell-Pages M. PCSK9 and LRP5 in macrophage lipid internalization and inflammation. Cardiovasc Res. 2021;117:2054–68. https://doi.org/10.1093/cvr/cvaa254.
125. Tang ZH, Peng J, Ren Z, et al. New role of PCSK9 in atherosclerotic inflammation promotion involving the TLR4/NF-κB pathway. Atherosclerosis. 2017;262:113–22. https://doi.org/10.1016/j.atherosclerosis.2017.04.023.

126. Leucker TM, Amat-Codina N, Chelko S, Gerstenblith G. Proprotein convertase subtilisin/kexin type 9 links inflammation to vascular endothelial cell dysfunction. bioRxiv. 2021:2021.01.15.426820. https://doi.org/10.1101/2021.01.15.426820.
127. Ding Z, Liu S, Wang X, et al. Cross-talk between LOX-1 and PCSK9 in vascular tissues. Cardiovasc Res. 2015;107(4):556–67. https://doi.org/10.1093/cvr/cvv178.
128. Moore KJ, Sheedy FJ, Fisher EA. Macrophages in atherosclerosis: a dynamic balance. Nat Rev Immunol. 2013;13(10):709–21. https://doi.org/10.1038/nri3520.
129. Miller YI, Choi S, Wiesner P, et al. Oxidation-specific epitopes are danger-associated molecular patterns recognized by pattern recognition receptors of innate immunity. Hazen S, McIntyre TM, eds. Circ Res. 2011;108(2):235–48. https://doi.org/10.1161/CIRCRESAHA.110.223875.
130. Kunjathoor VV, Febbraio M, Podrez EA, et al. Scavenger receptors class A-I/II and CD36 are the principal receptors responsible for the uptake of modified low density lipoprotein leading to lipid loading in macrophages. J Biol Chem. 2002;277(51):49982–8. https://doi.org/10.1074/jbc.M209649200.
131. Chistiakov DA, Melnichenko AA, Myasoedova VA, Grechko AV, Orekhov AN. Mechanisms of foam cell formation in atherosclerosis. J Mol Med. 2017;95(11):1153–65. https://doi.org/10.1007/s00109-017-1575-8.
132. Stewart CR, Stuart LM, Wilkinson K, et al. CD36 ligands promote sterile inflammation through assembly of a toll-like receptor 4 and 6 heterodimer. Nat Immunol. 2010;11(2):155–61. https://doi.org/10.1038/ni.1836.
133. Seimon TA, Nadolski MJ, Liao X, et al. Atherogenic lipids and lipoproteins trigger CD36-TLR2-dependent apoptosis in macrophages undergoing endoplasmic reticulum stress. Cell Metab. 2010;12(5):467–82. https://doi.org/10.1016/j.cmet.2010.09.010.
134. Binder CJ, Papac-Milicevic N, Witztum JL. Innate sensing of oxidation-specific epitopes in health and disease. Nat Rev Immunol. 2016;16(8):485–97. https://doi.org/10.1038/nri.2016.63.
135. Yu XH, Fu YC, Zhang DW, Yin K, Tang CK. Foam cells in atherosclerosis. Clin Chim Acta. 2013;424:245–52. https://doi.org/10.1016/j.cca.2013.06.006.
136. Lim HY, Thiam CH, Yeo KP, et al. Lymphatic vessels are essential for the removal of cholesterol from peripheral tissues by SR-BI-mediated transport of HDL. Cell Metab. 2013;17(5):671–84. https://doi.org/10.1016/j.cmet.2013.04.002.
137. Shankman LS, Gomez D, Cherepanova OA, et al. KLF4-dependent phenotypic modulation of smooth muscle cells has a key role in atherosclerotic plaque pathogenesis. Nat Med. 2015;21(6):628–37. https://doi.org/10.1038/nm.3866.
138. Llorente-Cortés V, Otero-Viñas M, Camino-López S, Costales P, Badimon L. Cholesteryl esters of aggregated LDL are internalized by selective uptake in human vascular smooth muscle cells. Arterioscler Thromb Vasc Biol. 2006;26(1):117–23. https://doi.org/10.1161/01.ATV.0000193618.32611.8b.
139. Pryma CS, Ortega C, Dubland JA, Francis GA. Pathways of smooth muscle foam cell formation in atherosclerosis. Curr Opin Lipidol. 2019;30(2):117–24. https://doi.org/10.1097/MOL.0000000000000574.
140. Chellan B, Rojas E, Zhang C, Hofmann Bowman MA. Enzyme-modified non-oxidized LDL (ELDL) induces human coronary artery smooth muscle cell transformation to a migratory and osteoblast-like phenotype. Sci Rep. 2018;8(1):1 14. https://doi.org/10.1038/s41598-018-30073-w.
141. Shi C, Pamer EG. Monocyte recruitment during infection and inflammation. Nat Rev Immunol. 2011;11(11):762–74. https://doi.org/10.1038/nri3070.
142. Tabas I, Bornfeldt KE. Macrophage phenotype and function in different stages of atherosclerosis. Hazen S, McIntyre TM, eds. Circ Res. 2016;118(4):653–67. https://doi.org/10.1161/CIRCRESAHA.115.306256.

143. Forrester SJ, Kikuchi DS, Hernandes MS, Xu Q, Griendling KK. Reactive oxygen species in metabolic and inflammatory signaling. Circ Res. 2018;122(6):877–902. https://doi.org/10.1161/CIRCRESAHA.117.311401.
144. Kattoor AJ, Pothineni NVK, Palagiri D, Mehta JL. Oxidative stress in atherosclerosis. Curr Atheroscler Rep. 2017;19(11):42. https://doi.org/10.1007/s11883-017-0678-6.
145. Bochkov VN, Oskolkova OV, Birukov KG, Levonen AL, Binder CJ, Stöckl J. Generation and biological activities of oxidized phospholipids. Antioxid Redox Signal. 2010;12(8):1009–59. https://doi.org/10.1089/ars.2009.2597.
146. Chang MK, Binder CJ, Miller YI, et al. Apoptotic cells with oxidation-specific epitopes are immunogenic and proinflammatory. J Exp Med. 2004;200(11):1359–70. https://doi.org/10.1084/jem.20031763.
147. Bochkov V, Gesslbauer B, Mauerhofer C, Philippova M, Erne P, Oskolkova OV. Pleiotropic effects of oxidized phospholipids. Free Radic Biol Med. 2017;(111):6–24. https://doi.org/10.1016/j.freeradbiomed.2016.12.034.
148. Bochkov VN, Philippova M, Oskolkova O, et al. Oxidized phospholipids stimulate angiogenesis via autocrine mechanisms, implicating a novel role for lipid oxidation in the evolution of atherosclerotic lesions. Circ Res. 2006;99(8):900–8. https://doi.org/10.1161/01.RES.0000245485.04489.ee.
149. Schröder K. Redox control of angiogenesis. Antioxid Redox Signal. 2019;30(7):960–71. https://doi.org/10.1089/ars.2017.7429.
150. Wolf D, Ley K. Immunity and inflammation in atherosclerosis. Circ Res. 2019;124(2):315–27. https://doi.org/10.1161/CIRCRESAHA.118.313591.
151. Baumer Y, McCurdy S, Weatherby TM, et al. Hyperlipidemia-induced cholesterol crystal production by endothelial cells promotes atherogenesis. Nat Commun. 2017;8(1) https://doi.org/10.1038/s41467-017-01186-z.
152. Okura Y, Brink M, Itabe H, Scheidegger KJ, Kalangos A, Delafontaine P. Oxidized low-density lipoprotein is associated with apoptosis of vascular smooth muscle cells in human atherosclerotic plaques. Circulation. 2000;102(22):2680–6. https://doi.org/10.1161/01.CIR.102.22.2680.
153. Doran AC, Yurdagul A, Tabas I. Efferocytosis in health and disease. Nat Rev Immunol. 2020;20(4):254–67. https://doi.org/10.1038/s41577-019-0240-6.
154. Vengrenyuk Y, Nishi H, Long X, et al. Cholesterol loading reprograms the microRNA-143/145-Myocardin axis to convert aortic smooth muscle cells to a dysfunctional macrophage-like phenotype. Arterioscler Thromb Vasc Biol. 2015;35(3):535–46. https://doi.org/10.1161/ATVBAHA.114.304029.
155. Kasikara C, Doran AC, Cai B, Tabas I. The role of non-resolving inflammation in atherosclerosis. J Clin Invest. 2018;128(7):2713–23. https://doi.org/10.1172/JCI97950.
156. Salic K, Morrison MC, Verschuren L, et al. Resolvin E1 attenuates atherosclerosis in absence of cholesterol-lowering effects and on top of atorvastatin. Atherosclerosis. 2016;250:158–65. https://doi.org/10.1016/j.atherosclerosis.2016.05.001.
157. Akers EJ, Nicholls SJ, Di Bartolo BA. Plaque calcification: do lipoproteins have a role? Arterioscler Thromb Vasc Biol. 2019;39(10):1902–10. https://doi.org/10.1161/ATVBAHA.119.311574.
158. Ridker PM, Everett BM, Thuren T, et al. Antiinflammatory therapy with Canakinumab for atherosclerotic disease. N Engl J Med. 2017;377(12):1119–31. https://doi.org/10.1056/nejmoa1707914.
159. Tardif J-C, Kouz S, Waters DD, et al. Efficacy and safety of low-dose colchicine after myocardial infarction. N Engl J Med. 2019;381(26):2497–505. https://doi.org/10.1056/nejmoa1912388.
160. Ridker PM, Danielson E, Fonseca FAH, et al. Rosuvastatin to prevent vascular events in men and women with elevated C-reactive protein. N Engl J Med. 2008;359(21):2195–207. https://doi.org/10.1056/NEJMoa0807646.

161. Cannon CP, Blazing MA, Giugliano RP, et al. Ezetimibe added to statin therapy after acute coronary syndromes. N Engl J Med. 2015;372(25):2387–97. https://doi.org/10.1056/nejmoa1410489.
162. Bartels ED, Christoffersen C, Lindholm MW, Nielsen LB. Altered metabolism of LDL in the arterial wall precedes atherosclerosis regression. Circ Res. 2015;117(11):933–42. https://doi.org/10.1161/CIRCRESAHA.115.307182.
163. Sulkava M, Raitoharju E, Levula M, et al. Differentially expressed genes and canonical pathway expression in human atherosclerotic plaques-Tampere vascular study. Sci Rep. 2017(7):1–10. https://doi.org/10.1038/srep41483.
164. Falk E, Nakano M, Bentzon JF, Finn AV, Virmani R. Update on acute coronary syndromes: the pathologists' view. Eur Heart J. 2013;34(10):719–28. https://doi.org/10.1093/eurheartj/ehs411.
165. Narula N, Dannenberg AJ, Olin JW, et al. Pathology of peripheral artery disease in patients with critical limb ischemia. J Am Coll Cardiol. 2018;72(18):2152–63. https://doi.org/10.1016/j.jacc.2018.08.002.
166. O'Neill WC, Han KH, Schneider TM, Hennigar RA. Prevalence of nonatheromatous lesions in peripheral arterial disease. Arterioscler Thromb Vasc Biol. 2015;35(2):439–47. https://doi.org/10.1161/ATVBAHA.114.304764.
167. Soor GS, Vukin I, Leong SW, Oreopoulos G, Butany J. Peripheral vascular disease: who gets it and why? A histomorphological analysis of 261 arterial segments from 58 cases. Pathology. 2008;40(4):385–91. https://doi.org/10.1080/00313020802036764.
168. Torii S, Mustapha JA, Narula J, et al. Histopathologic characterization of peripheral arteries in subjects with abundant risk factors: correlating imaging with pathology. JACC Cardiovasc Imaging. 2019;12(8P1):1501–13. https://doi.org/10.1016/j.jcmg.2018.08.039.
169. McDermott MM, Kramer CM, Tian L, et al. Plaque composition in the proximal superficial femoral artery and peripheral artery disease events. JACC Cardiovasc Imaging. 2017;10(9):1003–12. https://doi.org/10.1016/j.jcmg.2016.08.012.
170. Ho CY, Shanahan CM. Medial arterial calcification: an overlooked player in peripheral arterial disease. Arterioscler Thromb Vasc Biol. 2016;36(8):1475–82. https://doi.org/10.1161/ATVBAHA.116.306717.
171. McNally MM, Univers J. Acute limb ischemia. Surg Clin North Am. 2018;98(5):1081–96. https://doi.org/10.1016/j.suc.2018.05.002.
172. Duval S, Keo HH, Oldenburg NC, et al. The impact of prolonged lower limb ischemia on amputation, mortality, and functional status: the FRIENDS registry. Am Heart J. 2014;168(4):577–87. https://doi.org/10.1016/j.ahj.2014.06.013.
173. Howard DPJ, Banerjee A, Fairhead JF, Hands L, Silver LE, Rothwell PM. Population-based study of incidence, risk factors, outcome, and prognosis of ischemic peripheral arterial events: implications for prevention. Circulation. 2015;132(19):1805–15. https://doi.org/10.1161/CIRCULATIONAHA.115.016424.
174. Bonaca MP, Gutierrez JA, Creager MA, et al. Acute limb ischemia and outcomes with vorapaxar in patients with peripheral artery disease. Circulation. 2016;133(10):997–1005. https://doi.org/10.1161/CIRCULATIONAHA.115.019355.
175. Coats P, Wadsworth R. Marriage of resistance and conduit arteries breeds critical limb ischemia. Am J Physiol Hear Circ Physiol. 2005;288(3):1044–50. https://doi.org/10.1152/ajpheart.00773.2004.
176. Haghighat L, Ionescu CN, Regan CJ, Altin SE, Attaran RR, Mena-Hurtado CI. Review of the current basic science strategies to treat critical limb ischemia. Vasc Endovasc Surg. 2019;53(4):316–24. https://doi.org/10.1177/1538574419831489.
177. McDermott MM, Ferrucci L, Gonzalez-Freire M, et al. Skeletal muscle pathology in peripheral artery disease a brief review. Arterioscler Thromb Vasc Biol. 2020;40:2577–85. https://doi.org/10.1161/ATVBAHA.120.313831.

178. Tuomisto TT, Rissanen TT, Vajanto I, Korkeela A, Rutanen J, Ylä-Herttuala S. HIF-VEGF-VEGFR-2, TNF-α and IGF pathways are upregulated in critical human skeletal muscle ischemia as studied with DNA array. Atherosclerosis. 2004;174(1):111–20. https://doi.org/10.1016/j.atherosclerosis.2004.01.015.
179. Baczynska D, Michalowska D, Barc P, Skora J, Karczewski M, Sadakierska-Chudy A. The expression profile of angiogenic genes in critical limb ischemia popliteal arteries. J Physiol Pharmacol. 2016;67(3):353–62.
180. Choksy S, Pockley AG, Wajeh YE, Chan P. VEGF and VEGF receptor expression in human chronic critical limb ischaemia. Eur J Vasc Endovasc Surg. 2004;28(6):660–9. https://doi.org/10.1016/j.ejvs.2004.09.001.
181. Inampudi C, Akintoye E, Ando T, Briasoulis A. Angiogenesis in peripheral arterial disease. Curr Opin Pharmacol. 2018;39:60–7. https://doi.org/10.1016/j.coph.2018.02.011.
182. Hassanshahi M, Khabbazi S, Peymanfar Y, et al. Critical limb ischemia: current and novel therapeutic strategies. J Cell Physiol. 2019;234(9):14445–59. https://doi.org/10.1002/jcp.28141.
183. Caradu C, Couffnhal T, Chapouly C, et al. Restoring endothelial function by targeting desert hedgehog downstream of Klf2 improves critical limb ischemia in adults. Circ Res. 2018;123(9):1053–65. https://doi.org/10.1161/CIRCRESAHA.118.313177.
184. Gonzalez-Freire M, Moore AZ, Peterson CA, et al. Associations of peripheral artery disease with calf skeletal muscle mitochondrial DNA heteroplasmy. J Am Heart Assoc. 2020;9(7):e015197. https://doi.org/10.1161/JAHA.119.015197.
185. Beckman JA, Creager MA. Vascular complications of diabetes. Circ Res. 2016;118(11):1771–85. https://doi.org/10.1161/CIRCRESAHA.115.306884.
186. Aquino R, Johnnides C, Makaroun M, et al. Natural history of claudication: long-term serial follow-up study of 1244 claudicants. J Vasc Surg. 2001;34(6):962–70. https://doi.org/10.1067/mva.2001.119749.
187. Askew CD, Green S, Walker PJ, et al. Skeletal muscle phenotype is associated with exercise tolerance in patients with peripheral arterial disease. J Vasc Surg. 2005;41(5):802–7. https://doi.org/10.1016/j.jvs.2005.01.037.
188. Robbins JL, Schuyler Jones W, Duscha BD, et al. Relationship between leg muscle capillary density and peak hyperemic blood flow with endurance capacity in peripheral artery disease. J Appl Physiol. 2011;111(1):81–6. https://doi.org/10.1152/japplphysiol.00141.2011.
189. Baum O, Torchetti E, Malik C, et al. Capillary ultrastructure and mitochondrial volume density in skeletal muscle in relation to reduced exercise capacity of patients with intermittent claudication. Am J Physiol Regul Integr Comp Physiol. 2016;310(10):R943–51. https://doi.org/10.1152/ajpregu.00480.2015.
190. White SH, McDermott MM, Sufit RL, et al. Walking performance is positively correlated to calf muscle fiber size in peripheral artery disease subjects, but fibers show aberrant mitophagy: an observational study. J Transl Med. 2016;14(1):1–15. https://doi.org/10.1186/s12967-016-1030-6.
191. Duscha BD, Robbins JL, Jones WS, et al. Angiogenesis in skeletal muscle precede improvements in peak oxygen uptake in peripheral artery disease patients. Arterioscler Thromb Vasc Biol. 2011;31(11):2742–8. https://doi.org/10.1161/ATVBAHA.111.230441.
192. Beckman JA, Duncan MS, Damrauer SM, et al. Microvascular disease, peripheral artery disease, and amputation. Circulation. 2019;140(6):449–58. https://doi.org/10.1161/CIRCULATIONAHA.119.040672.

Chapter 2
Risk Factors of Patients with Peripheral Arterial Disease

Michael J. Gimbel III

Peripheral arterial disease (PAD) is a prevalent condition with an estimated 200 million people affected worldwide. There are many different presentations for PAD which may go unrecognized by patients and providers. It is critical to recognize this condition in order to implement measures to reduce cardiovascular morbidity and mortality and to reduce its progression. In patients with claudication and reduced ankle brachial index (ABI) <0.85 or those with prior revascularization for ischemia, about 20% will undergo elective revascularization and 4% urgent revascularization at 2-year follow-up. Cardiovascular death, myocardial infarction, and stroke will occur in 11% of these patients during the same 2 years [1, 2]. Faringa et al. reported in patients with an ABI <0.90 a 10-year mortality of 40%. The comorbid conditions that increased the risk of death were renal dysfunction, heart failure, ST segment changes, age >65 years, hyperlipidemia, ABI <0.60, Q waves, diabetes, cerebrovascular disease, and pulmonary disease [3]. In the VOYAGER-PAD study, in patients who had lower extremity revascularization, the 3-year incidence of death from cardiovascular causes, ischemic stroke, acute limb ischemia, major amputation from vascular causes, or ischemic stroke was almost 20% despite aggressive revascularization and medical therapy [4]. An even higher-risk population would include patients with diabetic foot wounds and PAD. Kim et al. looked at this group and found that 38% of these patients underwent major amputation. Osteomyelitis, congestive heart failure, leukocytosis, and dementia considerably increased the risk for amputation in this patient population [5].

Recognition of significant PAD may not be as simple as it would seem. In the Rotterdam Study, the vast majority of people with normal ABI (>0.9) had no claudication. However, of those with an abnormal ABI (<0.9), only 6.3% had

M. J. GimbelIII (✉)
Cardiovascular Medicine, PC, Davenport, IA, USA
e-mail: gimbel@cvmedpc.com

N. W. Shammas (ed.), *Peripheral Arterial Interventions*, Contemporary Cardiology, https://doi.org/10.1007/978-3-031-09741-6_2

claudication [6]. Likewise, a study on elderly women showed only 18.3% had claudication with low ABI [7]. So symptoms of PAD cannot be solely relied on to detect PAD, and one must have a higher index of suspicion, especially in those who have risk factors. Diagnosing PAD can be done with rest/exercise ABI testing, Doppler evaluation, and CT or MR angiography with varying levels of sensitivity and specificity.

Non-modifiable Risk Factors of PAD

Age

PAD increases in prevalence as we age. In patients in their 40s, approximately 2% had vascular disease. This increases steadily to 22.3% of patients in their 80s [1]. Males appear to have more claudication than females, but differences in incidence are less clear. The Framingham Study showed an incidence of claudication among males of 7.1 per 1000 and 3.6 per 1000 among women [8]. This increased prevalence of claudication is not consistently shown, but overall, the data do suggest that claudication is more common in men. This does not mean that PAD is more common in men than women, however. The Framingham Offspring Study had the incidence of claudication of 1.9% among men and 0.8% among women. However, the incidence of PAD diagnosed by abnormal ABI was 3.9% for men and 3.3% for women [9].

Family History

Family history of atherosclerotic disease is another risk factor that increases the risk of cardiovascular disease in general and PAD in particular. The National Heart, Lung, and Blood Institute Twin Study evaluated 94 monozygotic and 90 dizygotic white male twins [10]. 33% and 31% of monozygotic and dizygotic twins had concordantly reduced ABIs. The overall prevalence of reduced ABIs in the population studied was 8.2%, suggesting a four times increased risk of PAD among the twins. Another analysis of the Framingham Offspring Study looked at 2286 participants from 999 families [11]. They used two separate statistical analyses to determine the heritability of PAD. They found that after adjusting for cardiovascular risk factors, the estimated heritability of PAD was 22 and 21%. In the GENOA study [12], they looked at the heritability of low ABIs in 1310 African Americans and 796 non-Hispanic white people in a hypertensive sibling study. After adjusting for other cardiovascular disease risk factors, they noted an increased risk of 19.5% and 21.2% in the respective groups.

Renal Dysfunction

Renal dysfunction also increases the risk of developing PAD. The Atherosclerosis Risk in Communities (ARIC) study [13] had >15,000 patients in the United States, of which 14,280 had appropriate creatinine clearance and no history of PAD by ABIs or claudication. After a mean follow-up of 13.1 years, 1016 developed PAD. They found that those with CKD defined as eGFR 15–59 mL/min per 1.73 m^2 were at 1.5 times increased risk of developing PAD compared to those with normal renal function. This is not dissimilar from the observed risk found in the NHANES III analysis which had an OR of 2 for those with CKD [14]. Guerrero [15] looked at 73 patients with stage IV–V renal dysfunction that were not yet on dialysis. They did ABIs and transcranial and carotid ultrasound. 14 (19%) of the patients had ABI <0.91. Of these, 11 (15%) had claudication. Since the average age of the population was 58, this is much higher than the expected incidence based on age. There was also a significantly increased risk of mortality at 5 years for those with CKD and PAD of 64% vs 20% for those without CKD.

Ethnicity

There is also a difference in prevalence of PAD in different ethnicities. Allison et al. [16] combined seven studies to look at the prevalence of PAD in different ethnicities in the United States. This showed that the rate of PAD in black men was about twice the rate of non-Hispanic whites at any age. Rates for other studied groups (Hispanics, Asian Americans, and Native Americans) were similar to non-Hispanic whites. The data for women was similar, but Native American rates were elevated to rates similar with black women. The others were similar and lower at every age. The CHS study [17] measured ABIs in 5084 patients and after a multivariate analysis found non-white race had an odds ratio of 2.36.

Modifiable Risk Factors for PAD

There are risk factors that patients and providers can address to try to reduce complications of PAD. The most common of these are smoking tobacco, hypertension, hyperlipidemia, and diabetes. By aggressively treating these, we would hope to reduce overall cardiovascular risk and morbidity/mortality. Unfortunately, it seems that patients with PAD are undertreated as compared to those with CAD and cerebrovascular disease. Krishnamurthy et al. [18] looked at patients with PAD alone or in combination with CAD and/or cerebrovascular disease or polyvascular disease. 1318 patients had only PAD, whereas 3141 had polyvascular disease. The

PAD-only patients were younger, more commonly women, and more likely to be smoking. They had less diabetes, hyperlipidemia, ESRD, and COPD. Even after the patients had revascularization procedures, the PAD-only group was less likely to be on an ACE/ARB (53% vs 64%) or B-blocker (47% vs 77%) or be prescribed a statin (62% vs 80%). This tells us there is significant room for improvement in the said risk factor modification.

Tobacco Use

Smoking is one of the strongest predictors of risk for the development of PAD. It is also important that is at least partially modifiable. Murabito [19] looked at the data from the Framingham Heart Study to look at the risk factors that contributed to the development of claudication. The odds ratio for smoking was 1.4. In the Rotterdam Study [20] of 6450 patients over age 55, when looking at the increased risk of developing PAD as measured by low ABI, the highest odds ratio was noted for smoking at 2.8. The risk of amputation in patients is 10–11 times higher in smokers than non-smokers [21, 22]. One of the difficulties with attributing risk to smoking is that it is not merely a binary risk. There is stratification according to current smoking status, past smoking, and amount of smoking, i.e., pack-years. The Edinburgh Artery Study looked at 1592 patients aged 55–74 who were followed for 5 years. After 5 years, 5.1% had developed PAD but not CAD. 11.1% had developed CAD but not PAD. Only 1.1% developed both. They looked at those classified as never smokers, moderate smoking (0–25 pack-years), and heavy smoking (>25 pack-years). The odds ratio for moderate smokers compared to never smokers of developing PAD was 1.87 and for heavy smokers was 3.94. The ratios for developing CAD were lower for each group, particularly in the heavy smokers at 1.59 and 1.66, respectively.

Quitting smoking is a very challenging undertaking for many patients. As stated above, smoking significantly increases the risk of PAD. 1215 Japanese men aged 60–79 were evaluated according to smoking status (never, current, quit >20 years, and pack-years) and ABI [23]. The odds ratio of low ABI (<0.90) for smokers to never smokers was 3.7 and 4.2 for men with >45 pack-years of smoking. For men who had quit smoking for more than 20 years, the prevalence of low ABI was similar to never smokers. As stated above, the risk of amputation in smokers with PAD is 10–11 times higher than non-smokers. Stopping smoking does reduce the likelihood of symptomatic progression of PAD, but does not reduce the risk of amputation over the following 2–3 years [22]. This was likely at least partially a result of relatively short follow-up. A study in Sweden [24] looked at the risks 10 years after the onset of claudication. In current smokers, the incidence of myocardial infarction was 53% vs 11% in non-smokers. The overall survival rate was 42% in current smokers vs 82% in former smokers. This shows that smoking cessation has a large impact on not only progression of PAD but also other vascular and non-vascular beds.

Hypertension

Hypertension was also noted to increase the risk of claudication in the Framingham Heart Study. It showed that stage I hypertension increased the risk of developing claudication by 1.5 and stage II hypertension increased the risk by 2.2 [19]. In the Rotterdam Study, the odds ratio for hypertension was not as high at 1.2 [20]. As hypertension is the most common cardiovascular risk factor [25], it impacts the highest number of patients. Of patients at diagnosis for hypertension, 2–5% of them have intermittent claudication, increasing with age [26]. Likewise, 35–55% of patients at the time of diagnosis with PAD have hypertension [26]. A large meta-analysis of 123 studies showed a 10 mmHg decrease in systolic blood pressure was associated with a 20% reduction in major cerebrovascular events, 17% reduction in coronary heart disease, 17% reduction in stroke, and 13% reduction in all-cause mortality. It does appear that some care should be taken in how aggressively PAD patients have their hypertension treated. In a post hoc analysis of the INternational VErapamil-SR/Trandolapril STudy [27], 2699 patients with CAD and PAD were followed for 2.7 years. The primary outcome of all-cause death, non-fatal MI, or non-fatal stroke occurred in 16.3% of the patients with PAD vs 9.2% without PAD. Interestingly, as the systolic blood pressure dropped below 130 mmHg, the incidence of the primary endpoint began to rise in the PAD patients, but not in the others. The J-shaped curve implies lower systolic BPs could be harmful in PAD patients.

Hyperlipidemia

Hyperlipidemia was not as potent of a risk factor when looking at the Framingham Heart Study in that it only increased risk with an odds ratio of 1.2 [19]. However, therapy for lipid-lowering improving outcomes is overall strong. One study that goes contrary to this was an evaluation of bezafibrate. This randomized, double-blind, placebo-controlled study of 1568 men with lower extremity PAD showed no significant reduction of the incidence of coronary heart disease or stroke combined, but did show a reduction in the severity of intermittent claudication at 3 years. The Heart Protection Study evaluated 674 UK adults with PAD among other high-risk groups. They were randomly selected to 40 mg simvastatin vs placebo. After a mean of 5 years, those in the PAD group assigned to simvastatin had a 22% relative reduction in the rated of first vascular event. The REACH registry looked at 5861 patients with symptomatic PAD. 62.2% were on a statin at baseline. At 4 years, there was an 18% reduction in worsening claudication, new episode of critical limb ischemia, new percutaneous/surgical revascularization, or amputation noted. The IMPROVE-IT trial [28] looked at the addition of zetia to simvastatin post-ACS. 18,144 patients post-ACS were randomized to simvastatin 40 mg or simvastatin/zetia 40/10 mg daily and followed for 6 years. There was a significant decrease in cardiovascular death, MI, stroke, unstable angina leading to hospitalization, and coronary revascularization >30 days post-randomization. The data for lipid-lowering agents continues to rise with the study of PCSK-9 inhibitors. Evolocumab was studied in randomizing 27,564 patients with cardiovascular disease and LDL >70 on statin therapy to drug vs placebo and followed for a median duration of 2.2 years. The primary endpoint of cardiovascular death, MI, stroke, hospitalization for unstable angina, or coronary revascularization was reduced from 11.3 to 9.8%.

Diabetes

Diabetes is a particularly strong risk factor for PAD. Also looking at the Framingham Heart Study data, the odds ratio for increased risk with diabetes was 2.6 [19]. The only risk factor that they found with a higher risk was coronary artery disease at 2.7. The MetS-Greece Multicentre Study [29] looked at a cross-section of 4153 Greek people to assess the prevalence of PAD in patients with metabolic syndrome with and without diabetes. The odds ratio of those with metabolic syndrome without diabetes was 1.48, all metabolic syndrome was 1.94, and diabetes and metabolic syndrome was 3.04. Unfortunately, those who also have PAD are also at risk of increased risk of cardiovascular complications including death. In multiple studies looking at the increased risk of developing PAD and risk factors, having diabetes increased the risk of developing PAD two to four times [30]. As for those patients who do have diabetes and develop PAD, they were five times more likely to have an amputation and had three times the mortality than patients with PAD but no diabetes. The extent of other complications of diabetes, including albuminuria and retinopathy, has also been shown to increase the likelihood of PAD development and advancement. In the ADVANCE study, they followed 10,624 patients with type 2 diabetes for 5 years. They found that 6% of the patients developed PAD. Those having macroalbuminuria and photocoagulation therapy had the highest risk of major PAD, including chronic lower limb ulceration and amputation.

As we do classify diabetes as a modifiable risk factor, one wonders about the impact of improved diabetes control and outcomes in PAD. Unfortunately, this information is lacking. The UK Prospective Diabetes Study [31] looked at 3867 newly diagnosed patients with type 2 diabetes, average age of 54. They were placed into a conventional group with focus on diet and medications only if needed, sulfonylurea-based therapy, and insulin-based therapy. After 10 years, the HbA1c was 7.0% in both intensive groups and 7.9% in the conventional group, an 11% reduction. There were a 12% reduction in any diabetes-related complication and a 6% reduction in all-cause mortality. The majority of the risk reduction, 25%, was the reduction of microvascular complications including the need for retinal photocoagulation. No significant risk reduction was noted for peripheral vascular disease.

Newer therapies with SGLT2 inhibitors in patients with cardiovascular disease including PAD have shown a significant reduction in major cardiovascular adverse events in the diabetic patient irrespective of HbA1c at baseline. In the EMPA-REG study [32], the empagliflozin group had a lower rate of death from cardiovascular causes (3.7% vs 5.9% in the placebo group), hospitalization for heart failure (2.7% and 4.1%, respectively), and death from any cause (5.7% and 8.3%, respectively). PAD was present in 21% and 20.5% of the empagliflozin and placebo groups, respectively.

Obesity

Obesity has also been associated with PAD. Gorter et al. [33] looked at 1117 patients, of which 232 had PAD. Others had CAD, AAA, or cerebrovascular disease. The prevalence of metabolic syndrome overall was 46%, but was higher in the PAD group at 58%. Some studies have linked elevated BMI to PAD, but others have failed to show any association. Planas et al. [34] looked at 708 men aged 55–74 who were evaluated for PAD with ABI. 13.4% had PAD as defined by ABI <0.9. There was no association noted with BMI and PAD. A logistic regression model was fitted for smoking, DM, HTN, HDL cholesterol, and triglycerides and noted an increased waist-to-hip ratio was independently associated with PAD, odds ratio of 1.68. Data for improving outcomes with the reduction of BMI or wait-to-hip ratio, etc. have not been shown. However, lifestyle modifications with improved diet and exercise routines are universally recommended.

Inflammation

Inflammation has been one of the primary mechanisms proposed for the development of vascular disease from smoking, DM, metabolic syndrome, hyperlipidemia, and obesity. Evaluating 144 apparently healthy men in the Physicians' Health Study who went on to develop PAD were matched by age and smoking status with 144 who did not develop PAD [35]. Median CRP levels were significantly higher among those who developed PAD vs those who did not (1.34 vs 0.99 mg/L). The relative risk of developing PAD increased with each quartile of CRP as well from the lowest to highest of 1.0, 1.3, 2.0, and 2.3. CRP can also be a marker for the extent of PAD. 387 patients had baseline Hs-CRP and ABIs measured with ABIs repeated in 12 months [36]. The ABIs decreased with each tertile of Hs-CRP (0.70, 0.65, 0.57) and at 12-month follow-up (0.78, 0.70, 0.65). These associations held after correction for conventional risk factors. It was also associated with 24-month death or any cardiovascular event. This finding has not been universal, however. Musicant et al. looked at 332 patients in an NIH prospective study of PAD that had baseline CRP and D-dimer levels. They were followed every 6 months with clinical history and exam, ABIs, and carotid duplex imaging for a median of 38.4 months. Patients with elevated CRP or D-dimer were no more likely to have progression than the lowest tertile. An elevated D-dimer was associated with an increased risk of MI.

CRP and D-dimer are not the only biomarkers that have been evaluated. The InCHIANTI study [37] looked at several aspects of 955 patients over 60 years old, of which 107 had PAD. They evaluated ABI, comorbidities, cholesterol, HDL, albumin, alpha-2 macroglobulin, CRP, fibrinogen, IL-1beta, IL-1 receptor antagonist, IL-6, IL-6 receptor, IL-10, IL-18, TNF-alpha, and transforming growth factor beta. They adjusted for age, sex, BMI, smoking status, comorbidities, HDL, and total cholesterol. After these adjustments, patients with PAD had significantly higher levels of IL-1 receptor antagonist, IL-6, fibrinogen, and CRP. Interestingly, these associations were attenuated with additional adjustment for physical activity.

The changes in inflammatory markers with exercise have been more rigorously evaluated. Saetre et al. [38] evaluated 29 patients with PAD who underwent 8 weeks of a supervised exercise program. They measured walking differences, plasma E-selectin, ICAM-1, and VCAM-1 before and after the 8 weeks. They found significantly reduced levels of E-selectin and ICAM-1, but unchanged VCAM-1. Walking distances significantly improved as well. Signorelli et al. [39] looked at 40 people, 20 with PAD and claudication and 20 healthy controls. TNF-alpha, IL-6, E-selectin, L-selectin, P-selectin, VCAM-1, and ICAM-1 were measured at rest and immediately after treadmill exercise. All measurements were higher at baseline in the PAD patients. Levels were elevated from baseline in both groups after exercise, but the amount of change was significantly higher in the PAD patients compared to controls.

Summary

Evaluation and treatment of patients with possible PAD can be challenging. A thorough evaluation of a patient's risk of developing PAD may enable the diagnosis in someone at an earlier stage. This enables earlier interventions. Included in these interventions are aggressive management of DM, lipids, hypertension, and smoking cessation. Dietary modifications and exercise programs are of paramount importance as well. Other medical therapies, i.e., antiplatelet therapy, anticoagulant therapy, and revascularization, are also important and addressed elsewhere. With all of these different aspects involved, having a strong team of vascular specialists, exercise physiologists, diabetologists, and therapists is extremely advantageous. It is also important to remember that these interventions are aimed at not only treating PAD but also reducing death, MI, and stroke.

References

1. Savji N, Rockman CB, Skolnick AH, Guo Y, Adelman MA, Riles T, Berger JS. Association between advanced age and vascular disease in different arterial territories: a population database of over 3.6 million subjects. J Am Coll Cardiol. 2013;61(16):1736–43.
2. Bonaca MP, Scirica BM, Creager MA, Olin J, Bounameaux H, Dellborg M, Lamp JM, Murphy SA, Braunwald E, Morrow DA. Vorapaxar in patients with peripheral artery disease: results from TRA2{degrees}P-TIMI 50. Circulation. 2013;127(14):1522–9, 1529.e1–6.
3. Feringa HH, Bax JJ, Hoeks S, van Waning VH, Elhendy A, Karagiannis S, Vidakovic R, Schouten O, Boersma E, Poldermans D. A prognostic risk index for long-term mortality in patients with peripheral arterial disease. Arch Intern Med. 2007;167(22):2482–9.
4. Bonaca MP, Bauersachs RM, Anand SS, Debus ES, Nehler MR, Patel MR, Fanelli F, Capell WH, Diao L, Jaeger N, Hess CN, Pap AF, Kittelson JM, Gudz I, Mátyás L, Krievins DK, Diaz R, Brodmann M, Muehlhofer E, Haskell LP, Berkowitz SD, Hiatt WR. Rivaroxaban in peripheral artery disease after revascularization. N Engl J Med. 2020;382(21):1994–2004.
5. Kim SY, Kim TH, Choi JY, Kwon YJ, Choi DH, Kim KC, Kim MJ, Hwang HK, Lee KB. Predictors for amputation in patients with diabetic foot wound. Vasc Specialist Int. 2018;34(4):109–16.
6. Meijer WT, Hoes AW, Rutgers D, Bots ML, Hofman A, Grobbee DE. Peripheral arterial disease in the elderly: the Rotterdam study. Arterioscler Thromb Vasc Biol. 1998;18:185–92.
7. Vogt MT, Cauley JA, Kuller LH, Hulley SB. Prevalence and correlates of lower extremity arterial disease in elderly women. Am J Epidemiol. 1993;137:559–68.
8. Kannel WB, McGee DL. Update on some epidemiologic features of intermittent claudication: the Framingham study. J Am Geriatr Soc. 1985;33:13–8.
9. Murabito JM, Evans JC, Nieto K, Larson MG, Levy D, Wilson PW. Prevalence and clinical correlates of peripheral arterial disease in the Framingham offspring study. Am Heart J. 2002;143:961–96.
10. Carmelli D, Fabsitz RR, Swan GE, Reed T, Miller B, Wolf PA. Contribution of genetic and environmental influences to ankle-brachial blood pressure index in the NHLBI twin study: National Heart, Lung, and Blood Institute. Am J Epidemiol. 2000;151:452–8.
11. Murabito JM, Guo CY, Fox CS, D'Agostino RB. Heritability of the ankle-brachial index: the Framingham offspring study. Am J Epidemiol. 2006;164:963–8.
12. Kullo IJ, Turner ST, Kardia SL, Mosley TH Jr, Boerwinkle E, de Andrade M. A genome-wide linkage scan for ankle-brachial index in African American and non-Hispanic white subjects participating in the GENOA study. Atherosclerosis. 2006;187:433–8.
13. Wattanakit K, Folsom AR, Selvin E, Coresh J, Hirsch AT, Weatherley BD. Kidney function and risk of peripheral arterial disease: results from the atherosclerosis risk in communities (ARIC) study. J Am Soc Nephrol. 2007;18(2):629–36. https://doi.org/10.1681/ASN.2005111204. Epub 2007 Jan 10.
14. Moustapha A, Naso A, Nahlawi M, Gupta A, Arheart KL, Jacobsen DW, Robinson K, Dennis VW. Prospective study of hyperhomocysteinemia as an adverse cardiovascular risk factor in end-stage renal disease. Circulation. 1998;97:138–41.
15. Guerrero A, Montes R, Muñoz-Terol J, Gil-Peralta A, Toro J, Naranjo M, González-Pérez P, Martín-Herrera C, Ruiz-Fernández A. Peripheral arterial disease in patients with stages IV and V chronic renal failure. Nephrol Dial Transplant. 2006;21(12):3525–31. https://doi.org/10.1093/ndt/gfl470. Epub 2006 Aug 29.
16. Mohammedi K, Woodward M, Hirakawa Y, Zoungas S, Williams B, Lisheng L, Rodgers A, Mancia G, Neal B, Harrap S, Marre M, Chalmers J, ADVANCE Collaborative Group. Microvascular and macrovascular disease and risk for major peripheral arterial disease in patients with type 2 diabetes. Diabetes Care. 2016;39(10):1796–803.
17. Newman AB, Siscovick DS, Manolio TA, Polak J, Fried LP, Borhani NO, Wolfson SK. Ankle-arm index as a marker of atherosclerosis in the cardiovascular health study. Cardiovascular Heart Study (CHS) Collaborative Research Group. Circulation. 1993;88(3):837–45.

18. Krishnamurthy V, Munir K, Rectenwald JE, Mansour A, Hans S, Eliason JL, Escobar GA, Gallagher KA, Grossman PM, Gurm HS, Share DA, Henke PK. Contemporary outcomes with percutaneous vascular interventions for peripheral critical limb ischemia in those with and without poly-vascular disease. Vasc Med. 2014;19(6):491–9.
19. Murabito JM, D'Agostino RB, Silbershatz H, Wilson WF. Intermittent claudication. A risk profile from the Framingham heart study. Circulation. 1997;96(1):44–9.
20. Meijer WT, Grobbee DE, Hunink MG, Hofman A, Hoes AW. Determinants of peripheral arterial disease in the elderly: the Rotterdam study. Arch Intern Med. 2000;160(19):2934–8.
21. Dormandy J, Heeck L, Vig S. The natural history of claudication: risk to life and limb. Semin Vasc Surg. 1999;12(2):123–37. PMID: 10777239.
22. Dormandy J, Heeck L, Vig S. Predicting which patients will develop chronic critical leg ischemia. Semin Vasc Surg. 1999;12(2):138–41. PMID: 10777240.
23. Cui R, Iso H, Yamagishi K, Tanigawa T, Imano H, Ohira T, Kitamura A, Sato S, Shimamoto T. Relationship of smoking and smoking cessation with ankle-to-arm blood pressure index in elderly Japanese men. Eur J Cardiovasc Prev Rehabil. 2006;13(2):243–8. https://doi.org/10.1097/01.hjr.0000209818.36067.51. PMID: 16575279.
24. Jonason T, Bergstrom R. Cessation of smoking in patients with intermittent claudication. Effects on the risk of peripheral vascular complications, myocardial infarction and mortality. Acta Med Scand. 1987;221:253–60.
25. Lawes CM, Vander Hoorn S, Rodgers A, International Society of Hypertension. Global burden of blood-pressure-related disease, 2001. Lancet. 2008;371:1513–8.
26. Clement DL, De Buyzere ML, Duprez DA. Hypertension in peripheral arterial disease. Curr Pharm Des. 2004;10(29):3615–20. https://doi.org/10.2174/1381612043382819. PMID: 15579058.
27. Bavry AA, Anderson RD, Gong Y, Denardo SJ, Cooper-Dehoff RM, Handberg EM, Pepine CJ. Outcomes among hypertensive patients with concomitant peripheral and coronary artery disease: findings from the INternational VErapamil-SR/Trandolapril STudy. Hypertension. 2010;55(1):48–53.
28. Murphy SA, Cannon CP, Blazing MA, Giugliano RP, White JA, Lokhnygina Y, Reist C, Im K, Bohula EA, Isaza D, Lopez-Sendon J, Dellborg M, Kher U, Tershakovec AM, Braunwald E. Reduction in Total cardiovascular events with ezetimibe/simvastatin post-acute coronary syndrome: the IMPROVE-IT trial. J Am Coll Cardiol. 2016;67(4):353–61.
29. Athyros VG, Mikhailidis DP, Papageorgiou AA, Didangelos TP, Ganotakis ES, Symeonidis AN, Daskalopoulou SS, Kakafika AI, Elisaf M, METS-GREECE Collaborative Group. Prevalence of atherosclerotic vascular disease among subjects with the metabolic syndrome with or without diabetes mellitus: the METS-GREECE Multicentre Study. Curr Med Res Opin. 2004;20(11):1691–701. https://doi.org/10.1185/030079904x5599. PMID: 15587481.
30. Criqui MH, Aboyans V. Epidemiology of peripheral artery disease. Circ Res. 2015;116(9):1509–26.
31. Intensive blood-glucose control with sulphonylureas or insulin compared with conventional treatment and risk of complications in patients with type 2 diabetes (UKPDS 33). UK Prospective Diabetes Study (UKPDS) Group. Lancet. 1998;352(9131):837–53. Erratum in: Lancet 1999 Aug 14;354(9178):602. PMID: 9742976.
32. Zinman B, Wanner C, Lachin JM, et al. Empagliflozin, cardiovascular outcomes, and mortality in type 2 diabetes. N Engl J Med. 2015;373(22):2117–28. https://doi.org/10.1056/NEJMoa1504720. Epub 2015 Sep 17.
33. Gorter PM, Olijhoek JK, van der Graaf Y, Algra A, Rabelink TJ, Visseren FL, SMART Study Group. Prevalence of the metabolic syndrome in patients with coronary heart disease, cerebrovascular disease, peripheral arterial disease or abdominal aortic aneurysm. Atherosclerosis. 2004;173(2):363–9.
34. Planas A, Clara A, Pou JM, et al. Relationship of obesity distribution and peripheral arterial occlusive disease in elderly men. Int J Obes Relat Metab Disord. 2001;25:1068–70.

35. Ridker PM, Cushman M, Stampfer MJ, Tracy RP, Hennekens CH. Plasma concentration of C-reactive protein and risk of developing peripheral vascular disease. Circulation. 1998;97(5):425–8.
36. Vainas T, Stassen FR, de Graaf R, Twiss EL, Herngreen SB, Welten RJ, van den Akker LH, van Dieijen-Visser MP, Bruggeman CA, Kitslaar PJ. C-reactive protein in peripheral arterial disease: relation to severity of the disease and to future cardiovascular events. J Vasc Surg. 2005;42(2):243–51.
37. McDermott MM, Guralnik JM, Corsi A, Albay M, Macchi C, Bandinelli S, Ferrucci L. Patterns of inflammation associated with peripheral arterial disease: the InCHIANTI study. Am Heart J. 2005;150(2):276–81.
38. Saetre T, Enoksen E, Lyberg T, Stranden E, Jørgensen JJ, Sundhagen JO, Hisdal J. Supervised exercise training reduces plasma levels of the endothelial inflammatory markers E-selectin and ICAM-I in patients with peripheral arterial disease. Angiology. 2011;62(4):301–5.
39. Signorelli SS, Mazzarino MC, Di Pino L, Malaponte G, Porto C, Pennisi G, Marchese G, Costa MP, Digrandi D, Celotta G, Virgilio V. High circulating levels of cytokines (IL-6 and TNFalpha), adhesion molecules (VCAM-1 and ICAM-1) and selectins in patients with peripheral arterial disease at rest and after a treadmill test. Vasc Med. 2003;8(1):15–9.

Chapter 3
The Role of Exercise in Treating Symptomatic Claudication in Patients with Peripheral Arterial Disease

Nicolas W. Shammas

Exercise has been recognized as an important first step in treating patients with peripheral arterial disease (PAD) and claudication. Exercise does improve walking performance as a sole therapy or in combination with revascularization. There is a greater benefit when revascularization and exercise are combined [1]. In this chapter, we review data on exercise in symptomatic PAD patients with claudication.

Peripheral arterial disease (PAD) affects more than 200 million people worldwide and is associated with a poor quality of life, higher cardiovascular mortality, and higher major adverse limb events. A large percentage of patients with PAD are asymptomatic, and a smaller percentage has advanced limb ischemia. The remaining patients fall in the category of claudication or atypical limb pain. Claudication is defined as pain in the affected leg with exertion that resolves within 10 min of rest. The first-line treatment of claudicants, advanced limb ischemia patients, and asymptomatic patients is different. There is a consensus that patients with rest pain or ulcerations (chronic limb-threatening ischemia or CLTI) need to undergo revascularization to save their limbs as a first-line therapy. CLTI patients have a very high rate of amputation and cardiovascular death [2]. On the other hand, first-line treatment of asymptomatic patients is preventative with a focus on smoking cessation, exercise, high-dose statins, and antiplatelets. Revascularization for asymptomatic patients is not warranted in the majority of patients. Finally, exercise is now considered a first-line treatment for patients with claudication [1], with or without the addition of cilostazol. High-dose cilostazol 100 mg twice daily had a variable response in individual PAD patients, but there is an overall improvement in walking distance with this drug [3]. Failure of this initial conservative approach generally implies proceeding with revascularization. In patients, however, with very limiting

N. W. Shammas (✉)
Midwest Cardiovascular Research Foundation, Davenport, IA, USA

N. W. Shammas (ed.), *Peripheral Arterial Interventions*, Contemporary Cardiology, https://doi.org/10.1007/978-3-031-09741-6_3

symptoms and a significant compromise of their quality of life, a combined approach of preventative therapy, cilostazol, exercise, and revascularization may provide an optimal combined initial treatment strategy.

Definitions

Supervised exercise (SE): structured aerobic exercise under direct supervision in a facility.

Home-based exercise (HE): structured aerobic exercise performed at home.

Peak walking distance (PWD): maximum distance that can be walked before stopping because of limiting claudication on a treadmill test.

Peak walking time (PWT): maximum time that can be walked before stopping because of limiting claudication on a treadmill test.

6-min walk test (6 MW): maximum walking distance on a 6-min walking test.

Endurance shuttle walk test (ESWT): constant-load walk at submaximal capacity with endpoint is how long the subject can walk.

Medical Outcomes Short Form-36 (SF-36): questionnaire that assesses functional status and quality of life (QOL) and is non-disease-specific.

Walking Impairment Questionnaire (WIQ): self-reported measure of walking capacity and limitations. It incorporates speed and distance as well as stair climbing.

Vascular Quality of Life Assessment (VascuQOL): PAD-specific questionnaire. It assesses social and emotional well-being, activities, symptoms, and pain.

Peak walking performance: "the maximum distance or time walked, measured by an exercise treadmill, 6 MW, or shuttle walk within an individual study" [1].

Absolute claudication distance (ACD) is defined as the number of meters a patient walks before intolerable severe claudication occurs.

Vascular Effects of Exercise

Benefits of exercise in PAD patients include suppression of inflammatory processes, improving endothelial function and increasing nitric oxide synthase, remodeling of skeletal muscle by increasing capillary density, changing in microRNA expression, and increasing in arteriogenesis and angiogenesis. Angiogenesis is the budding of newly formed capillaries induced by hypoxia, whereas arteriogenesis is triggered by exercise and is the formation of functional collaterals from pre-existing arterio-arteriolar connections [4].

Exercise and/or Revascularization Versus Control

A meta-analysis of 27 randomized trials by Biswas et al. [1] showed that peak walking performance is better with exercise than control at 18-month follow-up. Depending on the measurement method, there was a net improvement of 8% (using 6MWD) to 54% (as measured by exercise treadmill testing). Furthermore, exercise improved claudication onset and QOL. Similarly, lower extremity revascularization (endovascular or surgical) resulted in superior peak waking distance and claudication onset on follow-up between 6 and 18 months. Using exercise treadmill, improvement in peak walking distance was about 54% based on strong evidence (level B) with additional strong evidence that this was sustained beyond 18 months. When exercise was compared to revascularization, a net benefit of peak walking performance using treadmill testing was 94% with exercise when compared to revascularization between 6 and 18 months. Weaker evidence suggested that in the first 6 months, revascularization performed better than exercise. Using the PAD-specific VascuQOL questionnaire, exercise and revascularization performed similarly. Finally, the combination of exercise and revascularization had the best improvement in peaking walking performance as measured by treadmill testing through 18 months of follow-up when compared to either exercise alone (156% net benefit) or revascularization alone (73% net benefit). Based on this most recent comprehensive meta-analysis, it appears that a revascularization-first approach to treat patients with limiting claudication will likely yield a quicker improvement in symptoms and along with exercise, a superior and sustained benefit will likely be seen on long follow-up [5]. Although the evidence is not strong, the combination therapy also led to less repeat revascularization at 12–18 months, whereas revascularization alone increased the need for repeat revascularization. Exercise combined with revascularization seems to yield the opposite outcome of less need for revascularization and therefore is a critical component of a comprehensive treatment of the patient [1, 5].

Exercise Programs for PAD Patients

The benefits of exercise are not immediate as normally seen with revascularization. A long-term commitment to exercise is critical to achieve the desired positive and durable results. Exercise can be performed in a supervised facility or at home [6, 7]:

(a) Supervised exercise training (SE).
(b) Home-based exercise training (HE).

Supervised exercise (SE) consists of at least 30–60 min of therapeutic exercise in patients with established symptomatic PAD and conducted in a hospital outpatient setting or physician's office supervised by qualified and trained individuals and under the direct supervision of a physician or an advanced practice provider trained in both basic and advanced life support. The trainer needs to determine the appropriate training modality and its intensity and educate the patient about what to expect from the exercise program. The program is a 12-week program with the option of extending this to 36 sessions. Transitioning the patient to a long-term program is important to continue to benefit from exercise.

Home-based exercise training (HE) is not as well defined as SE. The typical length is three to five sessions per week for 8–12 weeks. Long-term data beyond 36 weeks is not available. HE is flexible and generally better adhered to than SE and is more affordable. However, long-term data on HE and its impact is not clear although short-term improvements in functional capacity, QOL, and cardiovascular risk profile seem to be similar to SE despite the superiority of SE in improving maximal walking and claudication distances. HE however may carry some risks as in-person supervision is not available. Therefore, this is best suited for those who are stable and are mild- to moderate-risk patients.

There are several methods of exercise that have been evaluated. Data however comparing these methods remain of poor quality in general. These include supervised walking exercises, exercises to strengthen leg muscles, exercises that strengthen both arms and legs (Nordic), cycling, and arm ergometry. In a review of the types of exercise training on intermittent claudication, Janssen et al. [7] concluded that the various modalities of exercise were all beneficial in improving mean walking distance (MWD) and pain-free walking distance (PFWD). These different modes of exercise when compared to walking showed no clear differences for MWD or PFWD at 12 weeks or at the end of training. Also the walking impairment questionnaire (WIQ) distance score was not different between the two groups. The certainty of this evidence was judged by the authors to be low because of bias concerns and small sample size.

A sex-related difference in response to supervised exercise has been reported. Gommans et al. [8] reported on data from the prospective 2010 Exercise Therapy in Peripheral Arterial Disease (EXITPAD) study that randomized patients to SE or a walking advice. Analysis included 113 men and 56 women. ACD improved in both males and females but was significantly better in males during the first 3 months (Δ 280 m for men vs Δ 220 m for women; $p = 0.04$). Also the absolute walking distance was shorter for women after 1 year (565 m vs 660 m; $p = 0.032$). QOL and WIQ were similar however.

Cost-Effectiveness of Exercise for PAD

Bermingham et al. [9] reviewed data on cost-effectiveness of SE vs unsupervised exercise (USE). SE was cost-effective in 75% of model stimulations with an incremental cost-effectiveness ratio of £711 to £1608 per QALY gained. The authors concluded that SE should be made widely available and be a first-line treatment for

PAD patients with claudication. When compared to revascularization, SE was a more cost-effective primary treatment and was associated with more cost savings at a 5-year time (−€6412, 95% credibility interval (CrI) −€11,874 to −€1939) [10]. In order to reduce cost, a stepped-care model (SCM) that needs to be implemented with SE is the first strategy to treat claudicants. When this strategy was implemented among DUTCH patients, average cost of claudication treatment was 6% lower than a revascularization-first strategy [11]. Cost-effectiveness for revascularization needs to be looked at on the long term. The benefit of revascularization is lost on long-term follow-up (5 years). No improvement in QOL or walking capacity is seen following revascularization when compared to a non-invasive treatment approach at 5 years. The revascularization cost was also twice than that of the non-invasive conservative approach ($13,098 vs $6965, $p = 0.02$) [12].

Summary

Exercise is a very effective treatment for patients with intermittent claudication. Structured exercise is an ideal first approach to treatment but may not be affordable or convenient for some patients. HE is a good alternative. Both SE and HE require adherence to the program by the patient to optimize benefit, and the program should be at least for 3 months. The exercise program should be tailored to the patient, and several modalities of exercise are effective when compared to a supervised walking exercise. Although revascularization is effective in improving peak walking performance early after revascularization and likely more so in the very symptomatic patients, QOL and walking capacity are not superior to a non-invasive approach at 5 years and are costlier. A combination approach of SE and revascularization is promising as an initial first treatment, but the data is not strong, and more evidence is needed.

References

1. Biswas MP, Capell WH, McDermott MM, et al. Exercise training and revascularization in the management of symptomatic peripheral artery disease. JACC Basic Transl Sci. 2021;6(2):174–88. https://doi.org/10.1016/j.jacbts.2020.08.012. eCollection 2021 Feb.
2. Levin SR, Arinze N, Siracuse JJ. Lower extremity critical limb ischemia: a review of clinical features and management. Trends Cardiovasc Med. 2020;30(3):125–30. https://doi.org/10.1016/j.tcm.2019.04.002. Epub 2019 Apr 15.
3. Bedenis R, Stewart M, Cleanthis M, et al. Cilostazol for intermittent claudication. Cochrane Database Syst Rev. 2014;2014(10):CD003748. https://doi.org/10.1002/14651858.CD003748.pub4.
4. Vogel J, Niederer D, Jung G, Troidl K. Exercise-induced vascular adaptations under artificially versus pathologically reduced blood flow: a focus review with special emphasis on arteriogenesis. Cell. 2020;9(2):333. https://doi.org/10.3390/cells9020333.

5. Fakhry F, Spronk S, van der Laan L, et al. Endovascular revascularization and supervised exercise for peripheral artery disease and intermittent claudication: a randomized clinical trial. JAMA. 2015;314(18):1936–44. https://doi.org/10.1001/jama.2015.14851.
6. Treat-Jacobson D, McDermott MM, Beckman J, et al. Implementation of supervised exercise therapy for patients with symptomatic peripheral artery disease: a science advisory from the American Heart Association. Circulation. 2019;140:e700–10.
7. Jansen SC, Abaraogu UO, Lauret GJ, et al. Modes of exercise training for intermittent claudication. Cochrane Database Syst Rev. 2020;8:CD009638. https://doi.org/10.1002/14651858.CD009638.pub3.
8. Gommans LNM, Scheltinga MRM, van Sambeek MRHM, et al. Gender differences following supervised exercise therapy in patients with intermittent claudication. J Vasc Surg. 2015;62(3):681–8. https://doi.org/10.1016/j.jvs.2015.03.076.
9. Bermingham SL, Sparrow K, Mullis R. The cost-effectiveness of supervised exercise for the treatment of intermittent claudication. Eur J Vasc Endovasc Surg. 2013;46:707–14.
10. van den Houten MML, Lauret GJ, Fakhry F, et al. Cost-effectiveness of supervised exercise therapy compared with endovascular revascularization for intermittent claudication. Br J Surg. 2016;103(12):1616–25. https://doi.org/10.1002/bjs.10247. Epub 2016 Aug 11.
11. Hageman D, Fokkenrood HJP, Essers PPM, et al. Improved adherence to a stepped-care model reduces costs of intermittent claudication treatment in the Netherlands. Eur J Vasc Endovasc Surg. 2017;54(1):51–7. https://doi.org/10.1016/j.ejvs.2017.04.011. Epub 2017 May 20.
12. Djerf H, Millinger J, Falkenberg M, et al. Absence of long-term benefit of revascularization in patients with intermittent claudication: five-year results from the IRONIC randomized controlled trial. Circ Cardiovasc Interv. 2020;13(1):e008450. https://doi.org/10.1161/CIRCINTERVENTIONS.119.008450. Epub 2020 Jan 15.

Chapter 4
Pharmacologic Interventions in Patients with Peripheral Arterial Disease

Qais Radaideh and Nicolas W. Shammas

Peripheral arterial disease (PAD) is a global pandemic with more than 200 million people affected worldwide [1, 2]. The disease is asymptomatic in more than half of the patients. When symptomatic, patients can have claudication or advanced symptoms such as rest foot pain or ulcerations. Among symptomatic patients, 5–10% will progress to chronic limb-threatening ischemia (CLTI), a strong predictor for amputation and mortality [3]. CLTI affects two–three million people in the United States alone [4–6]. The Reduction of Atherothrombosis for Continued Health (REACH) registry showed that primary adverse limb outcome at 4 years in patients not taking statins was 26.2% vs 22.0% among those on statins ($p = 0.0013$) [2, 3].

PAD has a set of risk factors. Fowkes et al. [1] noted that in high-income versus low-income population, smoking (odds ratio 2.72 (95% CI: 2.39–3.09) vs 1.42 (1.25–1.62)), diabetes (1.88 [1.66–2.14] vs 1.47 [1.29–1.68]), hypertension (1.55 [1.42–1.71] vs 1.36 [1.24–1.50]), and hypercholesterolemia (1.19 [1.07–1.33] vs 1.14 [1.03–1.25]), respectively, were all important risk factors for PAD. In the United States, PAD affects 10–15% of the population and remains a growing problem [1, 7, 8] likely due to the rise of diabetes and the growing number of the aging population, both risk factors for PAD. The importance of modifying these risk factors is critical in reducing PAD and its cardiovascular morbidity and mortality.

PAD patients die mostly of myocardial infarction and stroke. In the REACH registry, the 1-year combined endpoint of cardiovascular death, myocardial infarction, stroke, and hospitalization was 21.14% for PAD patients [6]. All-cause death at 1 year was 16% as it has been shown in the Swedish national registry, and the worse the PAD, the worse the prognosis [9, 10]. Atherosclerosis is the primary underlying cause of these ischemic events in the PAD patient. Antithrombotic drugs, therefore, have become a cornerstone in the management of these patients to reduce

Q. Radaideh · N. W. Shammas (✉)
Midwest Cardiovascular Research Foundation, Davenport, IA, USA

N. W. Shammas (ed.), *Peripheral Arterial Interventions*, Contemporary Cardiology, https://doi.org/10.1007/978-3-031-09741-6_4

cardiovascular events but have no impact on symptom improvement. Higher-risk PAD patients [11] are more likely to benefit from antithrombotic therapy. In addition to these therapies, some oral diabetic drugs have emerged as important pharmacologic interventions in patients with diabetes and established cardiovascular disease, including PAD patients, to reduce the likelihood of cardiovascular mortality, non-fatal stroke, and non-fatal myocardial infarction.

In this chapter, we examine current data on antiplatelet, oral anticoagulant, and oral diabetic therapies in reducing cardiovascular events in the PAD patient as well as review pharmacologic interventions that reduce claudication in these patients.

Oral Antiplatelet Therapies

Aspirin

The role of aspirin in asymptomatic patients with diabetes and PAD was evaluated in the prevention of progression of arterial disease and diabetes (POPADAD) trial [12]. In this randomized, placebo-controlled study, 1276 adults with type 1 and 2 diabetes and abnormal ankle brachial index (ABI) were included. Patients were randomized to aspirin or placebo (with a 2 × 2 factorial design including antioxidant capsule). Similar major adverse events including death, amputation, non-fatal myocardial infarction (MI), and stroke were seen (18.2% vs 18.3%). Also, in the Aspirin for Asymptomatic Atherosclerosis trial [13], 3350 patients with abnormal but asymptomatic ABI were randomized to aspirin versus placebo. The primary endpoint was a composite of fatal or non-fatal coronary event or stroke or revascularization. After a mean follow-up of 8 years, there was no statistically significant difference between the two groups (13.7 events per 1000 person-years in the aspirin group vs 13.3 in the placebo group; hazard ratio [HR], 1.03; 95% CI: 0.84–1.27). Also, there was no statistical difference between the two groups in vascular events or all-cause mortality or major hemorrhage requiring admission to the hospital. Currently, it is a class III indication (not recommended) to prescribe aspirin in patients with asymptomatic PAD in the 2017 European Society of Cardiology guidelines [14]. The 2016 American College of Cardiology/American Heart Association guidelines [15] consider antiplatelet drugs in asymptomatic patients with PAD (ABI ≤0.90) to be reasonable to reduce the risk of MI, stroke, or vascular death. The ACC/AHA points out that the trial by Fowkes et al. [13] was not powered to analyze subgroups and the "uncertainty of the result does not rule out the possibility that aspirin could provide benefit in such patients, especially in those at increased risk of cardiovascular events." The ACC/AHA however acknowledges that in patients with asymptomatic PAD and borderline ABI (0.91–0.99), the role of antiplatelet therapy remains uncertain.

In contrast to the asymptomatic PAD patient, antiplatelet drugs including aspirin are recommended in the symptomatic PAD patient to prevent major cardiovascular events including MI, stroke, or vascular death. In a meta-analysis by the Antithrombotic Trialists' Collaboration [16], there was a 22% odds reduction for cardiovascular events, including MI, stroke, or vascular death. A dose of 75–150 mg led to a reduction in vascular events by 32%.

Clopidogrel

In the Clopidogrel Versus Aspirin in Patients at Risk of Ischemic Events (CAPRIE) [17] trial, there was an 8.7% relative risk reduction in MACE with clopidogrel compared to aspirin. A greater reduction of MACE was observed in the PAD subgroup with a relative risk of 0.76 [95% CI: 0.64–0.91]. Currently, the ACC/AHA guidelines [15] indicate that antiplatelet therapy with aspirin alone (range 75–325 mg per day) or clopidogrel alone (75 mg per day) is recommended to reduce MI, stroke, and vascular death in patients with symptomatic PAD. The ESC guidelines state that clopidogrel can be considered over aspirin therapy in symptomatic PAD patients (class IIb) [14].

The use of dual antiplatelet therapy is not recommended based on the Clopidogrel for High Atherothrombotic Risk and Ischemic Stabilization, Management, and Avoidance (CHARISMA) trial [18, 19] but may be considered for high-risk PAD patients with no increased risk of bleeding. A total of 9478 patients were included in CHARISMA and followed for 27.6 months. MACE was lower in the clopidogrel plus aspirin arm than in the placebo plus aspirin arm (7.3% vs 8.8%, $p = 0.01$), and no significant differences in the rate of severe bleeding (1.7% vs 1.5%, $p = 0.50$) were seen. An increase in moderate bleeding was, however, noted (2.0% vs 1.3%, $p = 0.004$).

Ticagrelor

The Prevention of Cardiovascular Events in Patients with Prior Heart Attack Using Ticagrelor Compared to Placebo on a Background of Aspirin-Thrombolysis in Myocardial Infarction 54 (PEGASUS-TIMI-54) trial suggested a greater benefit with ticagrelor plus aspirin versus aspirin alone in PAD patients with prior myocardial infarction [20]. In this trial and of 21,162 patients with prior MI (1–3 years) randomized to ticagrelor 90 mg twice daily, ticagrelor 60 mg twice daily, or placebo, all on a background of low-dose aspirin, 1143 patients had known PAD. Ticagrelor plus aspirin versus aspirin monotherapy conferred an absolute risk reduction of MACE (defined as CV death, MI, or stroke) in this PAD population by 4.1% and a significant reduction in risk of MALE (defined as acute limb ischemia or peripheral revascularization for ischemia) (HR, 0.65 [95% CI: 0.44–0.95]). The risk of major bleed however was higher in the ticagrelor group regardless of the presence of PAD (the absolute excess of TIMI major bleeding was 0.12%). The 60 mg dose had particularly favorable outcomes for CV and all-cause mortality.

The Examining Use of Ticagrelor in Peripheral Artery Disease (EUCLID) trial [11, 21] enrolled 13,885 patients with symptomatic PAD randomized to ticagrelor vs clopidogrel. Ticagrelor was not superior to clopidogrel in preventing MACE (HR, 1.02 [95% CI: 0.92–1.13]) or ALI (HR, 1.03 [95% CI: 0.79–1.33]). In both groups, acute limb ischemia (ALI) was 1.7% and major bleeding 1.6%.

In the Effect of Ticagrelor on Health Outcomes in Diabetes Mellitus Patients Intervention Study (THEMIS), 19,220 patients were randomized to ticagrelor versus placebo on a background of aspirin. Patients were included if they were more than 50 years or older with type 2 diabetes and stable CAD with either a prior percutaneous coronary intervention (PCI) or angiographic stenosis of 50% or more. Of these patients, 9% had PAD. Patients could not be included if they had prior MI or stroke. The prespecified endpoint of coronary, cerebral, and peripheral ischemic events was significantly reduced with ticagrelor compared with placebo. The composite of all-cause death, myocardial infarction, stroke, acute limb ischemia, or major amputation of vascular cause was lower (9.0%) compared with placebo (11.0%) in those with a history of PCI receiving ticagrelor and no benefit in those with no prior PCI. A 55% reduction in MALE was achieved with additional use of ticagrelor and aspirin vs aspirin only (HR, 0.45 [95% CI: 0.23–0.86]), at the expense of increased TIMI major bleeding (HR, 2.32 [95% CI: 1.82–2.94]).

In the Dual Antiplatelet Therapy (DAPT) trial [22], there were 649 patients with PAD who were randomized to thienopyridine plus aspirin therapy for an additional 18 months versus aspirin therapy alone. Extended DAPT was associated with consistent ischemic benefit at the expense of increase in major bleeding. Patients with PAD had higher rates of MI/stent thrombosis (6.03% vs 2.92%; $p < 0.001$), major adverse cardiovascular and cerebrovascular events (11.65% vs 4.62%; $p < 0.001$), and bleeding (4.86% vs 1.74%; $p < 0.001$) than those with no PAD. Extended DAPT showed a continued reduction in MI and stent thrombosis in the PAD patients (with PAD, HR: 0.63; 95% CI: 0.32–1.22; without PAD, HR: 0.53; 95% CI: 0.42, 0.66; interaction $p = 0.631$).

In the Prolonging Dual Antiplatelet Treatment After Grading Stent-Induced Intimal Hyperplasia Study (PRODIGY) trial [23], the presence of PAD was associated with poor prognosis. This trial showed that a prolonged versus shorter DAPT duration was associated with a greater reduction in MACE in patients with PAD compared with patients without PAD, particularly among those presenting with ACS. Prolonged (24 months) vs short DAPT (<6 months) conveyed a lower risk of the primary efficacy endpoint of the composite of death, myocardial infarction, or cerebrovascular accidents in patients with PAD (19 [16.1%] vs 35 [27.3%]; HR, 0.54; 95% CI: 0.31–0.95; $p = 0.03$) but not in patients without PAD (81 [9.3%] vs 63 [7.4%]; HR, 1.28; 95% CI: 0.92–1.77; $p = 0.15$). Bleeding was not statistically different between the long and short DAPT treatment (HR, 0.77; 95% CI: 0.27–2.21;

$p = 0.62$). It's important to note that DAPT and PRODIGY did not assess limb events. However, patients with PAD seem to benefit more from prolonged DAPT therapy.

Vorapaxar

Platelet activation is mediated by three main pathways: thromboxane A2, adenosine diphosphate acting on the P2Y12 receptor, and thrombin acting on the protease-activated receptors (PAR)-1; the latter is considered the most potent platelet activator.

Aspirin irreversibly inhibits the COX-1 enzyme, therefore blocking the production of TXA2. P2Y12 receptor antagonists block adenosine diphosphate from activating platelets. Vorapaxar is a PAR-1 and PAR-4 receptor blocker. Blocking more than one pathway leads to stronger inhibition of platelet activation but likely also more bleeding [24, 25].

Vorapaxar is the first oral PAR-1 antagonist approved in the United States and was shown to reduce major cardiovascular events in patients with history of MI and PAD. It is contraindicated in patients with history of central nervous system events. In the Thrombin Receptor Antagonist in Secondary Prevention of Atherothrombotic Ischemic Events-Thrombolysis in Myocardial Infarction 50 (TRA2°P-TIMI 50), patients with prior MI, ischemic stroke, or PAD were randomized to either vorapaxar or placebo. Both MACE (HR, 0.85 [95% CI: 0.73–0.99]) and MALE (HR, 0.70 [95% CI: 0.53–0.92]) were reduced with vorapaxar in patients with PAD [26]. Patients with both CAD and PAD had greater reductions in MACE than PAD alone, but a greater reduction in MALE was observed in PAD patients with prior history of revascularization. PAD patients with no prior history of CAD or PAD revascularization had no significant benefit from vorapaxar for reduction of MACE or MALE [27]. Finally, vorapaxar reduced hospitalizations for acute limb ischemia (ALI) (HR 0.58; 95% CI: 0.39–0.86; $p = 0.006$) and decreased need for PAD revascularization (HR 0.84; 95% CI: 0.73–0.97; $p = 0.017$) [28].

Oral Anticoagulants

Rivaroxaban

The Cardiovascular Outcomes for People Using Anticoagulation Strategies (COMPASS) trial randomized 27,395 patients with chronic atherosclerotic cardiovascular disease to a regimen of either rivaroxaban 5 mg twice daily or rivaroxaban 2.5 mg twice daily plus low-dose aspirin or low-dose aspirin alone [29].

After a mean follow-up of 23 months, the trial was stopped as the rivaroxaban 2.5 mg twice a day plus a baby aspirin versus aspirin alone was superior in reducing the primary outcome of cardiovascular death, stroke, or MI group (HR, 0.76 [95% CI: 0.66–0.86]). There were more major bleeding events with rivaroxaban plus aspirin than aspirin alone (HR, 1.70 [95% CI: 1.40–2.05]), though no significant difference in intracranial or fatal bleeding was detected between the two groups.

In a substudy from COMPASS limited to 7470 patients with PAD or carotid artery disease, rivaroxaban plus aspirin compared with aspirin alone reduced MACE (HR, 0.72 [95% CI: 0.57–0.90]), as well as MALE (HR, 0.54 [95% CI: 0.35–0.82]), albeit with an increase in major bleeding (HR, 1.61 [95% CI: 1.12–2.31]) [30].

In the Vascular Outcomes Study of ASA Along with Rivaroxaban in Endovascular or Surgical Limb Revascularization for PAD (VOYAGER-PAD) [31], a double-blind trial, 6564 patients with PAD and revascularization were randomly assigned to receive rivaroxaban (2.5 mg twice daily) plus aspirin or placebo plus aspirin. The primary efficacy outcome was a composite of acute limb ischemia, major amputation for vascular causes, myocardial infarction, ischemic stroke, or death from cardiovascular causes. At 3 years, rivaroxaban was associated with a significantly lower incidence of the primary endpoint than aspirin alone (17.3% and 19.9%, respectively (hazard ratio, 0.85, 95% confidence interval [CI]: 0.76–0.96; $p = 0.009$)) with no significant difference in Thrombolysis in Myocardial Infarction (TIMI) major bleed (2.65 and 1.87%, $p = 0.07$) but a higher incidence of International Society of Thrombosis and Hemostasis (ISTH) major bleeding (5.94 and 4.06%, $p = 0.007$).

Warfarin

Anticoagulation among patients with stable PAD was evaluated in different trials. In the Warfarin Antiplatelet Vascular Evaluation (WAVE) [32] trial, 2161 patients with symptomatic PAD were randomized to anticoagulation with Coumadin plus antiplatelet therapy versus antiplatelet therapy alone and followed for 35 months. The first co-primary outcome was MI, stroke, or death from cardiovascular causes; the second co-primary outcome was MI, stroke, severe ischemia of the peripheral or coronary arteries leading to urgent intervention, or death from cardiovascular causes. The first co-primary outcome occurred in 12.2 and 13.3% for warfarin and aspirin versus aspirin alone (relative risk, 0.92; 95% confidence interval [CI]: 0.73–1.16; $p = 0.48$). The second co-primary outcome occurred in 15.9% and 17.4%, respectively (relative risk, 0.91; 95% CI: 0.74–1.12; $p = 0.37$). Life-threatening bleeding occurred in 4.0% of the warfarin group compared to 1.25% of the aspirin only group (relative risk, 3.41; 95% CI: 1.84–6.35; $p < 0.001$). Warfarin and aspirin were not more effective than aspirin alone and were associated with an increase in major bleeding.

Edoxaban

In the Edoxaban in Peripheral Arterial Disease (ePAD) [33] study, 203 patients who underwent femoropopliteal endovascular therapy were randomized to receive aspirin plus edoxaban or aspirin plus clopidogrel. The primary safety endpoint was bleeding as classified by the TIMI and ISTH criteria; the efficacy endpoint was the rate of restenosis/reocclusion. The bleeding risk was not statistically different with treatment when assessed by either TIMI or ISTH. At 6 months, there was a numerically lower incidence of restenosis/reocclusion with edoxaban compared with clopidogrel, but this was not statistically significant (30.9% vs 34.7%; RR 0.89, 95% CI: 0.59–1.34, $p = 0.643$). This study, however, was not powered for efficacy but only for safety.

Cilostazol (Pletal)

Cilostazol is an oral antiplatelet agent (phosphodiesterase 3 inhibitor) which has been shown to be effective in reducing intermittent claudication (IC) [34]. Pentoxifylline has been used for reducing claudication, but data suggest that it is not more effective than placebo.

Dawson et al. [35] compared cilostazol to pentoxifylline. A total of 698 patients with moderate to severe IC were randomized to a standard dose of cilostazol 100 mg twice daily, a standard dose of pentoxifylline (400 mg three times daily), or placebo (three times daily). At 24 weeks, cilostazol had a 54% improvement in maximal walking distance from the baseline compared with increases of 30% in the pentoxifylline group ($p < 0.05$) and 34% in the placebo group ($p < 0.05$).

In a prospective, randomized, open-label, blinded endpoint study, Lida et al. [36] randomized 127 patients following treatment of femoropopliteal de novo disease to cilostazol (200 mg/day, $n = 63$) or ticlopidine (200 mg/day, $n = 64$) in addition to aspirin (100 mg/day). Vessel patency and freedom from TLR were significantly higher in the cilostazol group than the ticlopidine group. Also, Soga et al. [37] investigated the role of cilostazol in a cohort of 80 patients with IC due to a femoropopliteal lesion. Patients were randomized to cilostazol in addition to aspirin versus aspirin alone. The rate of restenosis was lower in the cilostazol group (43.6% vs 70.3%, $p = 0.02$), and freedom from target lesion revascularization and freedom from major adverse cardiovascular events were higher in the cilostazol group (87.2% vs 67.6%, $p = 0.046$, 76.8% vs 45.6%, $p = 0.006$, respectively)

The Sufficient Treatment of Peripheral Intervention by Cilostazol (STOP-IC) [38] study randomized 200 patients who underwent femoropopliteal angioplasty with nitinol stenting to aspirin either with or without cilostazol. At 12-month follow-up, the angiographic restenosis rate at 12 months was 20% (15/75) in the cilostazol group versus 49% (38/77) in the non-cilostazol group ($p = 0.0001$). The cilostazol group also had a significantly higher event-free survival at 12 months (83% vs 71%, $p = 0.02$).

Lipid-Lowering Drugs

Statins

The Heart Protection Study randomized over 20,536 to statin (simvastatin) or placebo [39]. Among the 6748 patients with PAD, there was a 22% relative reduction (95% CI: 15–29) in the rate of first major vascular events (26.4% simvastatin-allocated vs 32.7% placebo-allocated; $p < 0.0001$). Among all patients included, simvastatin group had a 16% relative reduction in rate of first peripheral vascular event compared to placebo.

In the retrospective REACH study [2], 5861 patients with PAD were evaluated. Among those using statins, there were 18% lower rate of adverse limb outcomes, including worsening symptoms, peripheral revascularization, and ischemic amputations. These findings suggest that statins reduce MALE in PAD patients.

PCSK9 Inhibitors

In the Further Cardiovascular Outcomes Research with PCSK9 Inhibition in Subjects with Elevated Risk (FOURIER) [8], 3642 patients had PAD (1505 with no prior MI or stroke). The primary endpoint of the trial was a composite of cardiovascular death, myocardial infarction, stroke, hospital admission for unstable angina, or coronary revascularization. One secondary outcome was major adverse limb events defined as acute limb ischemia, major amputation, or urgent peripheral revascularization for ischemia. Evolocumab significantly reduced the primary endpoint consistently in patients with PAD (hazard ratio [HR] 0.79; 95% confidence interval [CI]: 0.66–0.94; $p = 0.0098$) and without PAD (HR 0.86; 95% CI: 0.80–0.93; $p = 0.0003$). Evolocumab also reduced the risk of MALE in all patients (HR, 0.58; 95% CI: 0.38–0.88; $p = 0.0093$) with and without known PAD.

Oral Antidiabetic Drugs

GLP-1 Agonists

The role of GLP-1 agonists in the PAD patient has yielded mixed results. In the Exenatide Study of Cardiovascular Event Lowering (EXSCEL) trial [40], 2800 patients with PAD were included. PAD patients had higher rate of MACE when compared to placebo (13.6% vs 11.4%, respectively), higher all-cause mortality (adjusted hazard ratio 1.38 [95% CI: 1.20–1.60]; $p < 0.001$), and more frequent amputations (adjusted hazard ratio 5.48 [95% CI: 4.16–7.22]; $p < 0.001$). Treatment with exenatide showed no differences in MACE or amputation rates versus placebo. In contrast, in a recent analysis from the LEADER and SUSTAIN trials presented at the American Heart Association (AHA) in 2019, more MACE (LEADER, HR 1.27, 95% CI: 1.12, 1.44; SUSTAIN 6, HR 1.72, 95% CI: 1.36, 2.15) was observed in patients with PAD at baseline vs those without PAD. However, liraglutide (hazard ratio 0.77 (95% CI: 0.59, 1.02) and 0.89 (95% CI: 0.79, 1.00)) and semaglutide (hazard ratio 0.57 (95% CI: 0.3–1.07) and 0.78 (95% CI: 0.59–1.02)) appear to lower the risk of cardiovascular events in patients with and without PAD, respectively [41].

SGLT2 Inhibitors in Diabetics

In patients with type 2 diabetes mellitus and PAD, empagliflozin reduced mortality, heart failure, and progression of renal disease with no observed increase in the risk of lower limb amputation [42]. In this substudy of EMPA-REG, empagliflozin reduced cardiovascular death by 43% (HR, 0.57; 95% CI: 0.37–0.88) and all-cause mortality by 38% (HR, 0.62; 95% CI: 0.44–0.88) versus placebo, consistent with findings in patients with PAD. The reduction in cardiovascular death with empagliflozin in patients with T2DM and PAD translates to a number needed to treat of 29 patients over 3.1 years to prevent 1 event.

In the DECLARE-TIMI 58 trial [43], 17,160 patients with type 2 diabetes mellitus were enrolled. 1025 (6%) had PAD. Patients were randomized to dapagliflozin versus placebo. Overall, there were no significant differences in any limb outcome with dapagliflozin versus placebo including limb ischemic adverse events (HR, 1.07 [95% CI: 0.90–1.26]) and amputation (HR, 1.09 [95% CI: 0.84–1.40]).

In the CANagliflozin cardioVascular Assessment Study (CANVAS) trial, the effect of canagliflozin on amputation risk was evaluated and found to be increased [44, 45]. There were 1.8% subjects with atraumatic lower extremity amputations (minor 71%, major 29%) with a hazard ratio of 1.97 [95% CI: 1.41, 2.75] when compared to placebo. An increased risk of amputation was seen in those patients with prior history of amputation, peripheral vascular disease, and neuropathy. The amputation rate was 6.30 with canagliflozin vs 3.37 per 1000 participant-years among the placebo group.

Summary

The use of antiplatelets in symptomatic patients with PAD is recommended, and clopidogrel is preferred over aspirin.

The use of ticagrelor and aspirin in patients with PAD and prior history of myocardial infarction confers additional benefits than aspirin alone but at the expense of bleeding.

Vorapaxar reduces MACE and MALE in PAD patients with prior history of CAD or PAD revascularization and reduces hospitalizations for acute limb ischemia and the need for PAD revascularization.

Rivaroxaban 2.5 mg twice a day with a baby aspirin reduces MACE and MALE in high-risk CAD and PAD patients and in PAD patients post-revascularization.

Warfarin and aspirin are not more effective than aspirin alone, and warfarin is associated with an increase in major bleeding.

Cilostazol reduces claudication and restenosis post-vascular intervention.

Statins and PCSK9 inhibitors appear to reduce cardiovascular events in patients with PAD.

Empagliflozin reduces the risk of MACE in patients with atherosclerotic vascular disease and type 2 diabetes including PAD and reduces cardiovascular mortality with no increase in amputation.

Canagliflozin had higher amputation rates in the PAD diabetic patient, and dapagliflozin had no significant impact on limb outcome.

Liraglutide and semaglutide reduce MACE in diabetic patients with or without PAD, whereas exenatide showed no differences in MACE or amputation rates versus placebo in the PAD patient. Dulaglutide is indicated to reduce MACE in type 2 diabetics with atherosclerotic cardiovascular disease or multiple cardiovascular risk factors.

References

1. Fowkes FGR, Rudan D, Rudan I, et al. Comparison of global estimates of prevalence and risk factors for peripheral artery disease in 2000 and 2010: a systematic review and analysis. Lancet. 2013;382:1329–40.
2. Hirsch AT, Haskal ZJ, Hertzer NR, et al. ACC/AHA 2005 practice guidelines for the management of patients with peripheral arterial disease (lower extremity, renal, mesenteric, and abdominal aortic): a collaborative report from the American Association for Vascular Surgery/Society for Vascular Surgery, Society for Cardiovascular Angiography and Interventions, Society for Vascular Medicine and Biology, Society of Interventional Radiology, and the ACC/AHA Task Force on Practice Guidelines (Writing Committee to Develop Guidelines for the Management of Patients With Peripheral Arterial Disease). Circulation. 2006;113:e463–654. https://doi.org/10.1161/CIRCULATIONAHA.106.174526.
3. Kumbhani DJ, Steg PG, Cannon CP, et al. Statin therapy and long-term adverse limb outcomes in patients with peripheral artery disease: insights from the REACH registry. Eur Heart J. 2014;35:2864–72.
4. Hiatt WR, Hoag S, Hamman RF. Effect of diagnostic criteria on the prevalence of peripheral arterial disease. The San Luis Valley diabetes study. Circulation. 1995;91:1472–9.
5. Criqui MH, Aboyans V. Epidemiology of peripheral artery disease. Circ Res. 2015;116:1509–26.
6. Steg PG, Bhatt DL, Wilson PW, et al. One-year cardiovascular event rates in outpatients with atherothrombosis. JAMA. 2007;297:1197–206.
7. Nehler MR, Duval S, Diao L, et al. Epidemiology of peripheral arterial disease and critical limb ischemia in an insured national population. J Vasc Surg. 2014;60(3):686–95.e2.
8. Bonaca MP, Nault P, Giugliano RP, Keech AC, Pineda AL, Kanevsky E, Kuder J, Murphy SA, Jukema JW, Lewis BS, et al. Low-density lipoprotein cholesterol lowering with evolocumab and outcomes in patients with peripheral artery disease: insights from the FOURIER trial (further

cardiovascular outcomes research with PCSK9 inhibition in subjects with elevated risk). Circulation. 2018;137:338–50. https://doi.org/10.1161/CIRCULATIONAHA.117.032235.
9. Sigvant B, Hasvold P, Kragsterman B, et al. Cardiovascular outcomes in patients with peripheral arterial disease as an initial or subsequent manifestation of atherosclerotic disease: results from a Swedish Nationwide Study. J Vasc Surg. 2017;66:507–514.e1.
10. Ankle Brachial Index Collaboration. Ankle brachial index combined with Framingham risk score to predict cardiovascular events and mortality. A meta-analysis. JAMA. 2008;300: 197–208.
11. Gutierrez JA, Mulder H, Jones WS, Rockhold FW, Baumgartner I, Berger JS, Blomster JI, Fowkes FGR, Held P, Katona BG, et al. Polyvascular disease and risk of major adverse cardiovascular events in peripheral artery disease: a secondary analysis of the EUCLID trial. JAMA Netw Open. 2018;1:e185239. https://doi.org/10.1001/jamanetworkopen.2018.5239.
12. Belch J, MacCuish A, Campbell I, Cobbe S, Taylor R, Prescott R, Lee R, Bancroft J, MacEwan S, Shepherd J, et al. The prevention of progression of arterial disease and diabetes (POPADAD) trial: factorial randomised placebo controlled trial of aspirin and antioxidants in patients with diabetes and asymptomatic peripheral arterial disease. BMJ. 2008;337:a1840. https://doi.org/10.1136/bmj.a1840.
13. Fowkes FG, Price JF, Stewart MC, Butcher I, Leng GC, Pell AC, Sandercock PA, Fox KA, Lowe GD, Murray GD. Aspirin for Asymptomatic Atherosclerosis Trialists Aspirin for prevention of cardiovascular events in a general population screened for a low ankle brachial index: a randomized controlled trial. JAMA. 2010;303:841–8. https://doi.org/10.1001/jama.2010.221.
14. Aboyans V, Ricco J-B, Bartelink M-L, et al. 2017 ESC guidelines on the diagnosis and treatment of peripheral arterial diseases, in collaboration with the European Society for Vascular Surgery (ESVS): document covering atherosclerotic disease of extracranial carotid and vertebral, mesenteric, renal, upper and lower extremity arteries. Eur Heart J. 2018;39:763–816. https://doi.org/10.1093/eurheartj/ehx095.
15. Antithrombotic Trialists' Collaboration. Collaborative meta-analysis of randomised trials of antiplatelet therapy for prevention of death, myocardial infarction, and stroke in high risk patients. BMJ. 2002;324:71.
16. Gerhard-Herman MD, Gornik HL, Barrett C, et al. 2016 AHA/ACC guideline on the management of patients with lower extremity peripheral artery disease: a report of the American College of Cardiology/American Heart Association task force on clinical practice guidelines. J Am Coll Cardiol. 2017;69(11):e71–e126.
17. CAPRIE Steering Committee. A randomised, blinded, trial of clopidogrel versus aspirin in patients at risk of ischaemic events (CAPRIE). CAPRIE Steering Committee. Lancet. 1996;348:1329–39. https://doi.org/10.1016/s0140-6736(96)09457-3.
18. Cacoub PP, Bhatt DL, Steg PG, et al. Patients with peripheral arterial disease in the CHARISMA trial. Eur Heart J. 2009;30:192.
19. Bhatt DL, Flather MD, Hacke W, et al. Patients with prior myocardial infarction, stroke, or symptomatic peripheral arterial disease in the CHARISMA trial. J Am Coll Cardiol. 2007;49:1982.
20. Bonaca MP, Bhatt DL, Storey RF, Steg PG, Cohen M, Kuder J, Goodrich E, Nicolau JC, Parkhomenko A, López-Sendón J, et al. Ticagrelor for prevention of ischemic events after myocardial infarction in patients with peripheral artery disease. J Am Coll Cardiol. 2016;67:2719–28. https://doi.org/10.1016/j.jacc.2016.03.524.
21. Hiatt WR, Fowkes FGR, Heizer G, et al. Ticagrelor versus clopidogrel in symptomatic peripheral artery disease. N Engl J Med. 2017;376:32–40. https://doi.org/10.1056/NEJMoa1611688. Epub 2016 Nov 13.
22. Secemsky EA, Yeh RW, Kereiakes DJ, Cutlip DE, Steg PG, Massaro JM, Apruzzese PK, Mauri L, Dual Antiplatelet Therapy Study Investigators. Extended duration dual antiplatelet therapy after coronary stenting among patients with peripheral arterial disease: a subanalysis of the dual antiplatelet therapy study. JACC Cardiovasc Interv. 2017;10:942–54. https://doi.org/10.1016/j.jcin.2017.02.013.

23. Franzone A, Piccolo R, Gargiulo G, Ariotti S, Marino M, Santucci A, Baldo A, Magnani G, Moschovitis A, Windecker S, et al. Prolonged vs short duration of dual antiplatelet therapy after percutaneous coronary intervention in patients with or without peripheral arterial disease: a subgroup analysis of the PRODIGY randomized clinical trial. JAMA Cardiol. 2016;1:795–803. https://doi.org/10.1001/jamacardio.2016.2811.
24. Jennings LK. Mechanisms of platelet activation: need for new strategies to protect against platelet-mediated atherothrombosis. Thromb Haemost. 2009;102:248–57.
25. Coughlin SR. Thrombin signalling and protease-activated receptors. Nature. 2000;407:258–64.
26. Bonaca MP, Scirica BM, Creager MA, et al. Vorapaxar in patients with peripheral artery disease: results from TRA2°P-TIMI 50. Circulation. 2013;127:1522–9.
27. Deerhake ME, Tricoci P. Vorapaxar: the drug and its applications. https://www.acc.org/latest-in-cardiology/articles/2016/05/18/13/58/vorapaxar. Accessed 2 May 2021.
28. Alonso-Coello P, Bellmunt S, McGorrian C, et al. Antithrombotic therapy in peripheral artery disease: antithrombotic therapy and prevention of thrombosis, 9th ed: American College of Chest Physicians evidence-based clinical practice guidelines. Chest. 2012;141:e669S–90S.
29. Eikelboom JW, Connolly SJ, Bosch J, Dagenais GR, Hart RG, Shestakovska O, Diaz R, Alings M, Lonn EM, Anand SS, et al. Rivaroxaban with or without aspirin in stable cardiovascular disease. N Engl J Med. 2017;377:1319–30. https://doi.org/10.1056/NEJMoa1709118.
30. Anand SS, Bosch J, Eikelboom JW, Connolly SJ, Diaz R, Widimsky P, Aboyans V, Alings M, Kakkar AK, Keltai K, et al. Rivaroxaban with or without aspirin in patients with stable peripheral or carotid artery disease: an international, randomised, double-blind, placebo-controlled trial. Lancet. 2018;391(10117):219–29. https://doi.org/10.1016/S0140-6736(17)32409-1. Epub 2017 Nov 10.
31. Bonaca MP, Bauersachs RM, Anand SS, Debus ES, Nehler MR, Patel MR, et al. Rivaroxaban in peripheral artery disease after revascularization. N Engl J Med. 2020;382(21):1994–2004.
32. Anand S, Yusuf S, Xie C, Pogue J, Eikelboom J, Budaj A, et al. Oral anticoagulant and antiplatelet therapy and peripheral arterial disease warfarin antiplatelet vascular evaluation trial investigators. N Engl J Med. 2007;357(3):217–27. https://doi.org/10.1056/NEJMoa065959.
33. Moll F, Baumgartner I, Jaff M, Nwachuku C, Tangelder M, Ansel G, Adams G, Zeller T, Rundback J, Grosso M, et al. Edoxaban plus aspirin vs dual antiplatelet therapy in endovascular treatment of patients with peripheral artery disease: results of the ePAD trial. J Endovasc Ther. 2018;25:158–68. https://doi.org/10.1177/1526602818760488.
34. Thompson PD, Zimet R, Forbes WP, Zhang P. Meta-analysis of results from eight randomized, placebo-controlled trials on the effect of cilostazol on patients with intermittent claudication. Am J Cardiol. 2002;90:1314–9.
35. Dawson DL, Cutler BS, Hiatt WR, et al. A comparison of cilostazol and pentoxifylline for treating intermittent claudication. Am J Med. 2000;109:523–30.
36. Iida O, Nanto S, Uematsu M, Morozumi T, Kitakaze M, Nagata S. Cilostazol reduces restenosis after endovascular therapy in patients with femoropopliteal lesions. J Vasc Surg. 2008;48:144–9.
37. Soga Y, Yokoi H, Kawasaki T, et al. Efficacy of cilostazol after endovascular therapy for femoropopliteal artery disease in patients with intermittent claudication. J Am Coll Cardiol. 2009;53:48–53.
38. Lida O, Yokoi H, Soga Y, et al. Cilostazol reduces angiographic restenosis after endovascular therapy for femoropopliteal lesions in the sufficient treatment of peripheral intervention by Cilostazol study. Circulation. 2013;127:2307–15.
39. Heart Protection Study Collaborative Group. Randomized trial of the effects of cholesterol-lowering with simvastatin on peripheral vascular and other major vascular outcomes in 20,536 people with peripheral arterial disease and other high-risk conditions. J Vasc Surg. 2007;45:645–54; discussion 653–654.
40. Badjatiya A, Merrill P, Buse JB, et al. Clinical outcomes in patients with type 2 diabetes mellitus and peripheral artery disease: results from the EXSCEL trial. Circ Cardiovasc Interv.

2019;12(12):e008018. https://doi.org/10.1161/CIRCINTERVENTIONS.119.008018. Epub 2019 Nov 22.

41. Verma S, Rasmussen S, Saevereid HA, Ripa MS. Abstract 11456: liraglutide and semaglutide reduce cardiovascular events in patients with type 2 diabetes and peripheral arterial disease originally published 11 Nov 2019. Circulation. 2019;140:A11456.
42. Verma S, Mazer CD, Al-Omran M, Inzucchi SE, Fitchett D, Hehnke U, George JT, Zinman B. Cardiovascular outcomes and safety of Empagliflozin in patients with type 2 diabetes mellitus and peripheral artery disease. Circulation. 2018;137:405–7.
43. Bonaca MP, Wiviott SD, Zelniker TA, et al. Dapagliflozin and cardiac, kidney, and limb outcomes in patients with and without peripheral artery disease in DECLARE-TIMI 58. Circulation. 2020;142:734–47.
44. Neal B, Perkovic V, Mahaffey KW, et al. Canagliflozin and cardiovascular and renal events in type 2 diabetes. N Engl J Med. 2017;377:644–57.
45. Matthews DR, Li Q, Perkovic V, et al. Effects of canagliflozin on amputation risk in type 2 diabetes: the CANVAS program. Diabetologia. 2019;62:926–38.

Chapter 5
Blood Vessel Compliance, Barotrauma and Angioplasty-Induced Dissection Following Treatment of the Patient with Peripheral Artery Disease

Alexandra Stathis, Michiel T. Voûte, and Ramon L. Varcoe

Blood Vessel Wall Structure and Compliance

The arterial wall is composed of three concentric layers, the tunica intima, media and adventitia. The intima consists of a single layer of endothelium on the luminal surface, a subendothelial connective tissue matrix and the internal elastic lamina (IEL) [1]. The collagen, laminin-rich IEL as well as the smooth muscle and elastin of the media give the artery the flexibility to adapt to stretch and movement accommodating the diameter changes associated with pulsatile flow [2, 3]. It is these features that constitute vessel compliance.

Compliance may be reduced by several factors; however, age, calcification and atherosclerotic disease are the most common [4, 5]. As the artery ages, the intima and media become thickened due to the accumulation of additional matrix fibres and calcification of elastic fibres [6]. Moreover, arteries increase in diameter and elongate, further reducing compliance [7].

Pathophysiology of Intimal and Medial Calcification

Atherosclerotic plaque formation begins in the subendothelial layer of intima, immediately deep to the endothelium [8]. A fibrous cap of smooth muscle cells and connective tissue fibres develops over a central necrotic core which contains

A. Stathis · M. T. Voûte · R. L. Varcoe (✉)
Department of Surgery, Prince of Wales Hospital, Sydney, NSW, Australia

Faculty of Medicine, University of New South Wales, Sydney, NSW, Australia

The Vascular Institute, Prince of Wales Hospital, Sydney, NSW, Australia
e-mail: r.varcoe@unsw.edu.au

N. W. Shammas (ed.), *Peripheral Arterial Interventions*, Contemporary Cardiology, https://doi.org/10.1007/978-3-031-09741-6_5

lipid-rich cells, apoptotic macrophages, amorphous debris and matrix fibre remnants [9]. That cap may thicken and calcify the intima over time creating the appearance of plaque calcification during procedural imaging [10]. Concurrently, the necrotic core may enlarge causing luminal reduction and stenosis. Advanced plaque expansion which involves a significant proportion of the blood vessel circumference and the associated calcification is known to reduce elasticity and compliance [11].

Calcification of the media layer occurs with ageing and is associated with chronic kidney disease (CKD) and diabetes mellitus [12, 13]. It is independent of atherosclerosis, despite the two processes commonly occurring together as they have similar risk factors [14]. The process begins when hydroxyapatite crystals are deposited on to degraded elastin fibres inciting an osteoblast-like differentiation of the adjacent vascular smooth muscle cells (VSMC) [15]. This VSMC differentiation is also observed as part of normal ageing and the increased oxidative stress which may occur with CKD, smoking and diabetes [16].

It is common for atherosclerotic plaque stenosis to require angioplasty revascularisation in the context of coexisting blood vessel wall calcification and reduced compliance. Dissection is a frequent complication, with the potential to limit the durability of that procedure.

Barotrauma and the Immediate Cellular Response to Angioplasty

Percutaneous transluminal angioplasty (PTA) uses high-pressure expansion to dilate the stenotic plaque and achieve luminal gain. During inflation, the intima, media and adventitia are mechanically stretched by the outward force exerted from the balloon [17, 18]. With low-pressure inflation, the inherent elastic properties of the blood vessel (compliance) allow it to return to the original luminal diameter when the balloon deflates [18, 19]. However, with high pressure and increased stretch, the elastic properties of the artery are overcome, cleaving the intima and often media [19, 20]. These disrupted layers of blood vessel wall heal and remodel, ultimately facilitating an increased luminal diameter which restores blood supply to the extremity [18, 20].

It is important for angioplasty to disrupt the atherosclerotic plaque and the elastic properties of the inner layers of arterial wall if it is to result in permanent remodeling [18, 21]. This involves a physical trauma at the plaque-artery interface, stretching and tearing of the endothelium and alteration of the blood vessel substructure [20]. With that angioplasty-induced barotrauma come denudation of the endothelium and the immediate release of thrombogenic and vasoactive factors which promote platelet aggregation, thrombus formation and inflammation [22, 23]. Damage at the media level results in the necrosis of VSMC and matrix fibres, macrophage activation and release of cytokines and growth factors

[23]. This triggers a cascade response which ultimately results in the migration of VSMC from the media to intima, where they proliferate, undergo metaplasia and produce additional extracellular matrix [23, 24]. This process, and the cellular/matrix lesion which results, is called neointimal hyperplasia (NIH). In its early stages, it is considered a healthy response which facilitates blood vessel healing.

Mid-Term Cellular Response and Remodeling

Vascular remodeling can be described as negative (luminal reduction) or positive (luminal enlargement) [25, 26] and under normal conditions relies on an intact endothelium. Glagov et al. were the first to demonstrate that human coronary arteries undergo compensatory positive remodeling in response to decreased blood flow [26], with the same mechanism now also described in peripheral vessels [27]. However, angioplasty trauma mediated through cytokine and chemokine release may also lead to tissue remodeling and structural change. Normally, the intact endothelial layer inhibits platelet aggregation; however, angioplasty-induced barotrauma damages and denudes that inner layer of cells with an immediate release of thrombogenic and vasoactive factors that promote platelet aggregation and localised inflammation [23]. The degranulation of platelets releases chemokines and cytokines that lead to the migration and proliferation of VSMC located in the media. Furthermore, if the angioplasty trauma leads to stretching and tearing of the media, it may result in localised VSMC necrosis and release of additional growth factors. Together, these trigger a complex interaction between VSMC, platelets, endothelial cells, leukocytes and cellular mediators that culminate in remodeling and formation of neointimal hyperplasia (NIH) [24]. The mitogenic substances released by the degranulating platelet plug, together with those by the damaged media, result in the migration of VSMC from the media to intima. A significant proportion of those migratory VSMC proliferate and form new extracellular matrix (ECM) within the neointima [28]. If over-exuberant, NIH can lead to a pathophysiological compromise of the lumen, a description synonymous with negative remodeling which may lead to restenosis and the return of ischemic symptoms.

In addition to migration and proliferation of VSMC, there is evidence to suggest the barotrauma from angioplasty results in permanent functional change of the endothelium. It is known that regions of chronic denudation feature a layer of fibronectin, which can prevent the regrowth of endothelial cells [24, 29]. The increased production of the extracellular matrix protein fibronectin is driven by the release of transforming growth factor β1 (TGF- β1) from aggregated platelets [24, 29–31]. This process highlights the impact of the ECM on endothelial recovery following balloon angioplasty. In regions where the endothelium has recovered, the presence of actin stress filaments within them suggests that those overlying the NIH are operating in an altered functional state [32].

The Concept of Controlled Versus Uncontrolled Dissection

The goal of PTA is to create a series of small, controlled, blood vessel wall dissections that facilitate permanent luminal gain by enabling radial expansion [18] while avoiding large, flow-limiting dissections that might result in acute occlusion or lead to restenosis (Fig. 5.1) [19]. Histopathology studies demonstrate that microdissection and arterial wall disruption occur to some degree after every angioplasty [17, 33, 34]. However, there are aspects of the individual disease and procedural technique that can help predict the likelihood of uncontrolled dissection which may have detrimental clinical consequences. The nature of the atherosclerotic plaque may influence the angioplasty result and type of dissection observed. Calcified lesions are less compliant and more susceptible to dissection, even at lower force [20, 35]. Circumferential plaque is thought to evenly distribute the forces of angioplasty, resulting in small fractures and dissections at the thinner portions of the plaque [17, 20, 35], whereas eccentric lesions are more likely to dissect entirely from the blood vessel wall and at the margin of plaque and the normal underlying media [22]. Angioplasty of calcified vessels may result in cleavage of the plaque, putting the underlying vessel under high stress and increasing the risk of significant intimal dissection [20]. Moreover, sections of non-compliant artery may disproportionately transfer the angioplasty force in a proximal and distal direction causing stretch and increasing the risk of uncontrolled dissection in those adjacent zones [20, 35]. Angioplasty techniques used during treatment may also play a role.

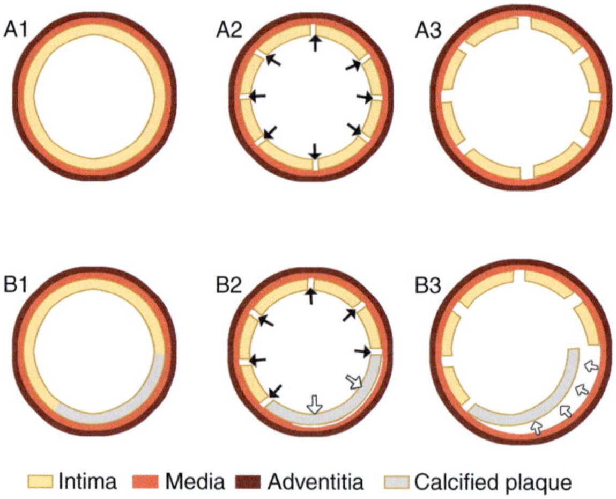

Fig. 5.1 Controlled and uncontrolled dissection. Controlled dissection induced by balloon angioplasty (A1–A3). A2 demonstrates the microdissections which result from balloon inflation (black arrows) and A3 the final result with circumferential dilatation of the luminal area (A3). Uncontrolled dissection (B1–B3) with calcified plaque in the intimal layer (grey shaded area), balloon inflation transfers shearing force to the plaque edge (B2, white arrows) leading to uncontrolled macrodissection which may have negative clinical consequences (B3, white arrows)

Subintimal wire passage prior to balloon inflation and the use of adjunctive atherectomy are two procedural aspects known to increase the risk of dissection [36], whereas prolonged angioplasty inflation times and the use of long (versus multiple short) balloon lengths are known to reduce it [37–39].

Stents for Mechanical Support

Nitinol self-expanding bare metal stents were developed to overcome some of the limitations observed with PTA. By providing mechanical scaffolding, they stabilise the treated blood vessel segment and overcome elastic recoil by exerting ongoing force on the vessel wall. However, that same chronic outward force results in a chronic low-grade vascular injury which can lead to the development of NIH deposited between the stent interstices. This NIH may also limit the durability of any stent-based intervention. A next generation of nitinol stents coated in antiproliferative drugs such as paclitaxel have been developed to limit the NIH response and reduce the incidence of in-stent restenosis. They have been shown to be superior to PTA and bare metal stents in multiple randomised trials [40, 41].

Modes of Failure Following Balloon Angioplasty

As described, angioplasty-induced barotrauma leads to a cellular response, and the blood vessel remodeling which follows can result in acute or delayed target lesion restenosis/failure. Uncontrolled macrodissection can also lead to poor clinical outcomes. Those may also occur in the acute setting within 24 h of PTA or take the form of a recurrent stenosis weeks or months after the index procedure.

Acute Occlusion

Acute occlusion occurs during or immediately after (<24 h) an angioplasty procedure. It is caused by mechanical obstruction which may result from any combination of occlusive dissection, thrombus formation, intraplaque haemorrhage, vasospasm and elastic recoil [42]. In practice, it is difficult to distinguish between these multiple mechanical factors, and it is common for there to be significant overlap. However, intravascular imaging with ultrasound or optical coherence tomography may be useful to determine the dominant mechanism.

Hypercoagulability factors are also known to play a role [43]. These range from the disruption of plaque contents which leads to tissue factors within the lipid core encountering the circulating blood to inadequate intra-procedural heparinisation. There are also a group of patients who are resistant to heparin and/or antiplatelet agents making them more susceptible to thrombus formation, even with correct dosage administration [44, 45].

A dissection which results in pressurised blood flow into the false lumen may propagate, spiral, compromise the true lumen and result in complete obstruction of flow. Stents and tack devices may be useful to treat flow-limiting dissection and overcome elastic recoil. However, they are not without their own limitations. The introduction of a foreign body into the circulation may result in platelet aggregation and thrombus formation unless antiplatelet agents are used and they remain vulnerable to metal fatigue-related fracture [46, 47].

Restenosis

It is well established that the barotrauma exerted on the blood vessel wall by an inflated angioplasty balloon may lead to negative remodeling and recurrent stenosis [23]. It is also a common view amongst peripheral interventionalists that dissection itself is a predictor of negative remodeling and target lesion failure [48]. It is uncertain whether the dissection is a marker for more advanced patterns of disease leading to reduced vessel compliance which predisposes to both the dissection and progressive disease or whether the dissection itself triggers a more exuberant form of NIH and elastic recoil that results in that recurrent stenosis. In the coronary literature, angiographic dissection has been classified and found to be associated with worse clinical outcomes [49, 50]. While it is known that physicians are more likely to implant stents with more severe forms of dissection, we know less about whether peripheral artery dissections lead to early restenosis and loss of patency [51, 52]. One observational study by Kobayashi et al. divided dissection types into 3 groups (A, no dissection; B, mild dissection; C, severe dissection) and followed 319 patients longitudinally after undergoing PTA for femoropopliteal disease. They found that 3-year primary patency was significantly reduced in those patients with severe dissection, but not mild (66.0% in group A, 63.8% in group B and 32.5% in group C; $p < 0.001$). This finding was more pronounced in longer length disease which was another independent predictor of reduced patency. They recommended that stents were not required for mild and short dissections, but that they continue to be used for severe dissection, particularly over longer lengths. Another study by Fujihara et al. used the NHLBI angiographic grading system to evaluate outcomes in 621 patients being treated for de novo disease of the superficial femoral artery [52]. They found that severe dissection was a significant risk factor for restenosis, which rose progressively from types C to F, and that after 2-year follow-up, the severe dissection group (types C–F) showed a significantly lower patency rate ($p < 0.001$) and higher clinically driven TLR ($p < 0.001$) compared to the non-severe group (no dissection and type A–B dissection). Together, these studies support the view of many experts in the field that severe dissection is a predictor of early restenosis and target lesion failure.

The Classification of Dissection

A detailed classification of angioplasty-induced dissection is helpful to provide uniform consistency in reporting and use in clinical trials and to guide discussion around treatment. Several classification systems have been proposed, many of which have been developed as tools to guide coronary interventions. Translation to a peripheral artery application is feasible as most systems can be made to apply to both arterial regions. However, experts disagree as to the relevance of some coronary dissection characteristics to peripheral arteries which have several distinct and important differences. Herein, we discuss the systems in common use.

Classification Systems: Angiography

The National Heart, Lung, and Blood Institute Percutaneous Transluminal Coronary Angioplasty (NHLBI PTCA) Registry published its manual of operations in 1985, describing the morphological presentations of arterial dissections that occur during percutaneous coronary interventions [53]. In the mid-1980s, cine-loop fluoroscopy was the dominant imaging modality used to diagnose and classify dissections, with less availability of intravascular ultrasound. The classification system developed by the NHLBI reflected that period. It distinguished six categories ranging from simple linear to spiral morphologies (A–F). It included contrast extravasation as a separate category and those with a persistent filling defect and total occlusion of the target vessel. These are illustrated in Table 5.1.

NHLBI has been the predominant classification method used for peripheral artery dissection for many years; however, some suggest that it is overly complex to be applied in routine daily practice and may incorporate features that are not relevant to peripheral artery angioplasty. For example, extravasation of contrast may be a very important finding in the coronary vascular bed but is usually a benign feature of peripheral artery interventions. This led to the simplified classification system developed specifically for peripheral artery interventions by Kobayashi et al [54]. It consists of three categories based on digital subtraction angiography (Table 5.2): group A where there was no angiographic dissection; group B, where there was mild dissection (the width of the dissection was less than one-third of the lumen); and group C, severe dissection, where the width of the dissection was more than one-third of the lumen. Spiral dissection was included in group C. Its simple design was intended to facilitate wide adoption in everyday practice; however, its lack of detail limited its utility in differentiating features which experts recognise as having clinical prognostic value and its use in clinical research as a method of categorisation.

Table 5.1 The National Heart, Lung, and Blood Institute (NHLBI) dissection classification system of procedural coronary artery dissections [53]

Type	Description	Depiction
A	Minor radiolucency within the lumen during contrast injection with no persistence of contrast after luminal clearance	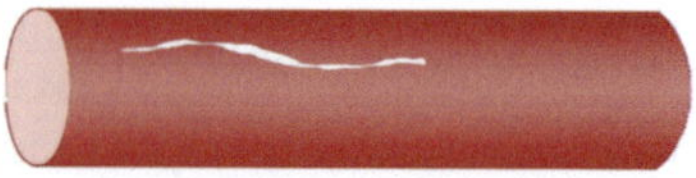
B	Linear dissection with parallel tracts or double lumen, with no persistence of contrast	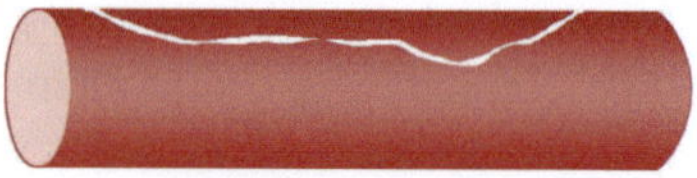
C	Extra-luminal 'cap' of contrast with persistence after clearance of luminal contrast	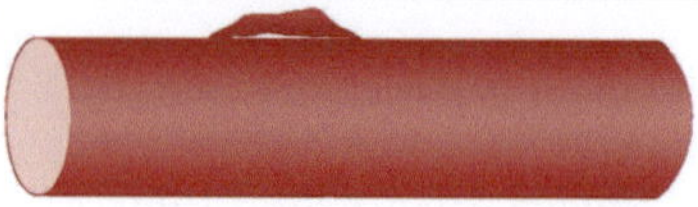
D	Spiral-shaped dissection, usually with filling defects within the false lumen	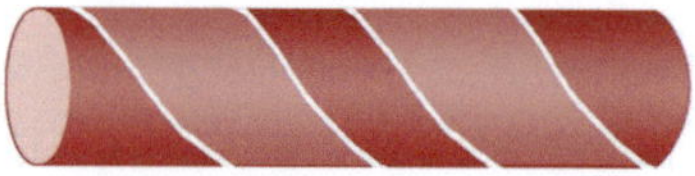
E	New persistent filling defect in the arterial lumen	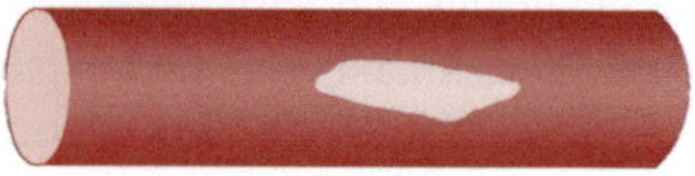
F	Dissection with total occlusion of the arterial lumen and no distal antegrade flow	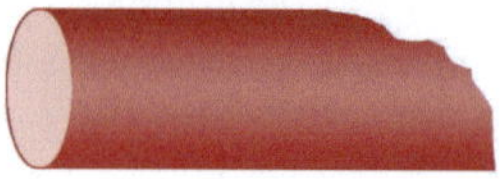

Table 5.2 Classification of angiographic dissections after balloon angioplasty for superficial femoral artery disease

Category	Degree of dissection
A	No angiographic dissection
B	The width of the dissection was less than one-third of the lumen
C	The width of the dissection is more than one-third of the lumen, or there is a spiral dissection

From Kobayashi et al. [54]

Classification Systems: Intravascular Ultrasound (IVUS)

Angiographic assessment of peripheral arteries during percutaneous intervention has several limitations. It relies upon a two-dimensional image of the arterial lumen. The detail of the blood vessel wall is limited to calcification and contrast entering a false lumen even with multiple orthogonal views. It provides little detail of plaque morphology, is challenged in the evaluation of thrombus and often underestimates blood vessel diameter and also the presence/severity of dissection itself.

The use of IVUS as an adjunctive imaging modality has grown in popularity since the 1990s. It provides information not available from angiography and is particularly useful in the evaluation of dissection, where it gives an accurate determination of depth and degree of arterial injury. Moreover, high-resolution IVUS can visualise the nature of material which is compromising the lumen, to differentiate between plaque, thrombus and intramural haematoma.

A Dutch study investigated the use of IVUS for the evaluation of dissection, performing both qualitative and quantitative analyses [55]. The qualitative analysis evaluated vascular wall damage, classifying the degree of injury as atherosclerotic plaque radial tear of the intimal surface, dissection (a radial tear separating the lesion from the underlying arterial wall) and/or medial rupture. The extent of dissection was then quantified and classified into one of the four groups (absent, minor, moderate and severe) as determined by 30° incremental arcs of the blood vessel circumference in cross section (Table 5.3). While this system provides a good framework to classify the degree and extent of dissection, it is limited in its description of other features thought to be clinically important, such as length, luminal diameter reduction and spiral morphology.

The more contemporary iDissection grading system is an alternative IVUS-based method proposed by Shammas et al. in 2018 [56]. It consists of six dissection grades which combine depth of injury (from the intima to adventitia) with circumference of dissection (<180° or ≥180°), features known to influence clinical outcomes (Table 5.4). However, those authors acknowledged that the grading system did not consider the length of the dissection and the presence of thrombus.

Table 5.3 Classification of dissections in femoropopliteal arteries after balloon angioplasty

Dissection	Extent of dissection as assessed by IVUS
Absent	No dissection
Mild	30°–90° arc of the circumference involved
Moderate	120°–180° arc of the circumference involved
Severe	210°–360° arc of the circumference involved

Adapted from Van der Lugt et al. [55]

Table 5.4 The iDissection classification scheme

Dissection	Circumference <180°	Circumference ≥180°
Intima	A1	A2
Media	B1	B2
Adventitia	C1	C2

Adapted from Shammas et al. [56]

It also failed to include spiral morphology and flow; however, it is a practical system that has the potential for wide adoption. The authors recommended a large, prospective registry to determine its role in predicting outcomes after arterial intervention.

While IVUS has been shown to identify dissections at higher frequency and in greater detail than conventional angiography, it is not available to all interventionalists and is more challenged in considering flow patterns, and its interpretation requires both skill and experience [36, 57]. It is therefore not universally applicable and is likely to remain an adjunctive imaging modality for the foreseeable future. It is our view that we will continue to rely on an angiographic classification system for dissection, one that is developed for peripheral arteries, underscored by expert opinion and validated as a predictor of clinical outcomes.

The DiSForM Classification System

The DiSForM (Diameter reduction, Spiral shape, Flow impairment or adverse Morphology) classification system was developed as a practical, universally applicable, angiography-based method of categorising arterial dissection designed specifically for peripheral arteries. It was developed utilising a three-stage Delphi consensus panel of experts to first determine angiographic features of clinical importance and then rank them for significance. Subsequently, a treatment algorithm was designed to assist interventionalists in managing angioplasty-induced dissection.

The features identified were luminal diameter reduction of ≥50%, spiral configuration, degree of flow impairment (by developing the FLIPI (FLow Impairment in Peripheral Intervention) grading system) and adverse morphology (length ≥2 cm and/or multiple dissections). The DiSForM classification system was based on the consensus of 17 expert interventional radiologists, interventional cardiologists, vascular surgeons and vascular medicine specialists who were asked to rate a series of combined dissection features for their likelihood to lead to acute occlusion and/or restenosis (Table 5.5). This then gives each individual dissection a pathological classification ($D_xS_xF_xM_x$) which can be used to aid treatment planning and evaluation, prognosis prediction, information exchange and the ongoing investigation of peripheral artery dissections. This classification system has features similar to the TNM system which is in common use for the classification of malignant tumors [58]. Examples of peripheral dissections classified using DiSForM are given in Fig. 5.2.

In the final Delphi round, the results of all possible $D_xS_xF_xM_x$ combinations were collated and analysed to validate its use as a decision-making tool and provide a treatment algorithm, which is given in Fig. 5.3.

Table 5.5 The DiSForM (Diameter reduction, Spiral shape, Flow impairment or adverse Morphology) classification system for peripheral artery dissection

DiSForM category	Parameter	Description of parameter as assessed on DSA[a]	
Di	Diameter reduction	D_0	Diameter reduction of <50%
		D_1	Diameter reduction of ≥50%
S	Spiral shape	S_0	Non spiral (linear) configuration
		S_1	Any spiral configuration
F	Flow impairment[b]	F_0	FLIPI 0: Normal antegrade flow
		F_1	FLIPI 1: Reduced antegrade flow
		F_2	FLIPI 2: Minor antegrade penetration
		F_3	FLIPI 3: No flow-through dissected segment, only collateral filling
M	Morphology	M_0	On single dissection <2 cm length
		M_1	Multiple <2 cm length dissections OR a single dissection ≥2 cm
		M_2	Multiple ≥2 cm dissections

[a] *DSA* digital subtraction angiography
[b] *FLIPI* flow impairment in peripheral intervention

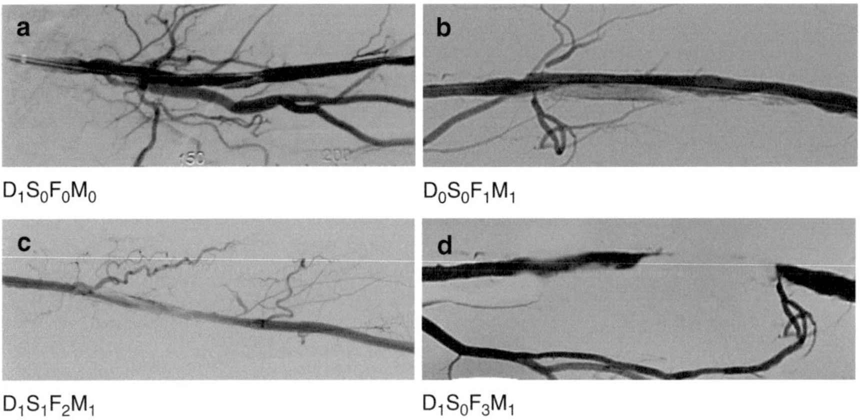

Fig. 5.2 **(a–d)** Dissection examples classified using the DiSForM classification system for peripheral artery dissections (note that flow must be rated on digital subtraction angiography and cannot be determined by a static image)

The strengths of the DiSForM classification system are that it is broadly applicable, does not rely on the availability of IVUS, is designed by experts in peripheral intervention specifically for use in that region and requires little additional training to incorporate into clinical practice. Future studies are planned to validate its utility as a tool for predicting short- and mid-term clinical outcomes.

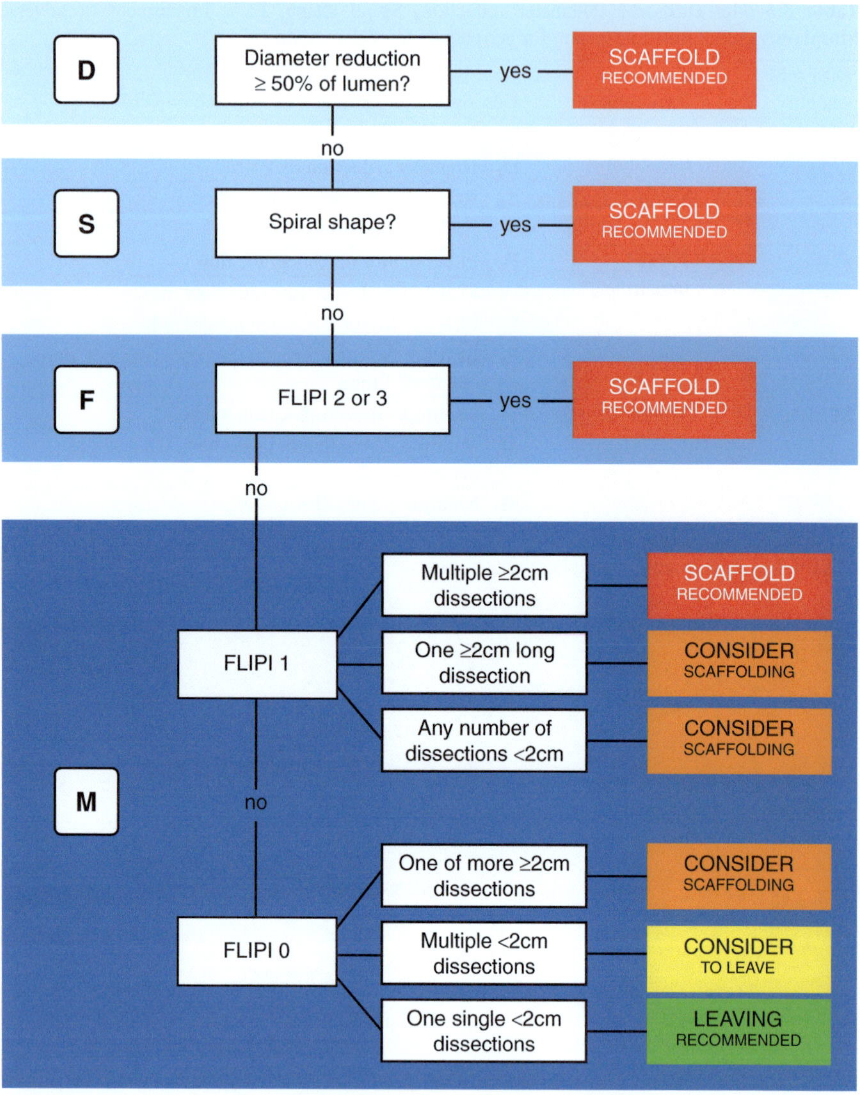

Fig. 5.3 Flowchart for the management of dissections in peripheral arterial interventions

Summary

Balloon angioplasty remains the cornerstone of endovascular treatment for occlusive arterial disease. Controlled dissection to facilitate luminal expansion is its main goal. However, that vascular injury may trigger a cellular response that leads to negative remodeling, restenosis and return of ischemic symptoms. Furthermore, uncontrolled dissection and deep blood vessel wall injury may result in acute occlusion and early target lesion failure. An understanding of the mechanisms of PTA and the pathophysiology which results is critical for interventionalists to guide PAD management and procedural decision-making.

Disclosures RV is a consultant for Abbott Vascular, Medtronic, Boston Scientific, Intact Medical, BD Bard, Surmodics and Intervene. No other authors have relevant disclosures.

References

1. Yurchenco PD, O'Rear JJ. Basal lamina assembly. Curr Opin Cell Biol. 1994;6:674–81.
2. Levy BI, Tedgui A. Biology of the arterial wall. Boston: Kluwer Academic Publishers; 1999.
3. Smith ML, Long DS, Damiano ER, Ley K. Near-wall micro-PIV reveals a hydrodynamically relevant endothelial surface layer in venules in vivo. Biophys J. 2003;85:637–45.
4. Cocciolone AJ, Hawes JZ, Staiculescu MS, Johnson EO, Murshed M, Wagenseil JW. Elastin, arterial mechanics, and cardiovascular disease. Am J Physiol Heart Circ Physiol. 2018;315:H189–205.
5. Willens HJDW, Herrington DM, Wade K, Kesler K, Mallon S, Brown WV, Reiber JHC, Raines JF. Relationship of peripheral arterial compliance and standard cardiovascular risk factors. Vasc Endovasc Surg. 2003;37:197–206.
6. Sims FH. The initiation of intimal thickening in human arteries. Pathology. 2000; 32:171–5.
7. Van Bortel LM, Spek JJ. Influence of aging on arterial compliance. J Hum Hypertens. 1998;12:583–6.
8. Lusis AJ. Atherosclerosis. Nature. 2000;407:233–41.
9. Otsuka F, Kramer MCA, Woudstra P, Yahagi K, Ladich E, Finn AV, de Winter RJ, Kolodgie FD, Wight TN. Natural progression of atherosclerosis from pathologic intimal thickening to late fibroatheroma in human coronary arteries: a pathology study. Atherosclerosis. 2015;241:772–82.
10. Amann K. Medial calcification and intima calcification are distinct entities in chronic kidney disease. Clin J Am Soc Nephrol. 2008;3:1599–605.
11. Maher E, Creane A, Sultan S, Hynes N, Lally C, Kelly DJ. Inelasticity of human carotid atherosclerotic plaque. Ann Biomed Eng. 2011;39:2445–55.
12. Paloian NJ, Giachelli CM. A current understanding of vascular calcification in CKD. Am J Physiol Renal Physiol. 2015;307:F891–900.
13. Goldsmith D, Ritz E, Covic A. Vascular calcification: a stiff challenge for the nephrologist: does preventing bone disease cause arterial disease? Kidney Int. 2004;66:1315–33.
14. Ho CY, Shanahan CM. Medial arterial calcification: an overlooked player in peripheral arterial disease. Arterioscler Thromb Vasc Biol. 2016;36:1475–82.
15. Lei Y, Sinha A, Nosoudi N, Grover N, Vyavahare N. Hydroxyapatite and calcified elastin induce osteoblast-like differentiation in rat aortic smooth muscle cells. Exp Cell Res. 2014;323:198–208.
16. Durham AL, Speer MY, Scatena M, Giachelli CM, Shanahan CM. Role of smooth muscle cells in vascular calcification: implications in atherosclerosis and arterial stiffness. Cardiovasc Res. 2018;114:590–600.
17. Zarins CK, Lu CT, Gewetz BL, Lyon RT, Rush DS, Glagov S. Arterial disruption and remodeling following balloon dilatation. Surgery. 1982;92:1086–95.
18. Castaneda-Zuniga WR, Amplatz K, Laerum F, Formanek A, Sibley R, Edwards J, Vlodaver Z. Mechanics of angioplasty: an experimental approach. Radiographics. 1981;1.
19. Becker GJ, Katen BT, Dake MD. Noncoronary angioplasty. Radiology. 1989;170:921–40.

20. Kinney TB, Chin AK, Rurik WG, Finn JC, Shoor PM, Hayden WG, Fogarty TJ. Transluminal angioplasty: a mechanical-pathophysiological correlation of its physical mechanisms. Radiology. 1984;153:85–9.
21. Waller BF, Miller J, Morgan R, Tejada E. Atherosclerotic plaque calcific deposits: an important factor in success or failure of transluminal coronary angioplasty (TCA). Circulation. 1988;78.
22. Cox JL, Gotlieb AI. Restenosis following percutaneous transluminal angioplasty: clinical, physiologic and pathological features. Can Med Assoc J. 1986;134:1129–32.
23. Mintz GS, Popma JJ, Pichard AD, Kent KM, Lowell F, Satler S, Wong C, Hong MK, Kovach JA, Leon MB. Arterial remodeling after coronary angioplasty; a serial intravascular ultrasound study. Circulation. 1996;94:35–43.
24. Tennant M, McGeachie JK. A biological basis for re-stenosis after percutaneous transluminal angioplasty: possible underlying mechanisms. ANZ J Surg. 1992;62:135–41.
25. Mulvany MJ, Baumbach GL, Aalkjaer C, Heagerty AM, Korsgaard N, Schiffrin EL, Heistad DD. Vascular remodeling. Hypertension. 1996;28:505–6.
26. Glagov S, Weisenberg E, Zarins CK, Stankunavicius R, Kolettis GJ. Compensatory enlargement of human atherosclerotic coronary arteries. N Engl J Med. 1987;316:1371–5.
27. Matsuo YTT, Mather V, Chung W, Barsness GW, Rihal CS, Gulati R, McCue E, Holmes DR, Eeckhout E, Lennon RJ, Lerman LO, Lerman A. Plaque characteristics and arterial remodeling in coronary and peripheral arterial systems. Atherosclerosis. 2012;223:265–71.
28. Ross R, Glomset JA. The pathogenesis of atherosclerosis: an update. N Engl J Med. 1986;314:488–500.
29. Madri JA, Reidy MA, Kochier O, Bell L. Endothelial cell behaviour after denudation injury is modulated by transforming growth factor B1 and fibronectin. Lab Invest. 1989;60:755–65.
30. Madri JA, Pratt BM, Tucker A. Phenotypic modulation of endothelial cells by transforming growth factor β depends upon the composition and organization of the extracellular matrix. J Cell Biol. 1988;106:1375–84.
31. Form DM, Pratt BM, Madri JA. Endothelial cell proliferation during angiogenesis: in vitro modulation by basement membrane components. J Cell Biol. 1986;106
32. Barja F, Blatter MC, James RW, Pometta D, Gabbiani G. Actin stress fiber content of regenerated endothelial cells correlates with intramural retention of intermediate plus low density lipoproteins in rat aorta after balloon injury. Atherosclerosis. 1989;76:181–91.
33. Spiliopoulos S, Karamitros A, Reppas L, Brountzos E. Novel balloon technologies to minimize dissection of peripheral angioplasty. Expert Rev Med Devices. 2019;16:581–8.
34. Fujihara M, Takahara M, Sasaki S, Nanto K, Utsunomiya M, Iida O, Yokoi Y. Angiographic dissection patterns and patency outcomes after balloon angioplasty for superficial femoral artery disease. J Endovasc Ther. 2017;24:367–75.
35. Cox JL, Gotlieb AI. Restenosis following percutaneous transluminal angioplasty: clinical, physiologic and pathological features. CMAJ. 1986;134:1129–32.
36. Shammas NW, Torey JT, Shammas WJ, Jones-Miller S, Shammas GA. Intravascular ultrasound assessment and correlation with angiographic findings demonstrating femoropopliteal arterial dissections post atherectomy: results from the iDissection study. J Invasive Cardiol. 2018;20:240–4.
37. Zorger N, Manke C, Lenhart M, et al. Peripheral arterial balloon angioplasty: effect of short versus long balloon inflation times on the morphologic results. J Vasc Interv Radiol. 2002;13:355–9.
38. Horie K, Tanaka A, Taguri M, et al. Impact of prolonged inflation times during plain balloon angioplasty on angiographic dissection in femoropopliteal lesions. J Endovasc Ther. 2018;25:683–91.
39. Tan M, Urasawa K, Koshida R, et al. Comparison of angiographic dissection patterns caused by long vs short balloons during balloon angioplasty of chronic femoropopliteal occlusions. J Endovasc Ther. 2018;25:192–200.

40. Dake MD, Ansel GM, Jaff MR, et al. Durable clinical effectiveness with paclitaxel-eluting stents in the femoropopliteal artery: 5-year results of the Zilver PTX randomized trial. Circulation. 2016;133:1472–83.
41. Gray WA, Keirse K, Soga Y, et al. A polymer-coated, paclitaxel-eluting stent (eluvia) versus a polymer-free, paclitaxel-coated stent (Zilver PTX) for endovascular femoropopliteal intervention (IMPERIAL): a randomised, non-inferiority trial. Lancet. 2018;392:1541–51.
42. de Feyter PJ, de Jaegere PP, Serruys PW. Incidence, predictors, and management of acute coronary occlusion after coronary angioplasty. Am Heart J. 1994;127:643–51.
43. Perler BA. Review of hypercoagulability syndromes: what the interventionalist needs to know. J Vasc Interv Radiol. 1991;2:183–93.
44. Gurbel PA, Tantry US. Aspirin and clopidogrel resistance: consideration and management. J Interv Cardiol. 2006;19:439–48.
45. Ranucci M, Isgrò G, Cazzaniga A, et al. Different patterns of heparin resistance: therapeutic implications. Perfusion. 2002;17:199–204.
46. Scheinert D, Scheinert S, Sax J, et al. Prevalence and clinical impact of stent fractures after femoropopliteal stenting. J Am Coll Cardiol. 2005;45:312–5.
47. Banerjee S, Sarode K, Mohammad A, et al. Femoropopliteal artery stent thrombosis: report from the excellence in peripheral artery disease registry. Circ Cardiovasc Interv. 2016;9:e002730.
48. Armstrong EJ, Brodmann M, Deaton DH, et al. Dissections after infrainguinal percutaneous transluminal angioplasty: a systematic review and current state of clinical evidence. J Endovasc Ther. 2019;26:479–89.
49. Huber MS, Mooney JF, Madison J, et al. Use of a morphologic classification to predict clinical outcome after dissection from coronary angioplasty. Am J Cardiol. 1991;68:467–71.
50. Rogers JH, Lasala JM. Coronary artery dissection and perforation complicating percutaneous coronary intervention. J Invasive Cardiol. 2004;16:493–9.
51. Tepe G, Zeller T, Schnorr B, et al. High-grade, non-flow-limiting dissections do not negatively impact long-term outcome after paclitaxel-coated balloon angioplasty: an additional analysis from the THUNDER study. J Endovasc Ther. 2013;20:792–800.
52. Fujihara M, Takahara M, Sasaki S, et al. Angiographic dissection patterns and patency outcomes after balloon angioplasty for superficial femoral artery disease. J Endovasc Ther. 2017;24:367–75.
53. NHLBI PTCA Registry: coronary artery angiographic changes after PTCA: manual of operations; 1985.
54. Kobayashi N, Hirano K, Yamawaki M, et al. Simple classification and clinical outcomes of angiographic dissection after balloon angioplasty for femoropopliteal disease. J Vasc Surg. 2018;67:1151–8.
55. van der Lugt A, Gussenhoven EJ, Mali WPTM, Reekers JA, Seelen JL, Tielbeek AV, Pieterman H. Effect of balloon angioplasty in femoropopliteal arteries assessed by intravascular ultrasound. Eur J Vasc Endovasc Surg. 1997;13:549–56.
56. Shammas NW, Torey JT, Shammas WJ. Dissections in peripheral vascular interventions: a proposed classification using intravascular ultrasound. J Invasive Cardiol. 2018;30:145–6.
57. Shammas NW, Shammas WJ, Jones-Miller S, et al. Femoropopliteal arterial dissections post flex vessel prep and adjunctive angioplasty: results of the flex iDissection study. J Invasive Cardiol. 2019;31:121–6.
58. Hermanek P, Sobin LH. TNM classification of malignant tumours. Berlin. Springer Science & Business Media; 2012.

Chapter 6
Controlling Dissections in Peripheral Arterial Interventions

Nicolas W. Shammas

Injury to the deeper layers of an infrainguinal artery is a potent trigger for restenosis, loss of patency, and the need for future target revascularization [1–3]. Dissections are an inevitable consequence of balloon angioplasty (PTA) and are the main mechanism to gain minimal luminal area (MLA) and prevent vessel recoil [4]. Recent research has focused on how to balance the occurrence of dissections and the gain in MLA without a detrimental disruption to the deeper layers of an artery. Also the interaction between residual narrowing, dissections' extent, dissection repair, and the use of antiproliferative therapy needs to be better explored because paclitaxel-coated balloons and dissection repair have been shown to partially mitigate some of the negative consequences of dissections. In this chapter, I will explore this concept more based on some findings from clinical trials.

Traditionally, the NHLBI classification has been used to classify dissections based on angiographic findings [5] (Table 6.1). This classification was adopted from the coronary literature and has several limitations. It only considers the single worst dissection regardless of number of dissections and does not consider the length, depth, and extent of dissections. Deeper injury is also not well appreciated using angiography, and therefore, this type of injury is not adequately or accurately captured by the NHLBI classification. These deeper injuries may not be visible or may appear low grade on angiogram. Larger arcs of dissections can also be missed on angiography and may not be well represented by the NHLBI classification. Despite its shortcomings, the NHLBI classification has been able to predict acute vessel

Modified from original publication "The Quest for Optimal Peripheral Angioplasty: Controlling Dissections" in the Journal of Arterial Venous and Lymphatic Interventions (https://javelinjournal.org/the-quest-for-optimal-peripheral-angioplasty-controlling-dissections/).

N. W. Shammas (✉)
Midwest Cardiovascular Research Foundation, Davenport, IA, USA

N. W. Shammas (ed.), *Peripheral Arterial Interventions*, Contemporary Cardiology, https://doi.org/10.1007/978-3-031-09741-6_6

Table 6.1 NHLBI classification for coronary dissections

Dissection	Description
Type A	Small radiolucent area within the lumen of the vessel disappearing with the passage of contrast material
Type B	Appearance of contrast medium parallel to the lumen of the vessel disappearing within a few cardiac cycles
Type C	Dissection protruding outside the lumen of the vessel persisting after passage of the contrast material
Type D	Spiral-shaped filling defect with delayed runoff of the contrast material in the distal vessel
Type E	Persistent luminal filling defect with delayed runoff of the contrast material in the distal vessel
Type F	Filling defect accompanied by total coronary occlusion

closure and loss of patency [6, 7]. NHLBI types C–F showed a significantly lower patency rate ($p < 0.001$) and higher clinically driven TLR ($p < 0.001$) compared to type A and B dissections.

Recently, a new angiographic-based classification was published which is dedicated to peripheral arteries. In the DISFORM study, Voute et al. [8] obtained expert consensus on features of dissections in the femoropopliteal artery that can potentially predict a poor outcome following intervention. An expert panel of 17 interventionalists ranked dissection features that have the potential to lead to acute technical failure and/or early restenosis and which combination of features would require repair of these dissections to improve outcome. Panelists recommended scaffolding in the presence of significant diameter reduction, spiral shape, flow impairment, or adverse morphology (Fig. 6.1). The Flow Impairment in Peripheral Intervention (FLIP) method was adopted (Table 6.2). The relationship of this classification to clinical outcome is yet unclear and needs to be determined in future studies.

Precise Imaging

Precise imaging within the vessel wall is critical to evaluate the degree and extent of dissections. The iDissection grading system uses intravascular ultrasound (IVUS) to classify dissections in infrainguinal interventions. The depth of dissection is graded as A (intima), B (media), and C (adventitia). The arc of dissection is graded as 1 (less than 180°) or 2 (more or equal 180°). This six-grade classification (A1, B1, C1, A2, B2, C2) is reliable and can quickly be performed during the procedure (Fig. 6.2, Table 6.3) [9].

The iDissection grading system was used for the first time in a small study evaluating the number, depth, and extent of dissections following atherectomy [10]. In this study, Jetstream atherectomy ($n = 13$) and B-laser ($n = 2$) were used. De novo and non-stent restenotic lesions were included. Angiography and IVUS (Eagle Eye

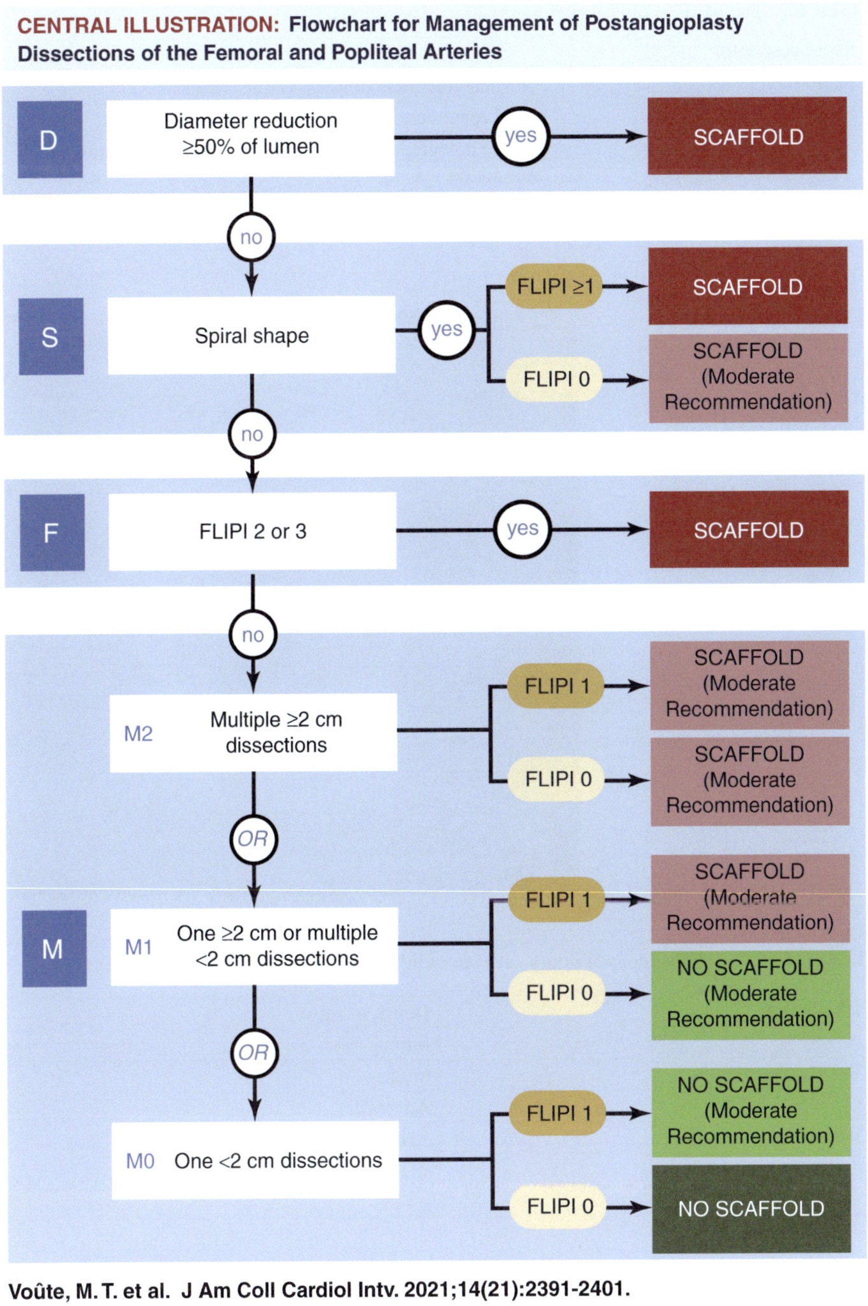

Fig. 6.1 Central illustration: flowchart for management of postangioplasty dissections of the femoral and popliteal arteries

Table 6.2 The FLIPI score for peripheral artery dissections

Score descriptor	
FLIPI 0	Normal antegrade flow
FLIPI 1	Mild reduction in antegrade flow
FLIPI 2	Minor antegrade contrast penetration, faint flow beyond the dissection
FLIPI 3	No flow-through, only collateral filling distal to the dissection

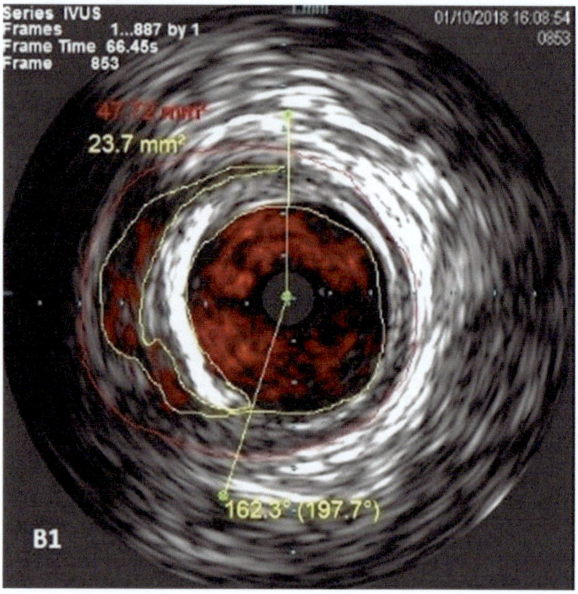

Fig. 6.2 Dissection involving the media and less than 180°. Based on iDissection classification, this is a B1 dissection

Table 6.3 iDissection, depth of injury, and arc of injury

iDissection	**Depth of injury**
A	Intima
B	Media
C	Adventitia
iDissection	**Arc of injury**
1	<180°
2	≥180°

Platinum, Philips) were performed at baseline, post-atherectomy, and post-adjunctive balloon angioplasty. Core angiographic (Midwest Cardiovascular Research Foundation, Davenport, IA) and intravascular ultrasound (Midwest Cardiovascular Research Foundation, Davenport, IA, and St John Hospital, Detroit, Michigan) laboratories evaluated all images. In this study, critical limb ischemia was present in 26.7% of patients, and 60% of lesions had grade 3 and 4 PACCS grade calcification. Adjunctive balloon angioplasty was performed in all patients (Shockwave 33.3%, drug-coated balloons 100%). Mean balloon pressures and inflation times were 10.3 atmospheres and 310 s. Procedural success (<30% residual narrowing at the end of procedure) was accomplished in all patients, and residual narrowing post-angioplasty was 19.7%. *Dissections were identified four to six times more on IVUS when compared to angiography* (post-atherectomy and adjunctive angioplasty IVUS to angiographic dissection ratios were 5.75–1 and 3.55–1, respectively) (Fig. 6.1). Wider dissections >180° were also noted on IVUS in 13% and 31% post-atherectomy and adjunctive PTA, respectively. Furthermore, deeper dissections involving the media and adventitia occurred in 39.1% and 33.3% post-atherectomy and adjunctive PTA, respectively. Finally, IVUS identified intramural hematoma in 13.3% of vessels post-atherectomy. These results showed clearly that Jetstream atherectomy can create a damage to the inner layer of the arterial wall and potentially this may offset some of its benefit in reducing restenosis from plaque removal.

The iDissection classification also was tested with the Flex VP (VentureMed Group) atherotome and was found to have a low number of deeper dissections. The FLEX Vessel Prep System (VentureMed Group) is a one-size-fits-all device with three atherotomes mounted on a self-expanding treating element designed to create multiple longitudinal, controlled-depth, continuous micro-incisions across the entire lesion length. IVUS-based analysis post-FLEX VP was recently published and confirmed less deep dissections (media and adventitia) than seen with historical data from some atherectomy devices [11]. In 15 patients treated with the FLEX VP followed by adjunctive balloon angioplasty (Shockwave 33.3%, PTA 26.7%, drug-coated balloon 40%) for de novo or non-stent restenotic femoropopliteal disease, procedural success was 86.7% (<30% residual narrowing at the end of procedure). Minimal luminal area increased from a median of 5.2 to 15.0 mm^2 ($p < 0.001$) with no change in reference lumen diameter or plaque burden area ($p = 0.32$). Of all new dissections ($n = 37$) post-FLEX VP and PTA, 18.9% were more than 180° in circumference, and 21.6% involved the media and adventitia. These numbers appear favorable compared to rotational and aspiration atherectomy, but head-to-head comparison data are not available. The low number of large flaps and deeper dissections may offer an explanation to the low provisional stenting seen with this device. The impact of these encouraging acute results on long-term outcomes is not yet known.

A recent study with the Auryon laser system has shown a very minimal number of C dissections based on the iDissection classification system [12]. In a prospective study of 29 patients, adventitial injury was assessed by IVUS following Auryon laser treatment and adjunctive balloon angioplasty. Core laboratory analysis was carried on all cases except for one patient (that crossed over to Jetstream atherectomy). Bailout stenting occurred in 21.4% patients (three for dissections, two for residual >30%, and one for both). By IVUS, there were 9 new dissections post-laser (1 adventitial; 3 ≥180°) and 21 new dissections post-laser and PTA (3 adventitial; 1 ≥180°). This small number of deep dissections can be attributed to the physics property of the long wavelength (355 nm) of the Auryon laser. The Auryon laser thermal injury dissipates quickly as it travels away from the tip of the catheter making deeper thermal injury less likely.

It is clear from precision imaging that various devices have the ability to remove a different amount of tissue from the treated vessels and lead to a range of deep damage to the inner layers of the artery. A balance between the extent of tissue excision and deep injury is likely to be of paramount interest when it comes to reducing long-term adverse events. The interaction of tissue removal, deep injury, dissection repair, and the application of antiproliferative therapy needs to be explored further.

The Relationship Between Deep Injury, Plaque Excision, Dissection Repair, and Antiproliferative Therapy

Several studies suggested an association between arterial dissections and high residual narrowing on poor outcomes in the treatment of infrainguinal arterial disease. However, the applications of antiproliferative therapy and dissections' repair seem to mitigate at least partially the subsequent adverse outcomes of dissections and high residual narrowing. Below are some studies that may give some insights into this interaction.

Aggressive Debulking, High Rate of Deeper Dissections, and Antiproliferative Treatment

The Jetstream atherectomy device is a high-power device in plaque excision and leads to low residual narrowing on its own (typically less than 50%). However, it also causes its share of deeper dissections into the vessel wall by IVUS although angiographically this may not always be apparent [9]. In the JET Registry [13], a prospective study of Jetstream atherectomy with no drug-coated balloons (DCB), the freedom from TLR was 79–80% at 1 year. In the JET-SCE [14], a retrospective study of all comers treated with the Jetstream atherectomy device, freedom from TLR was reduced to 69.8% at 1 year, but the cohort of patients receiving Jetstream + DCB had a freedom from TLR of 95.2%. Recently, data from the JET-RANGER [15] study presented at TCT 2021 have shown that freedom from TLR was 100% at 1 year in the cohort of patients who received the Jetstream atherectomy and either the Ranger DCB or IN.PACT DCB balloons. In the JET-RANGER, there was no bailout stenting in the Jetstream + DCB cohort based on lack of angiographic presence of a flow-limiting dissection or the presence of more than 30% residual narrowing. These studies point to the following:

(a) Aggressive debulking does not on its own lead to a better outcome.
(b) The administration of antiproliferative therapy had a strong mitigating factor on reducing the poor outcomes of deeper dissections with (JET-SCE) or without (JET-RANGER) repair in the setting of aggressive debulking device.

No Debulking, Deeper Dissections, Dissection Repair, and/or Antiproliferative Treatment

Angioplasty (PTA) leads to high rate of deeper dissections particularly in complex arterial disease. Also PTA is not a debulking tool, and its mechanism of vessel expansion is mostly through dissections. Therefore, PTA leaves a high residual narrowing and leads to a high rate of deeper dissections. This combination is likely to be a major predictor of loss of patency and high TLR in most femoropopliteal or tibial interventions.

Multiple studies have shown that this poor outcome with PTA alone can be impacted positively by the application of DCB balloons [16–18] and repair of dissections [19–23] with limited metal left behind irrespective of the dissection severity (types A to F). With this wide application of focal repair of dissections with and without DCB, freedom from TLR seems to markedly improve when compared to historic control. Several randomized studies comparing DCB to PTA have shown a superiority in patency and freedom from TLR when compared to PTA alone. In the PTA + DCB arm of the JET-RANGER [15], a 92% freedom from TLR was noted at the expense of bailout stenting in almost half these patients. Lesions included in this study were complex with high rate of moderate to severe calcium, long lesions, and total occlusions which explain the need for high bailout stenting. In the TOBA II trial [21], an excellent outcome was seen with or without DCB after PTA when a strategy of focal repair was applied. Even mild type A and B NHLBI dissections were repaired in this study. This was also reproduced in the TOBA III study [22]. The application of wide focal repair or bailout stent to flow-limiting dissections along with DCB seems to have a strong mitigating factor on poor outcomes following treatment of femoropopliteal lesions. This was also seen in THUNDER trial [24] where DCB led to a significant reduction in TLR irrespective of the presence of dissections. These studies also point to the following:

(a) PTA leads to a high rate of deeper dissections and leaves a large residual of plaque behind.
(b) DCB with bailout stenting mitigates the poor outcome of PTA.
(c) The application of a wide range of repair of dissections (types A to F) with or without DCB seems to have a positive impact on outcome.

Low-Level Debulking, Minimal Rate of Deep Dissections, and Antiproliferative Therapy

From the iDissection Auryon study [12], IVUS showed that the Auryon laser has a low level of debulking with residual narrowing over 50% after laser only, but no to minimal deep dissections. This serves as an interesting platform to determine how this impacts TLR with or without DCB. Bailout stenting, when occurred, was driven by either the occurrence of dissections or high rate of residual narrowing after adjunctive PTA following the laser.

In the EX-PAD-03 IDE study [25], bailout stenting was very low, and the freedom from TLR was lower than 5% at 6 months in all comers including femoropopliteal artery disease or tibial disease and irrespective of the lesion being de novo or restenotic (stent or not). Also in this study, only 60% of treated limbs received a DCB. The limited damage to the deeper layers of the vessel could have played an important role in reducing the TLR rate. Patency was also very favorable when compared to historic control. The Auryon SCE (In print JIC 2022) was a retrospective study that evaluated the impact of the Auryon laser on outcome in a real-world cohort of patients. In this study, a total of 56 patients (66 procedures, 71 lesions) were enrolled. 48.2% were diabetics and 25% had limb ischemia. Baseline stenosis was 91.4 ± 9.7%, post-laser 56.0 ± 17.3%, and post-final treatment 11.6 ± 11.2%. Lesion length was 117.1 ± 100.4 mm and treated length 177.3 ± 115.5 mm. Bailout stenting occurred in 12/66 procedures (18.2%). Post-laser, there was no D dissection, and post-laser + PTA, there was one D dissection. DCB usage was the following: 46.5% Lutonix, 28.2% IN.PACT, and 1.4% both. The probability of freedom from TLR was 100.0% at 6 months.

Orbital atherectomy has likely the same mechanism of action with softer debulking. The TRUTH study [26] has shown a low rate of deep dissections by IVUS following orbital atherectomy. In the COMPLIANCE trial [27], residual narrowing was very low with a low rate of bailout stenting at 5.3%. Patency at 1 year was high at 81.2% despite the presence of severe calcium and complex disease enrolled.

These studies point to the following:

(a) A soft debulking approach while preserving the deeper layer of the vessel has an excellent short-term and intermediate-term outcome despite a low rate of overall bailout stenting with or without drug-coated balloons.
(b) Long-term outcomes need to be evaluated to ensure no late loss of patency and increase in TLR.

Other Technologies to Reduce Dissections

Several technologies besides atherectomy and the FLEX VP were developed to control dissections as seen on angiography. These include cutting (Boston Scientific Corp.) and scoring balloons (AngioSculpt® scoring balloon (Philips); UltraScore Focal Force (BD/Bard)), the Serranator (Cagent Vascular), and the lithotripsy shockwave balloon (Shockwave Medical).

Cutting balloons (CB) continue to show angiographic dissections post-treatment of femoropopliteal lesions, and more than half of these dissections are NHLBI type C or higher (54.8%). High-grade angiographic dissections have been shown to correlate with loss of patency on follow-up. CB was shown by IVUS to be more effective than scoring balloons [28, 29] in modifying calcified plaque with a higher acute luminal gain and better stent symmetry. In calcified lesions, the larger luminal gain occurs in lesions with evidence of dissections and without significant change in vessel expansion (external elastic lumen surface area remains unchanged) or plaque-media cross-sectional area. On the other hand, CB in non-calcified lesions yields larger lumen area mostly by larger plaque reduction and less vessel expansion compared to PTA [30]. The depth and extent of dissections seen by IVUS following CB have not been well defined. CB as a sole intervention has not been shown to yield better outcome than PTA in treating restenotic or femoropopliteal disease.

The AngioSculpt scoring balloon (Philips) has three nitinol spiral elements mounted on the surface of a semi-compliant balloon. This allows a homogenous transmission of pressure over the plaque, theoretically reducing dissections irrespective of calcification. AngioSculpt, when assessed by IVUS, increased minimal luminal area post-stenting [31] and had a low rate of angiographic dissections and stenting [32–34]. It also had no impact on target lesion revascularization. The UltraScore Focused Force PTA balloon (Bard/BD) has two longitudinal wires intended to concentrate the force against the plaque for a controlled fracture at low pressure. IVUS-based patterns of dissections with this balloon are lacking.

Lithotripsy using the Shockwave balloon [35] uses sound waves to disrupt calcium in the vessel wall. Optical coherence tomography (OCT) has shown that lithoplasty modifies calcium with fracture as the predominant mechanism leading to significant favorable luminal area gain and stent expansion [35]. Applications of lithoplasty to calcified stenotic common femoral artery also showed excellent acute success with no dissections needing stenting. There were only 5 NHLBI type B non-flow-limiting dissections (out of 21 patients treated) and no perforation, distal embolization, or abrupt closure [36]. Patterns of dissections using IVUS with Shockwave lithoplasty have not been defined.

Dissection Repair

Dissection repair has been recently introduced as a strategy to improve outcomes of infrainguinal interventions. Repair of dissections in the TOBA BKA study showed a freedom from CD-TLR of 93.5% and patency of 78.4% at 1 year, significantly better than historic control [23]. In the TOBA II study [21], 213 patients with 100% dissected vessels following plain old balloon angioplasty or drug-coated balloons underwent repair of their dissections using the Tack Endovascular System. Of all dissections identified, 92.1% were repaired. Freedom from TLR and patency at 1 year were 86.5% and 79.3%, respectively. Bailout stent rate was 0.5%.

In conclusion, high-grade dissections and high residual narrowing predict higher TLR rates and reduced patency. Using IVUS, the depth and width of dissections can be more accurately classified. Several devices are now available to reduce deeper dissections with a wide range of plaque removal from none to soft debulking (>50% residual) to aggressive debulking (<50% residual). The interaction between the degree of debulking, deep dissections, application of antiproliferative therapies, and dissection repair needs to be further explored to determine their impact on long-term outcomes.

References

1. Tarricone A, Ali Z, Rajamanickam A, et al. Histopathological evidence of adventitial or medial injury is a strong predictor of restenosis during directional atherectomy for peripheral artery disease. J Endovasc Ther. 2015;22:712–5.
2. Miki K, Fujii K, Kawasaki D, Shibuya M, Fukunaga M, Imanaka T, Tamaru H, Sumiyoshi A, Nishimura M, Horimatsu T, Saita T, Okada K, Kimura T, Honda Y, Fitzgerald PJ, Masuyama T, Ishihara M. Intravascular ultrasound-derived stent dimensions as predictors of angiographic restenosis following nitinol stent implantation in the superficial femoral artery. J Endovasc Ther. 2016;23(3):424–32. https://doi.org/10.1177/1526602816641669. Epub 2016 Apr 4.
3. Shammas NW, Radaideh Q, Shammas WJ, Daher GE, Rachwan RJ, Radaideh Y. The role of precise imaging with intravascular ultrasound in coronary and peripheral interventions. Vasc Health Risk Manag. 2019;15:283–90. https://doi.org/10.2147/VHRM.S210928. eCollection 2019.
4. Finet G, Abrysch F, Rioufol G, Ohayon J, Lagache M. Qualitative and quantitative descriptions of the mechanisms of action of the angioplasty balloon on coronary stenosis. An endovascular ultrasonic study. Arch Mal Coeur Vaiss. 2000;93:1109–17.
5. Rogers JH, Lasala JM. Coronary artery dissection and perforation complicating percutaneous coronary intervention. J Invasive Cardiol. 2004;16(9):493–9.
6. Fujihara M, Takahara M, Sasaki S, Nanto K, Utsunomiya M, Iida O, Yokoi Y. Angiographic dissection patterns and patency outcomes after balloon angioplasty for superficial femoral artery disease. J Endovasc Ther. 2017;24(3):367–75. https://doi.org/10.1177/1526602817698634. Epub 2017 Mar 20.
7. Kobayashi N, Hirano K, Yamawaki M, Araki M, Sakai T, Sakamoto Y, Mori S, Tsutsumi M, Honda Y, Ito Y. Simple classification and clinical outcomes of angiographic dissection after balloon angioplasty for femoropopliteal disease. J Vasc Surg. 2018;67(4):1151–8. https://doi.org/10.1016/j.jvs.2017.08.092. Epub 2017 Dec 11.
8. Voûte MT, Stathis A, Schneider PA, Thomas SD, Brodmann M, Armstrong EJ, Holden A, Varcoe RL. Delphi consensus study toward a comprehensive classification system for angioplasty-induced femoropopliteal dissection: the DISFORM study. JACC Cardiovasc Interv. 2021;14(21):2391–401.
9. Shammas NW, Torey JT, Shammas WJ. Dissections in peripheral vascular interventions: a proposed classification using intravascular ultrasound. J Invasive Cardiol. 2018;30(4):145–6.
10. Shammas NW, Torey JT, Shammas WJ, Jones-Miller S, Shammas GA. Intravascular ultrasound assessment and correlation with angiographic findings demonstrating femoropopliteal arterial dissections post atherectomy: results from the iDissection study. J Invasive Cardiol. 2018;30(7):240–4.
11. Shammas NW, Shammas WJ, Jones-Miller S, Radaideh Q, Shammas GA. Femoropopliteal arterial dissections post flex vessel prep and adjunctive angioplasty: results of the flex iDissection study. J Invasive Cardiol. 2019;31(5):121–6.
12. Shammas NW, Torey JT, Shammas WJ, Jones-Miller S, Shammas GA. Intravascular ultrasound assessment and correlation with angiographic findings of arterial dissections following Auryon laser Atherectomy and adjunctive balloon angioplasty: results of the iDissection Auryon laser study. J Endovasc Ther. 2022;29(1):23–31. https://doi.org/10.1177/15266028211028200. Online ahead of print.
13. Gray WA, Garcia LA, Amin A, Shammas NW, JET Registry Investigators. Jetstream atherectomy system treatment of femoropopliteal arteries: results of the post-market JET registry. Cardiovasc Revasc Med. 2018;19(5 Pt A):506–11. https://doi.org/10.1016/j.carrev.2017.12.015. Epub 2017 Dec 27.
14. Shammas NW, Shammas GA, Jones-Miller S, Shammas WJ, Bou-Dargham B, Shammas AN, Banerjee S, Rachwan RJ, Daher GE. Long-term outcomes with Jetstream atherectomy with or without drug coated balloons in treating femoropopliteal arteries: a single center experience

(JET-SCE). Cardiovasc Revasc Med. 2018;19(7 Pt A):771–7. https://doi.org/10.1016/j.carrev.2018.02.003. Epub 2018 Feb 9.

15. Shammas NW, Purushottam B, Shammas WJ, et al. TCT-17 Jetstream atherectomy followed by paclitaxel-coated balloons versus balloon angioplasty followed by paclitaxel-coated balloons: twelve-month results of the prospective randomized JET-RANGER study. J Am Coll Cardiol. 2021;78(19):B8. https://doi.org/10.1016/j.jacc.2021.09.876.
16. Tepe G, Laird J, Schneider P, Brodmann M, Krishnan P, Micari A, Metzger C, Scheinert D, Zeller T, Cohen DJ, Snead DB, Alexander B, Landini M, Jaff MR, IN.PACT SFA Trial Investigators. Drug-coated balloon versus standard percutaneous transluminal angioplasty for the treatment of superficial femoral and popliteal peripheral artery disease: 12-month results from the IN.PACT SFA randomized trial. Circulation. 2015;131:495–502.
17. Krishnan P, Faries P, Niazi K, Jain A, Sachar R, Bachinsky WB, Cardenas J, Werner M, Brodmann M, Mustapha JA, Mena-Hurtado C, Jaff MR, Holden AH, Lyden SP. Stellarex drug-coated balloon for treatment of femoropopliteal disease: twelve-month outcomes from the randomized ILLUMENATE pivotal and pharmacokinetic studies. Circulation. 2017;136:1102–13.
18. Rosenfield K, Jaff MR, White CJ, Rocha-Singh K, Mena-Hurtado C, Metzger DC, Brodmann M, Pilger E, Zeller T, Krishnan P, Gammon R, Müller-Hülsbeck S, Nehler MR, Benenati JF, Scheinert D, LEVANT 2 Investigators. Trial of a paclitaxel-coated balloon for femoropopliteal artery disease. N Engl J Med. 2015;373:145–53.
19. Bosiers M, Scheinert D, Hendriks JM, et al. Results from the tack optimized balloon angioplasty (TOBA) study demonstrate the benefits of minimal metal implants for dissection repair after angioplasty. J Vasc Surg. 2016;64:109–16.
20. Geraghty P, Adams GL, Schmidt A, Lichtenberg M, Wissgott C, Armstrong EJ, Hertting K, on behalf of the TOBA II BTK Investigators. Twelve-month results of tack-optimized balloon angioplasty using the tack endovascular system in below-the-knee arteries (TOBA II BTK). J Endovasc Ther. 2020;27(4):626–36.
21. Gray WA, Cardenas JA, Brodmann M, et al. Treating post-angioplasty dissection in the femoropopliteal arteries using the tack endovascular system: 12-month results from the TOBA II study. JACC Cardiovasc Interv. 2019;12:2375–84.
22. Brodmann M, Wissgott C, Brechtel K, et al. Optimized drug-coated balloon angioplasty of the superficial femoral and proximal popliteal arteries using the tack endovascular system: TOBA III 12-month results. J Vasc Surg. 2020;72(5):1636–1647.e1. https://doi.org/10.1016/j.jvs.2020.01.078.
23. Brodmann M, Wissgott C, Holden A, et al. Treatment of infrapopliteal post-PTA dissection with tack implants: 12-month results from the TOBA-BTK study. Catheter Cardiovasc Interv. 2018;92:96–105.
24. Tepe G, Zeller T, Schnorr B, Claussen CD, Beschorner U, Brechtel K, Scheller B, Speck U. High-grade, non-flow-limiting dissections do not negatively impact long-term outcome after paclitaxel-coated balloon angioplasty: an additional analysis from the THUNDER study. J Endovasc Ther. 2013;20(6):792–800. https://doi.org/10.1583/13-4392R.1.
25. Shammas NW, Chandra P, Brodmann M, Weinstock B, Sedillo G, Cawich I, Micari A, Lee A, Metzger C, Palena LM, Rundback J, EX-PAD-03 Investigators. Acute and 30-day safety and effectiveness evaluation of Eximo Medical's B-laser™, a novel Atherectomy device, in subjects affected with infrainguinal peripheral arterial disease: results of the EX-PAD-03 trial. Cardiovasc Revasc Med. 2020;21(1):86–92. https://doi.org/10.1016/j.carrev.2018.11.022. Epub 2018 Nov 29.
26. Babaev A, Zavlunova S, Attubato MJ, Martinsen BJ, Mintz GS, Maehara A. Orbital atherectomy plaque modification assessment of the femoropopliteal artery via intravascular ultrasound (TRUTH study). Vasc Endovasc Surg. 2015;49(7):188–94. https://doi.org/10.1177/1538574415607361. Epub 2015 Oct 20.
27. Dattilo R, Himmelstein SI, Cuff RF. The COMPLIANCE 360° trial: a randomized, prospective, multicenter, pilot study comparing acute and long-term results of orbital atherectomy to balloon angioplasty for calcified femoropopliteal disease. J Invasive Cardiol. 2014;26(8):355–60.

28. Miyazaki T, Latib A, Ruparelia N, Kawamoto H, Sato K, Figini F, Colombo A. The use of a scoring balloon for optimal lesion preparation prior to bioresorbable scaffold implantation: a comparison with conventional balloon predilatation. EuroIntervention. 2016;11(14):e1580–8. https://doi.org/10.4244/EIJV11I14A308.
29. Matsukawa R, Kozai T, Tokutome M, Nakashima R, Nishimura R, Matsumoto S, Katsuki M, Masuda S, Meno H. Plaque modification using a cutting balloon is more effective for stenting of heavily calcified lesion than other scoring balloons. Cardiovasc Interv Ther. 2019;34(4):325–34. https://doi.org/10.1007/s12928-019-00578-w. [Epub ahead of print].
30. Okura H, Hayase M, Shimodozono S, Kobayashi T, Sano K, Matsushita T, Kondo T, Kijima M, Nishikawa H, Kurogane H, Aizawa T, Hosokawa H, Suzuki T, Yamaguchi T, Bonneau HN, Yock PG, Fitzgerald PJ, REDUCE Investigators. Restenosis reduction by cutting balloon evaluation. Mechanisms of acute lumen gain following cutting balloon angioplasty in calcified and noncalcified lesions: an intravascular ultrasound study. Catheter Cardiovasc Interv. 2002;57(4):429–36.
31. Fonseca A, Costa JR, Abizaid A, et al. Intravascular ultrasound assessment of the novel AngioSculpt scoring balloon catheter for the treatment of complex coronary lesions. J Invasive Cardiol. 2008;20:21–7.
32. Kiesz RS, Scheinert D, Peeters PJ, et al. Results from the international registry of the AngioSculpt scoring balloon catheter for the treatment of infrapopliteal disease. J Am Coll Cardiol. 2008;51(10 (suppl B)):75.
33. Scheinert D, Peeters P, Bosiers M, et al. Results of the multicenter first-in-man study of a novel scoring balloon catheter for the treatment of infra-popliteal peripheral arterial disease. Catheter Cardiovasc Interv. 2007;70:1034–9.
34. Bosiers M, et al. Use of the AngioSculpt scoring balloon for infrapopliteal lesions in patients with critical limb ischemia: 1-year outcome. Vascular. 2009;17(1):29–35.
35. Ali ZA, Brinton TJ, Hill JM, Maehara A, Matsumura M, Karimi Galougahi K, Illindala U, Götberg M, Whitbourn R, Van Mieghem N, Meredith IT, Di Mario C, Fajadet J. Optical coherence tomography characterization of coronary lithoplasty for treatment of calcified lesions: first description. JACC Cardiovasc Imaging. 2017;10(8):897–906. https://doi.org/10.1016/j.jcmg.2017.05.012.
36. Brodmann M, Schwindt A, Argyriou A, Gammon R. Safety and feasibility of intravascular lithotripsy for treatment of common femoral artery stenoses. J Endovasc Ther. 2019;26(3):283–7.

Chapter 7
The Role of Atherectomy in Vessel Prepping During Infrainguinal Arterial Interventions

Andrew N. Shammas and Nicolas W. Shammas

Vessel prepping (VP) is a strategy utilized during infrainguinal arterial endovascular interventions with several key benefits when used prior to definitive treatment. VP results in a reduction in vessel barotrauma, increases vessel compliance, allows optimal luminal gain, and decreases dissection rate. There are various options for VP including balloon angioplasty, atherectomy, lithotripsy (Shockwave Medical), specialty balloons, and the FLEX VP system (VentureMed). Quite often, the device selection appears to depend on operator comfort, training, availability, cost, reimbursement, and lesion morphology.

Atherectomy has been shown to be an effective VP device with multiple systems available to the operator (Fig. 7.1). Atherectomy utilizes debulking as a way to change vessel compliance. Although there is no well-powered randomized comparative data among various atherectomy devices, operators' preference and lesion characteristics seem to play a significant role in the choice of the device. Over the past several years, we have used a softer debulking strategy in less bulky or less calcified lesions. For instance, fatty, fibrofatty, and mild to moderately calcified lesions can be modified with a gentler debulking approach just enough to alter compliance and reduce subsequent barotrauma and deeper dissections. Another alternative to prepping these lesions would be the FLEX VP device or specialized balloons. We find a more aggressive debulking methods are more likely to be needed in complex disease such as chronic total occlusions (CTO), in-stent restenosis (ISR), and severely calcified lesions. In an aggressive debulking approach, a *residual narrowing* of about 30–40% lesion severity is targeted. On the other hand, we target a *reduction in lesion severity* by about 30% when using a softer debulking approach (for instance, a 90% lesion can be targeted to be about 60%). One advantage of a softer debulking strategy is less distal embolization and less dissections. An

A. N. Shammas · N. W. Shammas (✉)
Midwest Cardiovascular Research Foundation, Davenport, IA, USA

N. W. Shammas (ed.), *Peripheral Arterial Interventions*, Contemporary Cardiology, https://doi.org/10.1007/978-3-031-09741-6_7

aggressive debulking strategy can be associated with distal embolization, dissections, and need for bailout stenting although the latter is likely to be less than no debulking. Intravascular ultrasound (IVUS) can be very useful to guide therapy as this helps in determining lesion morphology and residual narrowing more accurately as well as helps in better sizing of the reference vessel diameter (Fig. 7.2).

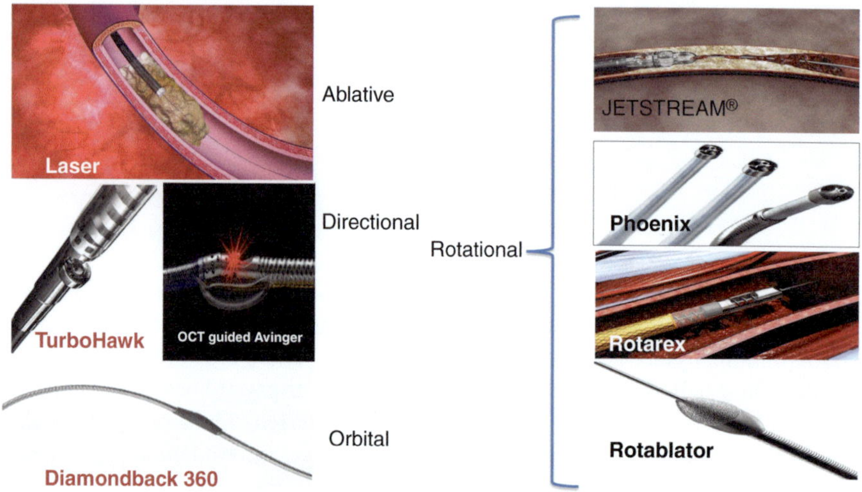

Fig. 7.1 Atherectomy devices

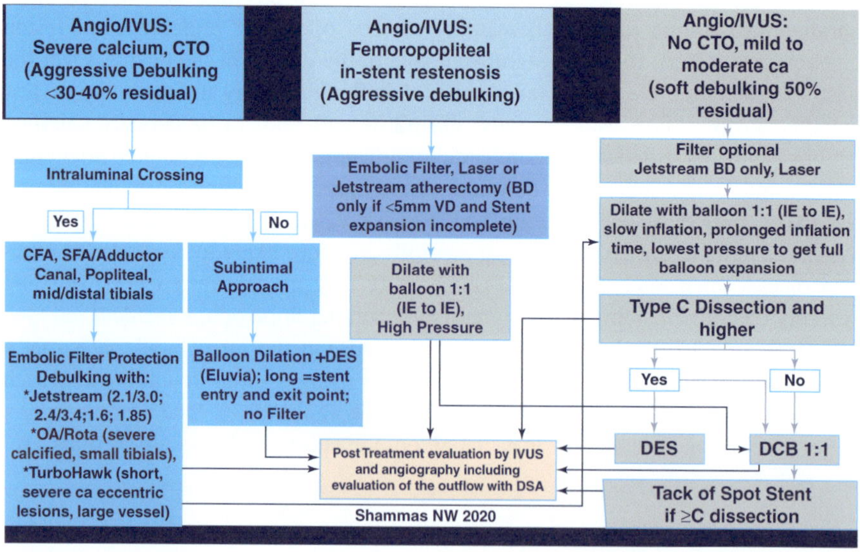

Fig. 7.2 Algorithm using intravascular ultrasound and atherectomy in approaching various lesion morphologies during infrainguinal arterial endovascular interventions (Reprinted with permission from HMP communications)

In general, atherectomy for vessel prepping includes laser, orbital, directional, and rotational devices. Below, we discuss how various atherectomy methods can achieve the debulking strategies described above. Table 7.1 illustrates a summary on how various atherectomy devices are likely to be more effective in specific lesion morphologies (Fig. 7.3).

Table 7.1 Suggested atherectomy device choices in different lesion subsets

🟢 = on label 🟠 = off label 🔴 = Do not use X = Effective XX = Very Effective

Atherectomy Type	Directional	Rotational	Laser Ablative		Orbital
Atherectomy Device	TurboHawk	Jetstream XC	Excimer	Auryon	Diamondback 360
Short Eccentric	XX 🟢	X 🟢	X 🟢	X 🟢	X 🟢
Thrombus	- 🔴	XX 🟢	XX 🟢	XX 🟢	- 🔴
Below the knee	X 🟢	X* 🟢	XX 🟢	X* 🟢	XX 🟢
Long calcified disease	XX 🟢	XX 🟢	X 🟢	XX 🟢	XX 🟢
In-stent restenosis	- 🔴	XX 🟠	XX 🟢	X* 🟢	- 🔴
Chronic total occlusion	XX 🟢	XX 🟢	XX 🟢	XX 🟢	XX 🟢

* More data needed

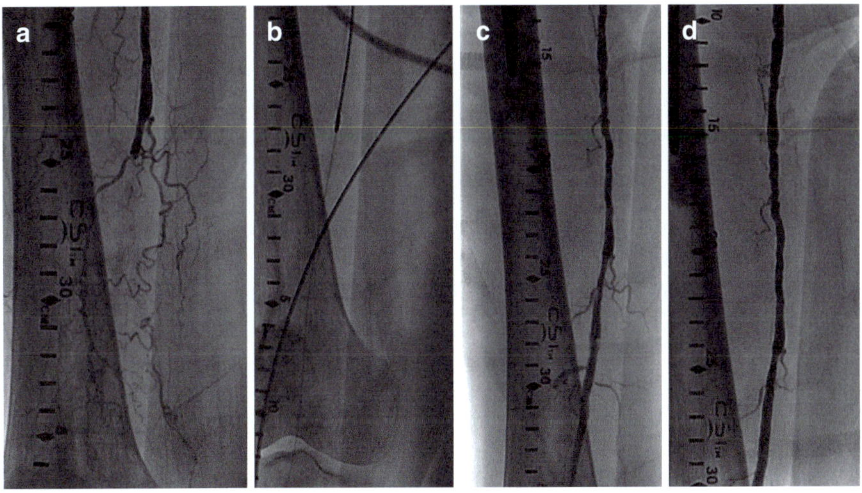

Fig. 7.3 (**a**) Chronic total occlusion of the superficial femoral artery. (**b**) Jetstream atherectomy catheter. (**c**) Post-atherectomy with the Jetstream rotational and aspiration device. (**d**) Final outcome post-PTA. No dissections or need for bailout stenting

Laser Atherectomy

Laser-based devices include the excimer laser (Philips) and the Auryon™ laser (AngioDynamics).

The CVX-300 excimer laser system (Philips) is indicated in fibrotic, calcific, and thrombotic infrainguinal lesions. Excimer or excited dimer is a form of ultraviolet light. The CVX-300 excimer uses xenon and chloride (XeCl) which under high pressure and electrical stimulation generates laser light in the ultraviolet range. The wavelength of the XeCl is 308 nm. Several studies have shown the effects of the excimer laser-based system on 1-year patency including the CELLO trial [1] which included 65 patients with moderate to severe calcified lesions of the femoropopliteal arteries. The percent diameter stenosis was reduced to 34.7 ± 17.8% from 77 ± 15%. This was further reduced to 21 ± 14.5% after balloon angioplasty (PTA) in 42 subjects and PTA plus stenting in 15 patients. The 12-month patency rate was 54%, and the freedom from TLR was 76.9%. Based on this study, the laser-based system appeared to be an effective plaque removal device, with no adverse events noted in this study. With adjunct therapy with PTA and stenting, procedural and long-term outcomes at 1 year appear reasonable but numerically suboptimal to the application of drug elution devices such as drug-coated balloons (DCB) or drug-eluting stents (DES).

The use of the excimer laser prior to PTA versus PTA alone was analyzed in the EXCITE ISR trial [2]. Patients with femoropopliteal in-stent restenosis (ISR) treated with laser and PTA had a greater freedom from TLR at 6 months when compared to PTA alone (61.8% vs 73.5% $p = 0.05$). The study also showed less residual stenosis in the laser plus PTA arm compared to the PTA arm alone (4.7% vs 13.6%, $p = 0.02$). The goal of VP in ISR is not to alter vessel compliance (as the vessel is confined within a stent) but to debulk excessive restenotic tissue particularly in chronic total occlusions (CTO). The Photoablation Using the Turbo-Booster and Excimer Laser for In-Stent Restenosis Treatment (PATENT) study [3], a European multicenter prospective study, evaluated the Turbo-Elite laser atherectomy catheter. Of the 90 ISR lesions, procedural success was 96.7% with percent stenosis reduced to 32.3% from 87.0%. Percent stenosis further reduced to 7.4% following adjunctive PTA which was performed in 79 of the lesions. Target lesion revascularization (TLR) at 6 and 12 months were 87.8% and 64.4%, respectively. The 30-day major adverse event (MAE) was 2.2%. Another important finding is the reduction of bail-out stenting in the laser and PTA arm.

The Auryon™ is hybrid technology with a laser and a blunt blade. The blade creates a slit that enables deeper catheter penetration into the tissue. The laser is a solid-state third harmonic Nd:YAG (neodymium-doped yttrium aluminum garnet) with a wavelength of 355 nm and a pulse duration less than 25 ns. The Auryon™ system has single-use catheters, with diameters ranging from 0.9 to 2.35 mm (4–7 French). The smaller catheters can be used for below-the-knee applications. The larger catheters (2 and 2.35 mm) have an aspiration system that seems to reduce distal embolization as was shown in the pivotal Investigation Device Exemption

(IDE) trial EX-PAD-03 study [4]. Having a solid-state medium, the Auryon™ system has a 15-s warm-up time, and no catheter calibration is required. Furthermore, the longer wavelength of 355 nm does not require saline flush since there is no interaction with contrast media. In the EX-PAD-03 trial, symptomatic (Rutherford 2–4) infrainguinal peripheral arterial disease patients were enrolled in a prospective, single-arm, international, multicenter, open-label trial at 8 US and 3 European sites. A total of 97 patients were enrolled and treated. Severe calcification was seen in 26.2% of patients. CTO was present in 21.5, and 20.6% were restenotic (of which 15.9% were ISR). The average reduction in residual stenosis post-laser alone prior to any adjunctive therapy was 33.6% and was not affected by lesion morphology. Patency by duplex evaluation at 30 days and 6 months was 96.8% and 85.6%, respectively, and was similar between those treated with drug-coated balloons and not [5]. Clinically driven target lesion revascularization (TLR) occurred in 3% of lesions, and no distal embolization was reported although only two patients had an embolic filter production. These results were encouraging and demonstrated that a soft ablation is effective in generating low bailout stenting and promising patency and TLR. It is speculated that these results are likely due to less damage to the deeper layers of the vessel wall given the short penetration distance of this laser and the softer debulking that seems to occur in all lesion subtypes treated.

Orbital Atherectomy

The orbital atherectomy (OA) system (Cardiovascular Systems, Inc.) utilizes a crown coated with diamond dust (Diamondback 360™) to sand moderate to severely calcified lesions. The benefits of the OA system in calcified lesions are the reduction of intimal calcium, as well as fracture of the deeper calcium layers due to transmission of mechanical rotational energy into the vessel wall [6]. The outcomes of this vessel preparation are the reduction of angiographic dissections due to the reduction in intimal calcium and improvement in vessel compliance.

The COMPLIANCE 360 study [7] was a randomized, prospective, and multicenter trial which evaluated the outcomes of OA plus PTA vs PTA alone. The study showed similar freedom from TLR when comparing OA plus PTA vs PTA alone at 81.2% and 78.3%, respectively. PTA alone showed significantly lower number of lesions being stented in the OA plus PTA arm vs PTA arm alone (5.3% vs 77.8%, $p < 0.001$). The OA plus PTA group also utilized a lower maximal balloon pressure when compared to the PTA alone (4.0 atm vs 9.1 atm, $p < 0.001$). At 12 months, freedom from TLR was similar between the two groups, 81.2% for OA plus PTA vs 78.3% for PTA alone ($p > 0.99$). While not significantly different, the PTA group had a significantly higher stenting rate which could have favored a lower long-term TLR in the PTA group. The study also suggested that OA was an effective vessel prep device in calcified femoropopliteal lesions. The overall results showed better luminal gain and less stenting.

The use of OA in vessel prepping was also evaluated in the CALCIUM 360 trial [8]. This randomized multicenter study evaluated the 1-year outcome in treating calcified lesions. The study utilized the Diamondback 360 Orbital atherectomy system followed by adjunct PTA versus PTA alone. A total of 50 patients were enrolled. The primary endpoint was defined as residual stenosis of ≤30% without bailout stenting type C through F dissection. OA plus PTA when compared to PTA alone had a numerically higher procedural success rate (93.1% vs 82.4%, $p = 0.27$) as well as lower use of bailout stenting (6.9% vs 14.3%, $p = 0.44$). At 1 year, there was an increased rate of freedom from TLR at 93.3% for OA plus PTA and 80% for the PTA group. There was a significant difference in freedom from all-cause mortality in the OA plus PTA groups vs PTA alone, at 100% and 68.4%, respectively, $p = 0.01$. While procedural success, rate of bailout stenting, and freedom of TLR were not statistically significant, the data suggest that OA when used for vessel preparation prior to definitive PTA in calcified infrapopliteal lesions may improve outcomes and reduce bailout stenting.

Rotational Atherectomy

The Jetstream atherectomy device (Boston Scientific) utilizes a combination of rotational cutting and aspiration. It is approved for infrainguinal peripheral arterial disease as well as thrombectomy. The Jetstream was evaluated in moderate and severely calcified vessel in the Jetstream Calcium study [9], which utilized intravascular ultrasound (IVUS) to evaluate the effectiveness of the device in calcified lesions. Study size included 55 patients. The study showed Jetstream use increased luminal area from 6.6 ± 3.7 to 10.00 ± 3.6 mm^2 ($p = 0.001$) where calcium removal was responsible for 86 ± 23% of the change. Patients who underwent PTA post-Jetstream saw a further increase from 7.1 to 11.9 mm^2 ($p = 0.001$). From this study, it was shown in moderate and severely calcified lesions, the Jetstream was effective at enhancing luminal area with further improvement post-PTA. It should be noted there were no flow-limiting dissection or adverse events 30-day post-procedure. This indicated that Jetstream could be an effective prepping device before PTA with excellent procedural outcomes.

The JET Registry study evaluated de novo and non-stent restenotic lesions in the femoropopliteal arteries [10]. Lesion length was 16.4 ± 13.6 mm, and pretreatment stenosis was 92.7% for patient who received a stent and 90.2% for non-stented lesions. Of 241 patients, 224 underwent PTA, and 84 of those received additional stenting. Post-Jetstream stenosis was 54.8 ± 22.0%. For those who underwent stenting, final stenosis was 6.6 ± 10.2% compared to 11.6 ± 11.7% in the adjunctive PTA group. Procedural success rate was 98.3%. At 30 days, MAE was 2%. At 12 months, TLR rate was 18.3%. Distal embolization occurred in three patients. This data suggest Jetstream atherectomy is an effective and safe treatment modality in de novo and non-stent restenosis lesions.

The JET-ISR study [11] evaluated Jetstream atherectomy in the setting of femoropopliteal ISR. In this multicenter prospective registry, the freedom from TLR at

6 months was 79.3% (95% CI 68.9–89.8%) and at 1 year 60.7% (95% CI 47.8–73.6%). No drug-coated balloons were used. Bailout stenting was seen in 6/60 (10%) lesions. Lesion length was 19.9 ± 13.5 cm, and 33/60 (55%) lesions were CTO. This suggests that for complex ISR and CTO lesions, vessel prepping with Jetstream produces good outcomes at 1 year with a reduced need for bailout stenting. Jetstream atherectomy in ISR remains off-label in the United States.

The Phoenix atherectomy system (Philips) is another rotational device that uses a front cutting device and internal helix screw designed to remove debulked material while cutting. The device is indicated in femoropopliteal and below-the-knee lesions. The EASE study [12] evaluated the safety and effectiveness of the device in de novo and restenotic infrainguinal arterial lesions. The study was a prospective, multicenter, nonrandomized investigational trial with sites located in the United States and Germany. 105 patients and 123 lesions were included in the primary analysis with a primary efficacy endpoint of post-atherectomy residual stenosis of ≤50%. Technical success was achieved in 95.1% of lesions with further reduction to ≤30% in 99.2%. There were a 5.7% major adverse event rate through 30 days and 16.8% through 6 months including arterial restenosis in seven cases, four type A and B dissections, three with intermittent claudication, two vessel perforations, one type C dissection, one in-stent restenosis, one stent occlusion, and one skin ulcer. TLR was 88% and TVR 86.1% at 6 months. Based on this data, the Phoenix system appears to be an effective debulking device when followed with adjunctive therapy. More comparative trials should be performed to fully assess the device as a debulking option prior to adjunctive therapy.

The Rotarex Rotational Excisional Atherectomy System (BD) also utilizes a rotating catheter and internal helix screw that removes debulked material simultaneously. The system utilizes blunt facets, as well as side windows to further remove debulked material. The device is approved in the United States and European markets. Bérczi et al. [13] evaluated the device in 18 patients and 19 limbs with acute or subacute occlusion of the femoropopliteal artery. Technical success was achieved in 15/19 vessel, with 17 of limbs utilizing adjunctive therapy with angioplasty or stent. The study reported two perforations in heavily calcified plaques, one arteriovenous fistula, and three distal embolizations. Wissgott et al. [14] evaluated the device in 40 patients with chronic occlusion of the iliac (n = 4) and femoropopliteal arteries (n = 36). In this study, technical success was 100% with 27/40 patients receiving adjunctive balloon and 7/40 requiring stenting. There was a 22.5% restenosis rate at 12 months. There was no distal embolization, amputations, or death. Two dissections were seen after balloon dilation.

Directional Atherectomy

There are multiple directional atherectomy (DA) devices that utilize a direct cutting method for plaque removal in the infrainguinal arteries. Devices including the SilverHawk, TurboHawk, and HawkOne (Medtronic) as well as newer devices such as the Pantheris (Avinger), which utilizes built-in optical coherence tomography (OCT), are available to operators.

The SilverHawk was evaluated in the DEFINITIVE LE trial [15], an 800-patient multicenter single-arm study. Technical success was 89% with 3.8% distal embolization, 2.3% dissection, 5.3% perforation, and 2.0% acute vessel occlusion. Bailout stenting was seen in 3.2% of lesions. At 1 year, primary patency was 84% with freedom from amputation at 97.1% [16].

The DEFINITIVE AR trial [17] investigated how directional atherectomy and anti-restenotic therapy (DAART), a combination of DA and drug-coated balloon therapy, performed when compared to DCB alone. Technical success was 89.6% for DAART therapy when compared to DCB alone at 64.2% ($p = 0.004$). The trial also showed lower rates of flow-limiting dissections in favor of DARRT at 2% vs DCB at 19% ($p = 0.01$). One-year data showed TLR of DAART at 7.3% and 8.0% for DCB ($p = 0.90$). The combination of DCB and DA delivered excellent technical success and reduced dissections, though 1-year data showed no significant difference in TLR. Following the DEFINITIVE AR trial, the ISAR-STATH study [18] evaluated the difference between DCB plus stenting and PTA plus stenting vs DA plus bailout stenting in superficial femoral lesions. This randomized trial included 155 patients with de novo lesions and showed that paclitaxel-based DCB and stenting had a 6-month angiographic diameter stenosis of 34 ± 31%, compared to PTA and stenting at 56 ± 29% ($p = 0.009$) and DA and bailout stenting at 55 ± 29% ($p = 0.007$). At 24 months, the DCB group had a decreased risk of TLR as well as no difference in target lesion thrombosis, mortality, or amputation. Angiographically, the ISAR-STATH study showed DCB and stenting were superior to DA and bailout stenting and BA with stenting.

The randomized trial of SilverHawk atherectomy and PTA versus PTA alone was the first trial that evaluated the added benefit of atherectomy when compared to PTA alone [19]. In this prospective, two-center randomized trial of PTA versus SilverHawk and PTA of infrainguinal arteries, 58 patients were included. Of these, 29 (36 vessels) were randomized to the atherectomy arm and 29 (48 vessels) to the PTA arm. There was no statistical difference in TLR (16.7% vs 11.1%) or TVR (21.4% vs 11.1%) or major adverse events between the PTA and atherectomy groups, respectively. Bailout stent placement was performed in 18 of 29 patients (62.1%) in the PTA arm and 8 of 29 patients (27.6%) in the atherectomy arm ($p = 0.017$). Distal embolization was more frequently seen in the atherectomy arm. This study was the first randomized study to show that atherectomy as a technique has a major impact on VP by reducing bailout stenting but did not affect the long-term outcome of the procedure.

The Pantheris OCT atherectomy device was evaluated in the VISION study [20], a single-arm, multicenter study with 158 subjects and 198 lesions. After use of the Pantheris device, the mean diameter stenosis decreased to 30.3 ± 11.8% from 78.7 ± 15.1%, $p < 0.001$. Further reduction to 22.4 ± 9.9% was seen after adjunctive therapy with PTA of 84 lesions and stenting in 10 lesions. At 6 months, a TLR rate of 6.4% was noted. The use of OCT appears to be key in the low adverse events. There were no significant perforations, a 0.5% catheter-related dissection rate, and a 2% rate of embolic events. Histological analysis showed less than 1% involvement of the adventitia in 82.1% of samples. The use of the OCT-guided device appears to be an effective plaque removal device with excellent procedural results. The device has the advantage of limiting adventitial damage, which is a key predictor in loss of patency post-intervention.

Atherectomy and Drug-Coated Balloons

Preclinical studies have shown that atherectomy enhances drug elution into the vessel wall which in return may improve the long-term outcomes of a procedure when compared to DCB alone. The dual advantage of improving acute procedural results and optimizing long-term outcome is a viable concept that was seen in some observational studies and small randomized trials, but more definitive large-scale trials are lacking. The JET-RANGER (NCT03206762) was designed to test this hypothesis with the Jetstream atherectomy and DCB vs DCB alone, but terminated early because of poor enrolment resulting from the DCB and mortality debate fueled by the Katsanos et al. meta-analysis [21] as well as the COVID-19 pandemic.

Severe calcium is a barrier to drug elution. Fanelli et al. [22] have shown that severe calcium has a negative impact on patency and TLR. In 60 patients with de novo lesions of the superficial femoral artery treated with DCB, dissections were more prevalent in patients with severe calcium. Higher circumferential degree of calcium (>270° vs <90°) resulted in more late lumen loss (0.75 ± 0.21 vs 0.45 ± 0.1) and loss of patency (50% vs 100%). Furthermore, TLR was higher in patients with severe calcium (TLR 25% vs 0%). In the Directional Atherectomy Followed by a Paclitaxel-Coated Balloon to Inhibit Restenosis and Maintain Vessel Patency—A Pilot Study of Anti-Restenosis Treatment (DEFINITIVE AR study) [17], a total of 19 patients with severely calcified lesions were treated with DA + DCB. Less rate of flow-limiting dissections was seen with DA + DCB (19% for DCB and 2% for DA + DCB (p = 0.01)). Patency by duplex ultrasound was 84.6% for DA + DCB, 81.3% for DCB (p = 0.78), and 68.8% for calcified lesions. In addition, Gandini et al. [23] randomized 48 patients with chronic superficial femoral artery in-stent occlusion to laser atherectomy + DCB (n = 24) versus DCB only (n = 24). Patency at 6 and 12 months (91.7% and 66.7%, respectively) were significantly higher than in the DCB group (58.3% and 37.5%, respectively) (p = 0.01). Also, TLR at 12 months was 16.7% in the laser + DCB group and 50% in the DCB only group (p = 0.01). Furthermore, observational data suggest a sustained long-term benefit of the combination of atherectomy and DCB when compared to atherectomy only. In 75 patients with de novo or restenotic femoropopliteal lesions, adjunctive PTA was performed on 50 patients (26 de novo, 13 in-stent restenosis, 3 non-stent restenosis, 8 mixed lesions) and adjunctive DCB (Lutonix® 24 (Bard/BD), IN.PACT® 1 (Medtronic)) on 25 patients (21 de novo, 1 in-stent restenosis, 2 non-stent restenosis, 1 mixed lesion). Freedom from TLR was significantly higher with atherectomy and adjunctive DCB compared to atherectomy with adjunctive PTA at 12 months

(94.7% vs 68.0%, $p = 0.002$) and 16 months (94.4% vs 54%; $p = 0.002$) [24]. Finally, in a single-center cohort, 89 patients (139 lesions) were treated with DCB, of whom 40 (29%) were treated with orbital atherectomy (OA) + DCB. Less bailout stenting was seen in those with OA + DCB (18% vs 39%, $p = 0.01$), but freedom from TLR (82% in both groups ($p = 0.6$)) and patency (81% DCB and 77% DCB + OA ($p = 0.8$)) were similar at 1 year [25]. One could conclude that OA + DCB with less bailout stenting yielded similar outcome to DCB with a higher rate of stenting.

Conclusion

The use of atherectomy as a plaque removal device appears to be an effective method prior to definitive treatment with PTA or drug-coated balloons in reducing angiographic dissections and bailout stenting. Atherectomy, however, does not appear to impact the long-term outcome of the procedure with the exception of in-stent restenosis when compared to PTA. Recently, Shammas et al. [26] showed that IVUS-based dissections can be significant with certain atherectomy devices, such as Jetstream atherectomy, in the femoropopliteal arteries. These dissections are not identified on angiography, which may partially explain the loss of patency in these vessels on long-term follow-up without the adjunctive treatment with a mitigating factor such as drug-coated balloons or stents. Other atherectomy devices have also been evaluated and have shown various degrees of dissection not visible on angiography [27]. Recently, the Auryon laser with its softer debulking capacity was shown to have a very low number of adventitial dissections which may partly explain the excellent intermediate-term patency and TLR on follow-up [28]. Finally, in the VISION study [20] where the adventitia has been mostly spared, the TLR rate was only 6.4% at 6 months. This certainly poses the important question whether too much of an aggressive debulking strategy is always needed and whether the choice of the atherectomy device can make a difference in the long-term outcome. Further studies are needed to prove this hypothesis.

VP using atherectomy requires that devices are tailored to certain lesion subsets as indicated in Table 7.1. Excimer laser atherectomy as a VP device appears to have success with limited adverse events in ISR lesions, in fatty and fibrofatty lesions, and in mild to moderate calcium. The Auryon laser appears to be quite effective in severe calcium and can also be used in other lesion subtypes including ISR. OA is an excellent device for severe calcium and particularly in below-the-knee lesions. Rotational atherectomy with the Jetstream device has been shown to yield good results in de novo and non-stent restenosis lesions as well as calcified lesions particularly in the femoropopliteal segments. It has also been shown to be safe in ISR although remains off-label in the United States for this application. Directional atherectomy is also effective for many lesions, but preferred overall for short and eccentric lesions [29] when compared to the laser, as it requires frequent removal and emptying of the nosecone and has a higher rate of distal embolization [30]. The

Pantheris OCT system appears to spare the adventitia because of OCT-guided debulking and performs well in multiple lesion subtypes at the expense of longer procedure time. It also requires an understanding of OCT imaging.

VP remains critical to the success of infrainguinal arterial endovascular treatment. Atherectomy is an important modality to VP, and devices are best tailored to lesion morphology. Other emerging technologies besides atherectomy are likely to play a significant role in VP without debulking such as the FLEX VP longitudinal microincision system (VentureMed Group), Shockwave lithoplasty (Shockwave Medical), or other specialty balloons. A common denominator among all vessel prepping devices is the ability to obtain excellent acute procedural results leaving the least metal behind. This is achieved by limiting dissections while maximizing luminal gain. Optimal imaging needs to play a critical role in understanding the best mechanism of VP devices in various lesion morphologies.

References

1. Dave RM, Patlola R, Kollmeyer K, et al. Excimer laser recanalization of femoropopliteal lesions and 1-year patency: results of the CELLO registry. J Endovasc Ther. 2009; 16:665–75.
2. Dippel EJ, Makam P, Kovach R, et al. Randomized controlled study of excimer laser atherectomy for treatment of femoropopliteal in-stent restenosis: initial results from the EXCITE ISR trial (Excimer Laser Randomized Controlled Study for Treatment of Femoropopliteal In-Stent Restenosis). JACC Cardiovasc Interv. 2015;8(1 Part A):92–101.
3. Schmidt A, Zeller T, Sievert H, et al. Photoablation using the turbo-booster and excimer laser for in-stent restenosis treatment: twelve-month results from the PATENT study. J Endovasc Ther. 2014;21(1):52–60.
4. Shammas NW, Chandra P, Brodmann M, et al. Acute and 30-day safety and effectiveness evaluation of Eximo Medical's B-Laser™, a novel atherectomy device, in subjects affected with infrainguinal peripheral arterial disease: results of the EX-PAD-03 trial. Cardiovasc Revasc Med. 2020;21:86–92. https://doi.org/10.1016/j.carrev.2018.11.022.
5. Rundback J, Chandra P, Brodmann M, et al. Novel laser-based catheter for peripheral atherectomy: 6-month results from the Eximo Medical B-Laser™ IDE study. Catheter Cardiovasc Interv. 2019;94:1010–7. https://doi.org/10.1002/ccd.28435.
6. Fitzgerald PJ, Ports TA, Yock PG. Contribution of localized calcium deposits to dissection after angio-plasty. An observational study using intravascular ultrasound. Circulation. 1992;86:64–70.
7. Dattilo R, Himmelstein SI, Cuff RF. The COMPLI-ANCE 360° trial: a randomized, prospective, multi-center, pilot study comparing acute and long-term results of orbital atherectomy to balloon angioplasty for calcified femoropopliteal disease. J Invasive Cardiol. 2014;26:355–60.
8. Shammas NW, Lam R, Mustapha J, et al. Comparison of orbital atherectomy plus balloon angioplasty vs. balloon angioplasty alone in patients with critical limb ischemia: results of the CALCIUM 360 randomized pilot trial. J Endovasc Ther. 2012;19:480–8.
9. Maehara A, Mintz GS, Shimshak TM, et al. Intravascular ultrasound evaluation of JETSTREAM atherectomy removal of superficial calcium in peripheral arteries. EuroIntervention. 2015;11(1):96–103.
10. Gray WA, Garcia LA, Amin A, et al. Jetstream atherectomy system treatment of femoropopliteal arteries: results of the post-market JET registry. Cardiovasc Revasc Med. 2018;19(5 Pt A):506–11.

11. Shammas NW, Petruzzi N, Henao S, et al. Jetstream atherectomy for the treatment of in-stent restenosis of the femoropopliteal segment: one-year results of the JET-ISR study. J Endovasc Ther. 2021;28(1):107–16.
12. Davis T, Ramaiah V, Niazi K, et al. Safety and effectiveness of the Phoenix atherectomy system in lower extremity arteries: early and midterm outcomes from the prospective multicenter EASE study. Vascular. 2017;25:563–75.
13. Bérczi V, Deutschmann HA, Schedlbauer P, Tauss J, Hausegger K. Early experience and midterm follow-up results with a new, rotational thrombectomy catheter. Cardiovasc Interv Radiol. 2002;25:275–81.
14. Wissgott C, Kamusella P, Andresen R. Treatment of chronic occlusions of the iliac or femoropopliteal arteries with mechanical rotational catheters. Rofo. 2011;183:945–51. https://doi.org/10.1055/s-0031-1273451. Epub 2011 Sep 5.
15. McKinsey JF, Zeller T, Rocha-Singh KJ, et al. Lower extremity revascularization using directional atherectomy: 12-month prospective results of the DEFINITIVE LE study. JACC Cardiovasc Interv. 2014;7:923–33.
16. Rastan A, McKinsey JF, Garcia LA, et al. One-year outcomes following directional atherectomy of infrapopliteal artery lesions: subgroup results of the prospective, multicenter DEFINITIVE LE trial. J Endovasc Ther. 2015;22:839–46.
17. Zeller T, Langhoff R, Rocha-Singh KJ, et al. Directional atherectomy followed by a paclitaxel-coated balloon to inhibit restenosis and maintain vessel patency: twelve month results of the DEFINITIVE AR study. Circ Cardiovasc Interv. 2017;10(9):e004848. https://doi.org/10.1161/CIRCINTERVENTIONS.116.004848.
18. Ott I, Cassese S, Groha P, et al. Randomized comparison of paclitaxel-eluting balloon and stenting versus plain balloon plus stenting versus directional atherectomy for femoral artery disease (ISAR-STATH). Circulation. 2017;135:2218–26.
19. Shammas NW, Coiner D, Shammas GA, et al. Percutaneous lower-extremity arterial interventions with primary balloon angioplasty versus Silverhawk atherectomy and adjunctive balloon angioplasty: randomized trial. J Vasc Interv Radiol. 2011;22:1223–8.
20. Schwindt AG, Bennett JG Jr, Crowder WH, et al. Lower extremity revascularization using optical coherence tomography-guided directional atherectomy: final results of the eValuatIon of the PantheriS optIcal cOherence tomography ImagiNg atherectomy system for use in the peripheral vasculature (VISION) study. J Endovasc Ther. 2017;24:355–66.
21. Katsanos K, Spiliopoulos S, Kitrou P, Krokidis M, Karnabatidis D. Risk of death following application of paclitaxel-coated balloons and stents in the femoropopliteal artery of the leg: a systematic review and meta-analysis of randomized controlled trials. J Am Heart Assoc. 2018;7(24):e011245. https://doi.org/10.1161/JAHA.118.011245.
22. Fanelli F, Cannavale A, Gazzetti M, et al. Calcium burden assessment and impact on drug-eluting balloons in peripheral arterial disease. Cardiovasc Interv Radiol. 2014;37(4):898–907.
23. Gandini R, Del Giudice C, Merolla S, et al. Treatment of chronic SFA in-stent occlusion with combined laser atherectomy and drug-eluting balloon angioplasty in patients with critical limb ischemia: a single center, prospective, randomized study. J Endovasc Ther. 2013;20:805–14.
24. Shammas NW, Shammas GA, Jones-Miller S, et al. Long-term outcomes with Jetstream atherectomy with or without drug coated balloons in treating femoropopliteal arteries: a single center experience (JET-SCE). Cardiovasc Revasc Med. 2018;19(7 Pt A):771–7.
25. Foley TR, Cotter RP, Kokkinidis DG. Midterm outcomes of orbital atherectomy combined with drug-coated balloon angioplasty for treatment of femoropopliteal disease. Catheter Cardiovasc Interv. 2017;89:1078–85.
26. Shammas NW, Torey JT, Shammas WJ, Jones-Miller S, Shammas GA. Intravascular ultrasound assessment and correlation with angiographic findings demonstrating femoropopliteal arterial dissections post atherectomy: results from the iDissection study. J Invasive Cardiol. 2018;30(7):240–4.
27. Shammas NW, Shammas WJ, Jones-Miller S, et al. Optimal vessel sizing and understanding dissections in infrapopliteal interventions: data from the iDissection below the knee study.

J Endovasc Ther. 2020;27(4):575–80. https://doi.org/10.1177/1526602820924815. Epub 2020 May 18.
28. Shammas NW, Shammas WJ, Torey JT, et al. Auryon™ Atherectomy of infrainguinal arterial disease: an IVUS-based single center prospective study. Presented virtually at LINC; 2021.
29. Shammas NW, Shammas GA, Jerin M. Differences in patient selection and outcomes between SilverHawk atherectomy and laser ablation in the treatment of femoropopliteal in-stent restenosis: a retrospective analysis from a single center. J Endovasc Ther. 2013;20:844–52. https://doi.org/10.1583/13-4411R.1.
30. Shammas NW, Dippel EJ, Coiner D, et al. Preventing lower extremity distal embolization using embolic filter protection: results of the PROTECT registry. J Endovasc Ther. 2008;15:270–6. https://doi.org/10.1583/08-2397.1.

Chapter 8
Vessel Preparation with Longitudinal and Controlled-Depth Micro-Incisions

John P. Pigott

Peripheral artery disease (PAD) involving the lower extremities is an increasingly prevalent problem. It is estimated that worldwide more than >200 million people have PAD [1]. The standard practice for endovascular treatment of peripheral artery disease is percutaneous transluminal angioplasty (PTA), including plain balloon (POBA) and drug-coated balloons (DCB). The safety and efficacy of PTA compared to surgical revascularizations have been established [2]. PTA is intended to increase luminal gain in the obstructed vessel. Although PTA and DCB are primary therapies, there is risk of uncontrolled dissections, including those that are flow-limiting. Severe dissections can require bailout stenting and have subsequent negative effects on long-term clinical outcomes, including restenosis and the need for future reinterventions [3]. The FLEX Vessel Prep (FLEX VP) System (VentureMed Group, Minneapolis, MN) is a proprietary technology that enables for controlled and predictable plaque modification in long, complex lesions of varying morphology. The FLEX VP System is designed to create longitudinal, controlled-depth, circumferential micro-incisions along the entire length of a lesion that reduce the number and severity of dissections and other complications often seen with other vessel preparation devices. These controlled-depth micro-incisions help reduce the circumferential tension along the entire length of stenoses, improving vessel compliance that enables enhanced luminal gain at lower balloon inflation pressures.

J. P. Pigott (✉)
VentureMed Group, Inc., Plymouth, MN, USA

Jobst Vascular Institute, Promedica Health Systems, Toledo, USA
e-mail: jpigott@venturemedgroup.com

N. W. Shammas (ed.), *Peripheral Arterial Interventions*, Contemporary Cardiology, https://doi.org/10.1007/978-3-031-09741-6_8

The Clinical Benefit of Reducing Dissections

PTA remains the primary intervention to treat peripheral arterial stenoses [4]. Balloon dilatation can result in uncontrolled dissections that separate the intima from the media of a vessel wall and/or cause injury to the adventitia [5, 6]. The acute vessel damage may range from a superficial plaque disruption to deep, flow-limiting dissections. Dissections are a clinical concern as dissection-induced damage to smooth muscle tissue increases the risk of stenosis due to induction of an inflammatory response, leukocyte recruitment, platelet activation, thrombosis, and neointimal hyperplasia [7–12].

Dissections have been reported across a wide range of superficial femoral artery (SFA) and popliteal angioplasties (7–84%) [13–18]. However, the reported occurrence and severity of dissection may be underestimated as data from clinical studies that utilize independent core lab review tend to report significantly higher extent and severity of dissections as compared to the dissection data reported from non-adjudicated clinical studies [19]. It has also been noted that intravascular imaging methods such as intravascular ultrasound (IVUS) or optical coherence tomography (OCT) allow for more precise identification of arterial dissections, as compared to conventional angiography, with a comparative analysis demonstrating that IVUS identified four to six times more dissections than angiography [20]. High-grade dissections post balloon angioplasty correlate with reduced patency and increased target lesion revascularization (TLR) [14, 20]. Mild-to-moderate-grade dissections also may be associated with lower patency and higher TLR rates (National Heart, Lung, and Blood Institute [NHLBI] Classification of Dissection) [4]. PTA-induced dissections have been identified as a contributing factor in acute procedure complications, such as bailout stenting, long-term clinical outcomes such as reduced patency, acute occlusions, thrombus formation, in-stent restenosis, and an increased need for future target lesion revascularization (TLR) [4, 14, 16, 20–24]. Minimizing dissection rate and severity are key to successful endovascular procedures.

Plaque morphology and lesion length play a key role in the severity of dissections after angioplasty. It is widely accepted that calcification is a more challenging lesion morphology to treat and often results in higher rates of severe dissections [16, 25–28]. In a study involving IVUS in coronary and peripheral arteries to assess dissections and calcium burden of the lesion, it was noted that 87% of dissections showed calcium deposits on the same side of the vessel wall as the dissection [25]. Unfortunately, our understanding of calcification's contribution to dissection rates during endovascular procedures is limited because severely calcified lesions that are associated with higher rates of dissections are routinely excluded as part of trial criteria [4, 28]. In addition, lesion length was found as independent predictor of severe dissection rate [14, 21].

Often dissections are treated with adjunctive therapies, such as stenting, to maximize luminal gain and improve flow dynamics. Another commonly used technique to treat dissections is prolonged balloon inflation. Contributing factors such as the location, depth, and magnitude of dissections determine the treatment algorithm. Minor dissections (Type A or B) may not require further treatment, while more severe (Types C through F) dissections may require a bailout stent. A retrospective analysis of the incidence of post-PTA dissections found an occurrence of 84% [14]. Lesions with Type C–F dissections had a 34% TLR at 6 months, as compared to a 14% TLR for Type A and B dissections or patients with zero dissections identified in the same study [14].

The THUNDER study evaluated the safety and efficacy of a paclitaxel-coated balloon and reported that lesions with Type A and B dissections had statistically similar rates of TLR at 6 months as lesions with Types C through E (33% and 44%, respectively). At 24 months, the TLR rates increased to 43% for Type A and B dissections and to 78% for Type C through E dissections [17]. The prevalence of dissections identified via angiography has been reported to be between 50 and 85% following balloon angioplasty in the SFA [14]. POBA complication rates have been reported to be as high as 30%, including high rates of uncontrolled dissections with higher rates observed in longer lesions with likelihood that angiographically identified dissections are under-reported [20, 29–32].

Current Methods for Vessel Preparation

Although PTA remains the most common endovascular intervention, the dissections that occur remain uncontrolled and have the potential to impact the patient's long-term outcomes. Advances in vessel preparation prior to PTA show promise in reducing the risk of severe dissections and long-term adverse consequences. Numerous technologies have been developed to modify the plaque prior to endovascular treatments in order to improve therapeutic response and reduce procedural complications. Additionally, vessel preparation and plaque modification may potentially facilitate the delivery of anti-restenotic drugs across the arterial wall [33, 34]. Current technologies include specialty angioplasty balloons, atherectomy, and intravascular lithotripsy.

Specialty Angioplasty Balloons

Specialty angioplasty balloons include additional features that modify plaque by focal force, static cutting, or scoring. These balloon-based scoring devices utilize the combination of external wires or atherotomes and balloon dilatation to attempt to create controlled dissections by exerting focal force to the lesion [32]. However, limitations of these devices include fixed scoring elements, application of symmetrical focal force even when lesions are asymmetrical, potential requirement for overlapping dilatations, and risk for injury to healthy tissue due to dilatation of more normal vessel segments. A pivotal trial for evaluating intervention of a specialty scoring balloon in 245 patients with SFA/PA lesions reported dissection and stent rates of 26% and 32%, respectively [35].

Atherectomy

Atherectomy is intended to provide lumen gain by removing (debulking) the plaque through cutting, shaving, grinding, or vaporizing. The four current types of atherectomy technologies are directional, rotational, orbital, and laser. Atherectomy has reported advantages in shorter lesions, severely calcified lesions, and longer non-occlusive lesions [36, 37]. However, limitations to atherectomy include the inability to control depth of plaque removal, risk of vessel perforations during debulking, damage to the media and adventitia, and risk of embolization [38–40]. Dissection rates related to atherectomy range from 2 to 17% [41–43]. In addition to clinical risks, atherectomy may both increase procedure times and require the use of additional procedural resources related to training, capital equipment, extra time with fluoroscopy, additional ancillary products like filter devices, and inventory of multiple size single-use devices [36].

Intravascular Lithotripsy (IVL)

IVL is intended to achieve plaque modification in calcified lesions by using sonic pressure waves to create microfractures or microfissures [22, 44]. IVL relies on energy absorption by calcium and thus may have suboptimal impact on lesions with mixed morphology and/or light calcification. Furthermore, the current device is limited to 300 pulses with longer lesions requiring overlapping treatments for complete coverage. Based on its design, IVL may be best suited for shorter, severely calcified lesions with circumferential calcium deposition [45].

Creating Longitudinal Micro-Incisions to Modify Plaque with Fewer Complications

The FLEX VP System is a novel approach to vessel preparation and plaque modification that uses proprietary non-balloon technology to create multiple, longitudinal, controlled-depth micro-incisions across the entire lesion length (Fig. 8.1). These circumferential controlled-depth micro-incisions are an integral part of the design that reduce the number and severity of dissections and other complications (Fig. 8.2). The FLEX VP System is indicated for use with PTA catheters to facilitate dilation of stenoses in the femoral and popliteal arteries and treatment of obstructive lesions of native or synthetic arteriovenous dialysis fistulae. The device is also indicated for the treatment of in-stent restenosis (ISR) of balloon-expandable and self-expanding stents in the peripheral vasculature. The FLEX VP is designed for mixed morphology lesions with a range of characteristics (e.g., long, calcified).

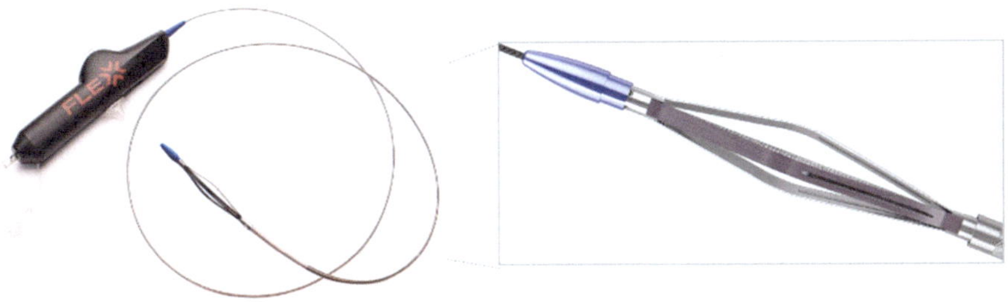

Fig. 8.1 FLEX Vessel Prep System product overview

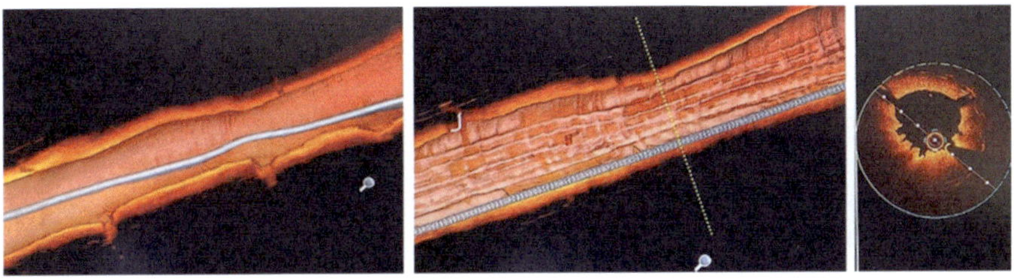

Fig. 8.2 Longitudinal optical coherence tomography reconstruction pre- (left) and post-FLEX VP (center, right) in a porcine model of superficial femoral artery in-stent restenosis demonstrating the micro-incisions (longitudinal view, center; cross-sectional view, right)

The FLEX VP is an over-the-wire sheathed catheter with a three-strut treatment element at the distal tip. It is compatible with a 6-French sheath and 0.014 in or 0.018 in guidewire and is available in two working lengths (40 cm or 120 cm). The proximal portion of each treatment element strut includes a 0.010 in height micro-surgical blade. Once the device is advanced past the lesion, the treatment element (TE) is deployed and expanded, and the catheter is drawn back, allowing the micro-surgical blades on the proximal end of each TE strut to independently engage in the lesion and create three parallel, circumferential continuous micro-incisions, with a consistent depth, along the entire length of the lesion. After the first pass, the TE is re-sheathed and advanced again through the lesion, rotated approximately 30 degrees before the treatment element is re-deployed and the retrograde pullback described above is repeated. This process is repeated based on the patient's disease characteristics. For example, a procedure with 4 passes of the device prepares the artery by performing 12 longitudinal micro-incisions in the lesions (as illustrated in Fig. 8.2 center and right panels). Additional features that benefit the clinician and adoption into current clinical practice include a braided shaft that is engineered to facilitate tracking the pullback performance; an atraumatic tip, with a 2 mm crossing profile that provides trackability and a low risk of perforation; a radiopaque marker band that facilitates placement of the FLEX VP System to treat any length lesion; and a single size that applies to most complex, mixed morphology lesions by self-sizing to the lumen diameter.

Clinical Data in Peripheral Arterial Disease

Clinical data has reported consistent outcome with FLEX VP treatment across long complex lesions [20, 46]. In over 700 peripheral arterial disease patients, average luminal gain following FLEX VP alone was 20–30% with average balloon opening pressure <5 atm and provisional stent rate of <20% in lesions with average length ranging from 136 to 245 mm (see Table 8.1 for study summary details).

Collectively, these data indicate that FLEX VP is effective in a broad range of PAD lesion lengths across real-world plaque morphologies, improves vessel compliance, is associated with reduced rate/grade/severity of dissections, and creates luminal gain without perforations or embolization.

Mechanism of Action

The longitudinal micro-incisions created by FLEX VP are key to the technology's mechanism of action in several ways. First, the treatment element struts are designed to independently "flex" (adaptively expand and compress) to the contour of the vessel wall morphology (Fig. 8.3). This is in contrast with other vessel preparation or plaque modification technologies that utilize concentric expansion of angioplasty balloons to apply focal force to the vessel wall. The independent, dynamic action of

Table 8.1 Summary of clinical studies

Subset	Patient (N)	Average lesion length (mm)	Lumen gain (%)	Balloon opening pressure (atm)	Provisional stent use (%)
Jobst retrospective study [47]	123	245 ± 102	22.4 ± 16[a]	4.8 ± 1.4[a]	17 (12)
BELONG feasibility study [48]	63	196 ± 127	N/A	N/A	11 (16.9)
iDissection study [20]	15[b]	63.6 ± 32.5	17	N/A	6 (40)
Acute outcomes [46]	255[c]	133.4 ± 87.5[d]	25.2 ± 16.4[a]	4.2 ± 1.5[a]	49 (19.2)
Post-market surveillance summary[e]	523[e]	136 ± 96[f]	31 ± 20%[a]	4.5 ± 1.6[a]	103 (19%)

[a] Subset analysis
[b] Patients also enrolled in Intact Vascular study
[c] Initial 255 patients of Post-Market Surveillance Study
[d] $N = 252$
[e] Data on file; $N = 538$ lesions in 523 patients
[f] $N = 531$

the protective struts of the FLEX VP System enables precise, controlled-depth micro-incisions that self-size to the lesion during the retrograde pullback. The FLEX VP is also indicated for ISR which can be difficult to treat due to the limitations of other vessel prep devices inside a stent (Fig. 8.4).

Minimizing disruption to the elastic lamina during vessel prep reduces the damage to the media and adventitia and associated risk of an inflammatory response leading to lower rates of restenosis [7–12]. FLEX VP evaluated in cadaveric tissue demonstrates minimal disruption to the elastic lamina while offering continuous engagement along the treated lesion (Figs. 8.5 and 8.6).

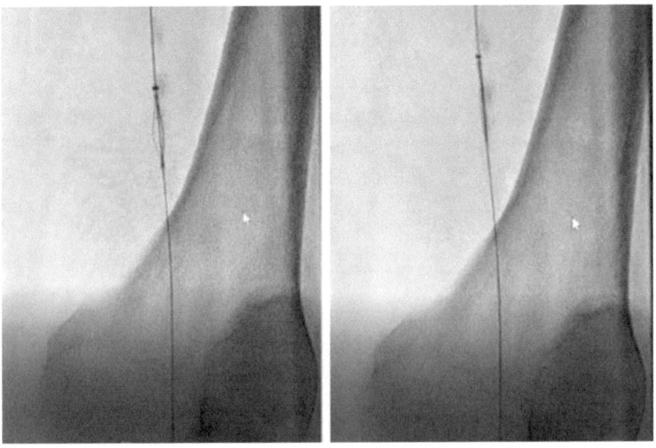

Fig. 8.3 FLEX VP treatment element shown expanded in a non-stenotic segment of the vessel (left) and FLEX VP treatment element self-sized and engaged in stenosis (right)

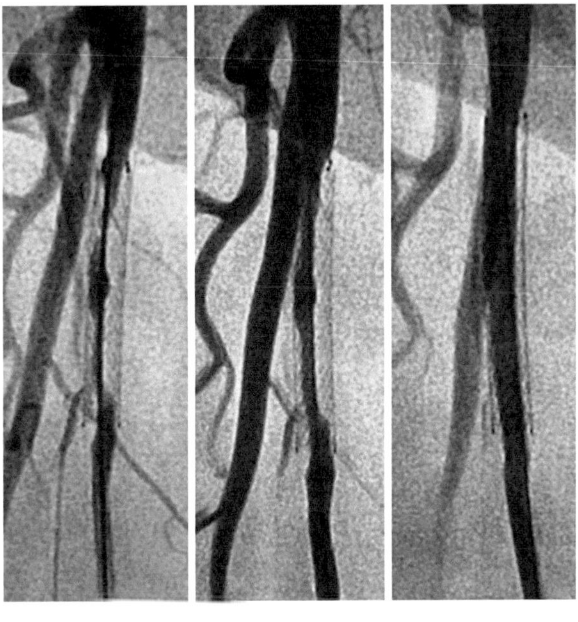

Fig. 8.4 Angiography images of in-stent restenosis in the SFA at baseline ISR (left), post-FLEX VP recanalization (middle), and final result post-DCB (right)

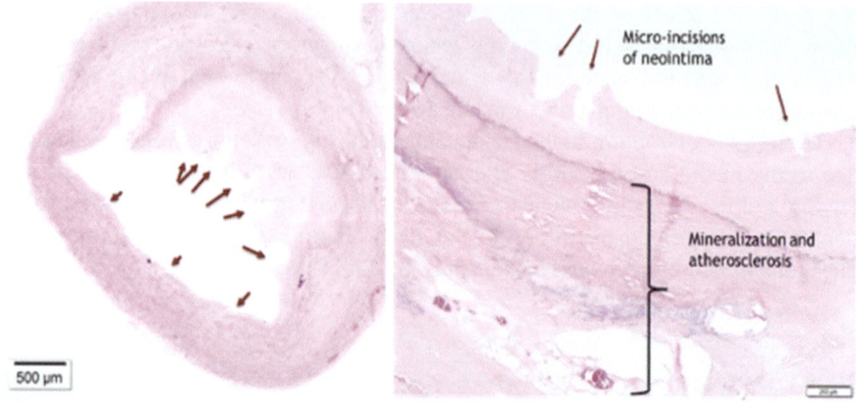

Fig. 8.5 Histology (hematoxylin and eosin stain; H&E) in a tibial cadaveric lesion with an asymmetrical neointima with partial luminal occlusion (left) and a calcified cadaveric SFA lesion (right) post-FLEX VP. Arrows indicate micro-incisions created by FLEX VP used to treat cadaveric popliteal stenosis. Micro-incision depth is equivalent to the blade height (0.25 mm)

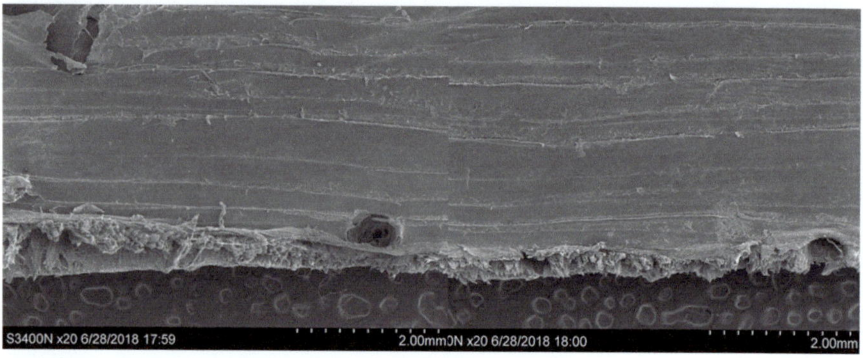

Fig. 8.6 Scanning electron microscopy (SEM) image of a cadaveric SFA treated with FLEX VP. Longitudinal lines (left to right) demonstrate consistent and parallel FLEX VP micro-incision engagement along the entire length of the lesion

Next, the circumferential placement and controlled depth of the micro-incisions improve vessel compliance and enable even lumen gain and controlled expansion of the artery during PTA or DCB. Figure 8.7 provides an optical coherence tomography (OCT) cross-sectional image of pre- and post-different vessel preparation technologies tested in an ISR porcine lesion. Vessel prep technology tested included scoring PTA, direction atherectomy, and FLEX VP. Note the lack of circumferential engagement in alternative technologies as compared to FLEX VP, which demonstrates a consistent circumferential engagement (Fig. 8.8).

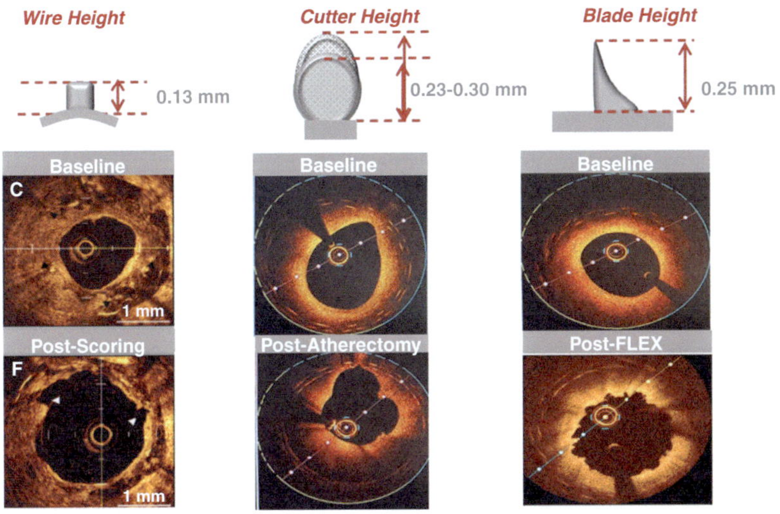

Fig. 8.7 OCT cross section of pre- (baseline, top image) and post- (bottom images) application of different vessel preparation technologies tested in an ISR porcine lesion. Vessel prep technology tested included wire-wrapped balloon scoring PTA directional atherectomy and FLEX VP

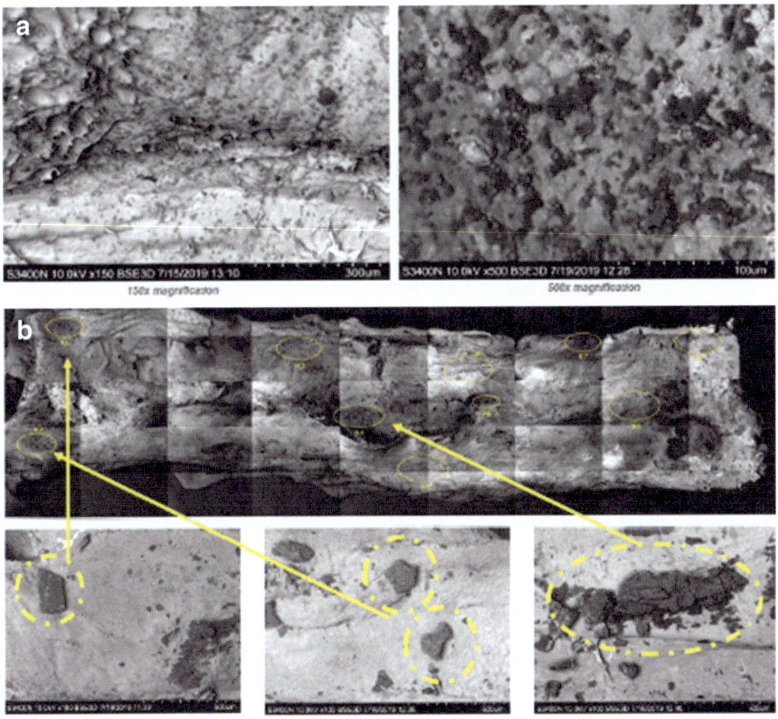

Fig. 8.8 Confirmation of drug deposition along FLEX VP micro-incisions. (**a**) Sirolimus drug microspheres deposited in the FLEX micro-incisions after DCB treatment in cadaveric lesions. (**b**) Shards of paclitaxel from a drug-coated balloon treating a cadaveric lesion post-FLEX VP

FLEX VP Micro-Incisions May Facilitate Drug Delivery

In addition to improving vessel compliance, FLEX VP micro-incisions potentially facilitate the diffusion of anti-restenotic drugs to the target lesions from drug-coated or drug-eluting technologies. SEM evaluation in human cadaver studies confirms the deposition of both sirolimus and paclitaxel anti-restenotic drugs into FLEX VP micro-incisions (Fig. 8.8).

A retrospective clinical study evaluating 12-month outcomes of patients with de novo SFA/PA lesions treated with FLEX VP prior to a DCB reported freedom from TLR rates (>93%) that were comparable to freedom from TLR rates reported for DCBs with published superior performance characteristics [49, 50]. Thus, these encouraging early patency results suggest that vessel preparation with circumferential, controlled-depth, continuous micro-incisions may facilitate DCB drug delivery [33, 34]. Results from this retrospective observational study are currently being investigated in the BELONG prospective study (NCT03721939).

Future Directions

In conclusion, the FLEX VP System provides safe plaque modification and vessel preparation via consistent circumferential controlled-depth micro-incisions in complex, mixed morphology PAD lesions. FLEX VP is currently indicated for use with PTA catheters to facilitate dilation of stenoses in the femoral and popliteal arteries and treatment of obstructive lesions of native or synthetic arteriovenous dialysis fistulae. In addition, FLEX VP is indicated for ISR treatment of balloon-expandable and self-expanding stents in the peripheral vasculature. Future directions include seeking expanded indications to include below-the-knee lesions. Other new indications being evaluated include venous, iliac, and coronary applications.

References

1. Shu J, Santulli G. Update on peripheral artery disease: epidemiology and evidence-based facts. Atherosclerosis. 2018;275:379–81.
2. Adam DJ, Beard JD, Cleveland T, Bell J, Bradbury AW, Forbes JF, et al. Bypass versus angioplasty in severe ischaemia of the leg (BASIL): multicentre, randomised controlled trial. Lancet. 2005;366(9501):1925–34.
3. Shammas NW, Coiner D, Shammas G, Jerin M. Predictors of provisional stenting in patients undergoing lower extremity arterial interventions. Int J Angiol. 2011;20(2):95–100.
4. Armstrong EJ, Shishehbor MH. Commentary: contemporary outcomes of endovascular interventions for peripheral artery disease: the LIBERTY to determine optimal treatment strategies. J Endovasc Ther. 2019;26(2):155–7.
5. Castaneda-Zuniga WR, Formanek A, Tadavarthy M, Vlodaver Z, Edwards JE, Zollikofer C, et al. The mechanism of balloon angioplasty. Radiology. 1980;135(3):565–71.

6. van der Lugt A, Gussenhoven EJ, Mali WP, Reekers JA, Seelen JL, Tielbeek AV, et al. Effect of balloon angioplasty in femoropopliteal arteries assessed by intravascular ultrasound. Eur J Vasc Endovasc Surg. 1997;13(6):549–56.
7. Welt FG, Rogers C. Inflammation and restenosis in the stent era. Arterioscler Thromb Vasc Biol. 2002;22(11):1769–76.
8. Mongiardo A, Curcio A, Spaccarotella C, Parise S, Indolfi C. Molecular mechanisms of restenosis after percutaneous peripheral angioplasty and approach to endovascular therapy. Curr Drug Targets Cardiovasc Haematol Disord. 2004;4(3):275–87.
9. Ohtani K, Egashira K, Ihara Y, Nakano K, Funakoshi K, Zhao G, et al. Angiotensin II type 1 receptor blockade attenuates in-stent restenosis by inhibiting inflammation and progenitor cells. Hypertension. 2006;48(4):664–70.
10. Araujo PV, Ribeiro MS, Dalio MB, Rocha LA, Viaro F, Dellalibera Joviliano R, et al. Interleukins and inflammatory markers in in-stent restenosis after femoral percutaneous transluminal angioplasty. Ann Vasc Surg. 2015;29(4):731–7.
11. Nakazawa KR, Wengerter SP, Power JR, Lookstein RA, Tadros RO, Ting W, et al. Preoperative inflammatory status as a predictor of primary patency after femoropopliteal stent implantation. J Vasc Surg. 2017;66(1):151–9.
12. Guimaraes TS, da Rocha LA, Becari C, Piccinato CE, Joviliano RD, Ribeiro MS, et al. The role of interleukins and inflammatory markers in the early restenosis of covered stents in the femoropopliteal arterial segment. Ann Vasc Surg. 2018;50:88–95.
13. Fanelli F, Cannavale A, Boatta E, Corona M, Lucatelli P, Wlderk A, et al. Lower limb multilevel treatment with drug-eluting balloons: 6-month results from the DEBELLUM randomized trial. J Endovasc Ther. 2012;19(5):571–80.
14. Fujihara M, Takahara M, Sasaki S, Nanto K, Utsunomiya M, Iida O, et al. Angiographic dissection patterns and patency outcomes after balloon angioplasty for superficial femoral artery disease. J Endovasc Ther. 2017;24(3):367–75.
15. Rosenfield K, Jaff MR, White CJ, Rocha-Singh K, Mena-Hurtado C, Metzger DC, et al. Trial of a paclitaxel-coated balloon for femoropopliteal artery disease. N Engl J Med. 2015;373(2):145–53.
16. Tepe G, Beschorner U, Ruether C, Fischer I, Pfaffinger P, Noory E, et al. Drug-eluting balloon therapy for femoropopliteal occlusive disease: predictors of outcome with a special emphasis on calcium. J Endovasc Ther. 2015;22(5):727–33.
17. Tepe G, Zeller T, Schnorr B, Claussen CD, Beschorner U, Brechtel K, et al. High-grade, non-flow-limiting dissections do not negatively impact long-term outcome after paclitaxel-coated balloon angioplasty: an additional analysis from the THUNDER study. J Endovasc Ther. 2013;20(6):792–800.
18. Werk M, Albrecht T, Meyer DR, Ahmed MN, Behne A, Dietz U, et al. Paclitaxel-coated balloons reduce restenosis after femoro-popliteal angioplasty: evidence from the randomized PACIFIER trial. Circ Cardiovasc Interv. 2012;5(6):831–40.
19. Bosiers M, Scheinert D, Hendriks JM, Wissgott C, Peeters P, Zeller T, et al. Results from the tack optimized balloon angioplasty (TOBA) study demonstrate the benefits of minimal metal implants for dissection repair after angioplasty. J Vasc Surg. 2016;64(1):109–16.
20. Shammas NW, Torey JT, Shammas WJ, Jones-Miller S, Shammas GA. Intravascular ultrasound assessment and correlation with angiographic findings demonstrating femoropopliteal arterial dissections post atherectomy: results from the iDissection study. J Invasive Cardiol. 2018;30(7):240–4.
21. Kobayashi N, Hirano K, Yamawaki M, Araki M, Sakai T, Sakamoto Y, et al. Simple classification and clinical outcomes of angiographic dissection after balloon angioplasty for femoropopliteal disease. J Vasc Surg. 2018;67(4):1151–8.
22. Kokkinidis DG, Jeon-Slaughter H, Khalili H, Brilakis ES, Shammas NW, Banerjee S, et al. Adjunctive stent use during endovascular intervention to the femoropopliteal artery with drug coated balloons: insights from the XLPAD registry. Vasc Med. 2018;23(4):358–64.
23. Laird JA, Schneider PA, Jaff MR, Brodmann M, Zeller T, Metzger DC, et al. Long-term clinical effectiveness of a drug-coated balloon for the treatment of femoropopliteal lesions. Circ Cardiovasc Interv. 2019;12(6):e007702.

24. Tan M, Urasawa K, Koshida R, Haraguchi T, Kitani S, Igarashi Y, et al. Comparison of angiographic dissection patterns caused by long vs short balloons during balloon angioplasty of chronic femoropopliteal occlusions. J Endovasc Ther. 2018;25(2):192–200.
25. Fitzgerald PJ, Ports TA, Yock PG. Contribution of localized calcium deposits to dissection after angioplasty. An observational study using intravascular ultrasound. Circulation. 1992;86(1):64–70.
26. Kaladji A, Vent PA, Danvin A, Chaillou P, Costargent A, Guyomarch B, et al. Impact of vascular calcifications on long femoropopliteal stenting outcomes. Ann Vasc Surg. 2018;47:170–8.
27. Mattesini A, Di Mario C. Calcium: a predictor of interventional treatment failure across all fields of cardiovascular medicine. Int J Cardiol. 2017;231:97–8.
28. Rocha-Singh KJ, Zeller T, Jaff MR. Peripheral arterial calcification: prevalence, mechanism, detection, and clinical implications. Catheter Cardiovasc Interv. 2014;83(6):E212–20.
29. Scheinert D, Micari A, Brodmann M, Tepe G, Peeters P, Jaff MR, et al. Drug-coated balloon treatment for femoropopliteal artery disease. Circ Cardiovasc Interv. 2018;11(10):e005654.
30. Thieme M, Von Bilderling P, Paetzel C, Karnabatidis D, Perez Delgado J, Lichtenberg M, et al. The 24-month results of the Lutonix global SFA registry: worldwide experience with Lutonix drug-coated balloon. JACC Cardiovasc Interv. 2017;10(16):1682–90.
31. Torsello G, Stavroulakis K, Brodmann M, Micari A, Tepe G, Veroux P, et al. Three-year sustained clinical efficacy of drug-coated balloon angioplasty in a real-world femoropopliteal cohort. J Endovasc Ther. 2020;27(5):693–705.
32. Singh H, Kirtane A, Moses J. AngioSculpt® scoring balloon catheter: an atherotomy device for coronary and peripheral interventions. Interv Cardiol. 2010;2:469–78.
33. Hwang CW, Levin AD, Jonas M, Li PH, Edelman ER. Thrombosis modulates arterial drug distribution for drug-eluting stents. Circulation. 2005;111(13):1619–26.
34. Tzafriri AR, Garcia-Polite F, Zani B, Stanley J, Muraj B, Knutson J, et al. Calcified plaque modification alters local drug delivery in the treatment of peripheral atherosclerosis. J Control Release. 2017;264:203–10.
35. Kronlage M, Werner C, Dufner M, Blessing E, Muller OJ, Heilmeier B, et al. Long-term outcome upon treatment of calcified lesions of the lower limb using scoring angioplasty balloon (AngioSculpt). Clin Res Cardiol. 2020;109(9):1177–85.
36. Korosoglou G, Lichtenberg M, Celik S, Andrassy J, Brodmann M, Andrassy M. The evolving role of drug-coated balloons for the treatment of complex femoropopliteal lesions. J Cardiovasc Surg. 2018;59(1):51–9.
37. Armstrong EJ, Kokkinidis DG. EDITORIAL: Eximo Medical's B-Laser for infrainguinal peripheral artery disease: the new kid on the block for lesion preparation in complex peripheral interventions? Cardiovasc Revasc Med. 2020;21(1):93–5.
38. Tarricone A, Ali Z, Rajamanickam A, Gujja K, Kapur V, Purushothaman KR, et al. Histopathological evidence of adventitial or medial injury is a strong predictor of restenosis during directional atherectomy for peripheral artery disease. J Endovasc Ther. 2015;22(5):712–5.
39. Krishnan P, Tarricone A, Purushothaman KR, Purushothaman M, Vasquez M, Kovacic J, et al. An algorithm for the use of embolic protection during atherectomy for femoral popliteal lesions. JACC Cardiovasc Interv. 2017;10(4):403–10.
40. Shrikhande GV, Khan SZ, Hussain HG, Dayal R, McKinsey JF, Morrissey N. Lesion types and device characteristics that predict distal embolization during percutaneous lower extremity interventions. J Vasc Surg. 2011;53(2):347–52.
41. Dattilo R, Himmelstein SI, Cuff RF. The COMPLIANCE 360 degrees trial: a randomized, prospective, multicenter, pilot study comparing acute and long-term results of orbital atherectomy to balloon angioplasty for calcified femoropopliteal disease. J Invasive Cardiol. 2014;26(8):355–60.
42. Zeller T, Krankenberg H, Steinkamp H, Rastan A, Sixt S, Schmidt A, et al. One-year outcome of percutaneous rotational atherectomy with aspiration in infrainguinal peripheral arterial occlusive disease: the multicenter pathway PVD trial. J Endovasc Ther. 2009;16(6):653–62.

43. Zeller T, Langhoff R, Rocha-Singh KJ, Jaff MR, Blessing E, Amann-Vesti B, et al. Directional Atherectomy followed by a paclitaxel-coated balloon to inhibit restenosis and maintain vessel patency: twelve-month results of the DEFINITIVE AR study. Circ Cardiovasc Interv. 2017;10(9):e004848.
44. Kassimis G, Raina T, Kontogiannis N, Patri G, Abramik J, Zaphiriou A, et al. How should we treat heavily calcified coronary artery disease in contemporary practice? From atherectomy to intravascular lithotripsy. Cardiovasc Revasc Med. 2019;20(12):1172–83.
45. Brodmann M, Schwindt A, Argyriou A, Gammon R. Safety and feasibility of intravascular lithotripsy for treatment of common femoral artery stenoses. J Endovasc Ther. 2019;26(3):283–7.
46. Zeller T, Lopez L, Pigott JP. Acute outcomes with a novel plaque modification system in real-world femoropopliteal lesions. J Endovasc Ther. 2019;26(3):333–41.
47. Oriwo B, Abbas J, Lurie F. 2-year experience using FLEX catheter as a preparatory device for drug-coated balloon and/or balloon angioplasty. International symposium on endovascular therapy, Hollywood, FL; 2019.
48. Dexpert J-P, Hayoz D, Engelberger R, Krieger C, M-AR M, Periard D. Arterial preparation by longitudinal micro-incisions before balloon angioplasty of the superficial femoral and popliteal artery: acute and 12-month results. J Endovasc Ther. 2022;29(3):420–6.
49. Brodmann M, Keirse K, Scheinert D, Spak L, Jaff MR, Schmahl R, et al. Drug-coated balloon treatment for femoropopliteal artery disease: the IN.PACT global study de novo in-stent restenosis imaging cohort. JACC Cardiovasc Interv. 2017;10(20):2113–23.
50. Kinstner CM, Lammer J, Willfort-Ehringer A, Matzek W, Gschwandtner M, Javor D, et al. Paclitaxel-eluting balloon versus standard balloon angioplasty in in-stent restenosis of the superficial femoral and proximal popliteal artery: 1-year results of the PACUBA trial. JACC Cardiovasc Interv. 2016;9(13):1386–92.

Chapter 9
Intravascular Lithotripsy for Calcified Peripheral Arterial Disease

Ari J. Mintz and Peter A. Soukas

Introduction

The presence of vascular calcification imparts specific difficulties for the cardiovascular interventionist to provide safe and effective therapies. Vascular calcification is often seen in patients with comorbidities, such as diabetes mellitus and chronic kidney disease, as well as in those with advanced age [1]. Moderate to severe vascular calcification is common, being present in up to one third of patients presenting with acute coronary syndromes and up to one half of patients undergoing peripheral artery revascularization [1, 2]. Extensive vascular calcification is associated with reduction in lesion crossing, device delivery, and adequate lesion preparation (including a decrease in the effect of antiproliferative therapies), which, in turn, is directly related to an increase in procedural failure [3, 4]. Recently, there has been increasing use of large-bore access for interventional therapies such as endovascular aneurysm repair (EVAR), thoracic endovascular aneurysm repair (TEVAR), and transcatheter aortic valve replacement (TAVR) with transfemoral access being the preferred site. Iliofemoral calcification is a predominant factor for the utilization of alternative access [5]. Current techniques in the management of noncompliant calcified lesions include high-pressure balloon angioplasty, specialty cutting and scoring balloons, and atherectomy devices, which are associated with increased risk of vessel dissection, acute closure, perforation, and no reflow phenomenon [6, 7].

A. J. Mintz
Columbia University Irving Medical Center, New York, NY, USA

P. A. Soukas (✉)
Lifespan Cardiovascular Institute, Providence, RI, USA

Division of Cardiology, Department of Medicine, Alpert Medical School of Brown University, Providence, RI, USA

N. W. Shammas (ed.), *Peripheral Arterial Interventions*, Contemporary Cardiology, https://doi.org/10.1007/978-3-031-09741-6_9

Intravascular lithotripsy (IVL) is a novel device therapy which modifies both intimal and medial calcified lesions using pulsatile sonic waves which are converted to mechanical energy. External shock wave lithotripsy has been used for decades in the treatment of renal calculi and gallstones [8, 9]. In a similar way, IVL utilizes electrohydraulically generated sonic waves which pass harmlessly through soft tissue and target high-density calcium in the intimal and medial walls of the artery. The pressures generated by the sonic waves fracture vascular calcium with effective dilating force of approximately 50 atmospheres (atm), thereby rendering the vessel more compliant and reducing elastic recoil [10].

IVL: Device Specifics

In 2016, Shockwave Medical, Inc. (Santa Clara, CA) received 510 k premarket approval for their peripheral IVL system for the treatment of calcified peripheral artery disease. This device, labelled the Shockwave M5, consisted of an over-the-wire system on an 0.014″ wire platform (Fig. 9.1). The balloon sizes ranged from 3.5 to 7.0 mm, in 0.5 mm increments, in a single available 60 mm length mounted on a 110 cm shaft. The M5+ catheters became available in 135 cm shaft length with the additional availability of an 8.0 mm device in April 2022. The M5 catheter has a slightly increased profile when compared to comparable-sized noncompliant balloons (0.050–0.066 in), similar in crossing profile to contemporary cutting balloons. The M5 catheters up to 6.0 mm are compatible with a 6-Fr sheath with 6.5, 7.0 mm, 8 mm requiring a 7-Fr sheath. The balloon is semi-compliant with five emitters located between two radiopaque markers. Balloon preparation is done in the standard over-the-wire fashion with the central lumen being flushed prior to loading of the 0.014 in guidewire. A mixture of 50/50 saline/contrast is used to prepare the balloon. Balloon sizing is based on a 1.1:1 balloon-to-reference lumen ratio with the

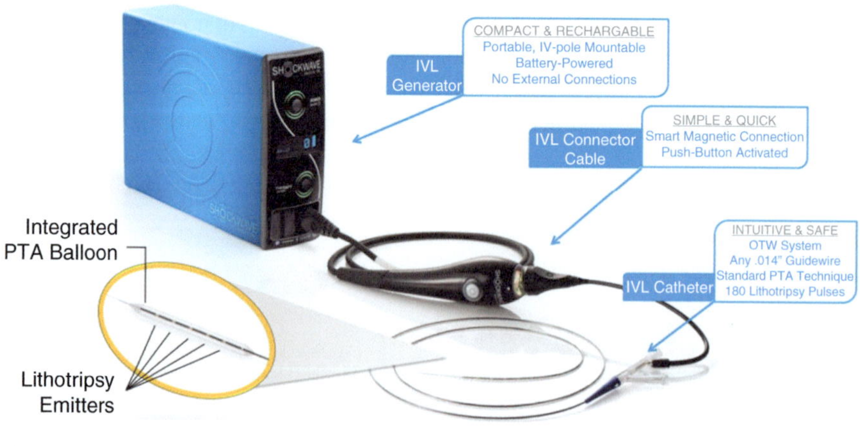

Fig. 9.1 Shockwave equipment and setup

balloon being inflated to subnominal pressures, typically starting at 4 atm and increasing to nominal pressure of 6 atm after several inflations. This ensures contact with the vessel wall and minimizes the risk of endothelial trauma. If contact with the vessel wall is not accomplished, the sonic waves will not reach the intimal or medial calcification as the energy does not traverse dead space. The M5 catheter is attached to the power generator which is programmed to deliver 30 pulses at a rate of 1 pulse per second. Each M5 catheter is capable of delivering a maximum of 300 pulses allowing for overlapping inflations of adjacent arterial segments. After each round of 30 pulses, it is imperative to deflate the balloon in order to remove microbubbles which are generated as a byproduct of the sonic waves. It is recommended that any single segment is treated with no more than 180 pulses. When overlapping inflations are done, it is important to ensure at least 1 cm of overlap in treated segments to avoid "geographic miss" of intentional treatment zones.

The Shockwave S4 is a smaller design catheter for below-the-knee angioplasty and was FDA approved for use in 2019. The balloon sizing is 2.5–4.0 mm in 0.5 mm increments with a single 40 mm length housing four emitters. The catheter comes in a 135 cm length and requires a minimum of 5 Fr sheath. Each catheter has the ability to provide 180 pulses in 20 pulse/cycle increments (Table 9.1). The coronary device, labelled Shockwave C2, is a shorter catheter specifically designed for intracoronary lithotripsy. This device obtained investigational device exemption in 2020 after several clinical trials provided data on safety and effective use [11, 12]. The C2 device is available in 2.5–4.0 mm balloons in 0.5 mm increments. The balloon length is 12 mm and available on a 138 cm catheter. The C2 requires a minimum of a 6 Fr guiding catheter. Each catheter is capable of delivering 80 pulses in 10 pulse/cycle increments to limit coronary artery occlusive time.

Table 9.1 Technical features of shockwave IVL catheters

Features	M5	S4	C2
Guide/Sheath size	6 Fr: 3.5 mm–6 mm 7 Fr: 6.5 mm, 7.0 mm	5 Fr	6 Fr guide
Balloon size (mm)	3.5, 4.0, 4.5, 5.0, 5.5, 6.0, 6.5, 7.0	2.5, 3.0, 3.5, 4.0	2.5, 3.0, 3.5, 4.0
Catheter length (cm)	135	135	138
Wire compatibility (in)	0.014	0.014	0.014
Balloon length (mm)	60	40	12
Number of emitters	5	4	2
Nominal pressure (atm)	6	6	6
Rated burst pressure (atm)	10	10	10
Pulses per catheter	300 pulses 30 pulses/cycle 1 pulse/s	180 pulses 20 pulses/cycle 1 pulse/s	80 pulses 10 pulses/cycle 1 pulse/s

atm atmosphere, *cm* centimeter, *Fr* French, *in* inch, *mm* millimeter

IVL in Peripheral Artery Disease

Although there is no standard definition for grading severity of calcification in peripheral arteries, several scoring systems have been proposed. The Society for Cardiovascular Angiography and Intervention (SCAI) in a 2018 consensus document defined severe calcification as >180° involving both sides of the vessel [13]. The Peripheral Arterial Calcification Scoring System (PACSS) takes into account the lesion length (greater than 5 cm) as well as location of calcification (intimal, medial, mixed, unilateral, bilateral) in the anteroposterior fluoroscopic projection. The PARC (Peripheral Academic Research Consortium) scoring system defines severe calcification as greater than 180° on both sides of the vessel and greater than one half of the total lesion length [14].

It is well described that in patients with peripheral artery disease, the presence of vascular calcification is associated with worse outcomes including higher Rutherford classification and higher rates of amputation [15]. The use of percutaneous transluminal angioplasty (PTA) with conventional angioplasty balloons in severely calcified peripheral artery disease is associated with low success rates due to acute recoil, suboptimal lesion expansion, and the potential of vessel injury, dissection, or even perforation [16]. Rotational and orbital atherectomy are able to achieve acute luminal gain by affecting superficial calcium, but medial calcium is unaffected [17]. IVL has been studied in an attempt to overcome the limitations of the previously available devices for calcium modification.

DISRUPT PAD I/II were multicenter, single-arm registries which enrolled a total of 95 patients with symptomatic peripheral artery disease (Rutherford 2–4), ankle-brachial index (ABI) <0.9, and angiographic evidence of calcific femoropopliteal stenosis of >70% with at least 1 patent runoff vessel to the foot [18, 19] (Table 9.2). Using the PARC definition, severe calcification was seen in over half of participants, and procedural success, defined as residual stenosis of <50%, was achieved in all patients. IVL showed a reduction in luminal stenosis from 76 to 23% with a mean acute luminal gain of 3.0 mm (1.2 ± 0.8 to 4.2 ± 0.6 mm) [18]. Clinically important outcomes from this showed that at 1 and 6 months, no target lesion revascularization (TLR) occurred and vessel patency rates were 100% and 82%, respectively. At 12 months, patency rates were 54% with TLR rates of only 21% [19]. In a subgroup analysis of DISRUPT PAD II, when optimal technique was performed, patency rates were elevated to 63%, there was an improvement of 15%, and TLR decreased to 8.6% at 12 months (Fig. 9.2). Optimal techniques include appropriate balloon sizing of 1.1:1 balloon-to-reference ratio and full lesion coverage of treatment zones with at least 1 cm of emitter overlap (Fig. 9.3).

IVL has also been shown effective in the treatment of below-the-knee disease in patients with critical limb ischemia (CLI) as well [20]. The DISRUPT BTK study reported 20 patients, Rutherford classes 3–5 (16 patients with CLI), with heavily calcified infrapopliteal lesions (angiographic stenosis 72.6%, mean lesion length

Table 9.2 Trials of IVL in peripheral artery disease

		DISRUPT PAD I/II (*N* = 95)	DISRUPT PAD III RCT (*N* = 306)		DISRUPT BTK (*N* = 20)
Design		Multicenter, single arm	Multicenter, prospective, randomized		Multicenter, single arm
Population			IVL	PTA	
	Rutherford 2	33.7%	17%	17%	–
	Rutherford 3	65.3%	77%	74%	20.0%
	Rutherford 4	1.1%	6%	8%	5.0%
	Rutherford 5	–	–	1%	75.0%
	Rutherford 6	–	–		–
Angiographic appearance			IVL	PTA	
	Severe calcification (PARC)	54.7%	82.9%	89.5%	47.6%
	RVD (mm)	5.3	5.3	5.4	3.2
	Lesion length (mm)	71.9	101	97	52.2
	CTO	18.9%	26%	31%	9.5%
Safety			IVL	PTA	
	Complications	1%	1.1%	15.1%	0.0%
	Grade > C dissections		0.0%	0.7%	
	Perforations Thromboembolic events		0.0%	0.7%	
Efficacy	Residual stenosis	24%	23.6%		26%
	Acute gain (mm)	3	3.4		1.5
Outcomes	30 days	Freedom from TLR: 100% Patency: 100%	Freedom from TLR at 12 months (IVL+DCB): 95.7% vs. 98.3% (PTA+DCB), P= .94		Freedom from TLR: 100% MAE: 0%
	6 months	Freedom from TLR: 96.8% Patency: 76.7%	Primary patency at 12 months (IVL+DCB): 80.5% vs. 68.0%, (PTA+DCB), P= .017		

CTO chronic total occlusion, *MAE* major adverse events [myocardial infarction, amputation, death], *PARC* peripheral academic research consortium, *RVD* reference vessel diameter, *TLR* target lesion revascularization

52.2 ± 35.8 mm). Procedural success was achieved in 95% of patients, with a residual percent stenosis of 26.2% and an acute lumen gain of 1.5 ± 0.5 mm. Two stents were implanted for residual stenosis, but none for flow-limiting arterial dissection, without major adverse events.

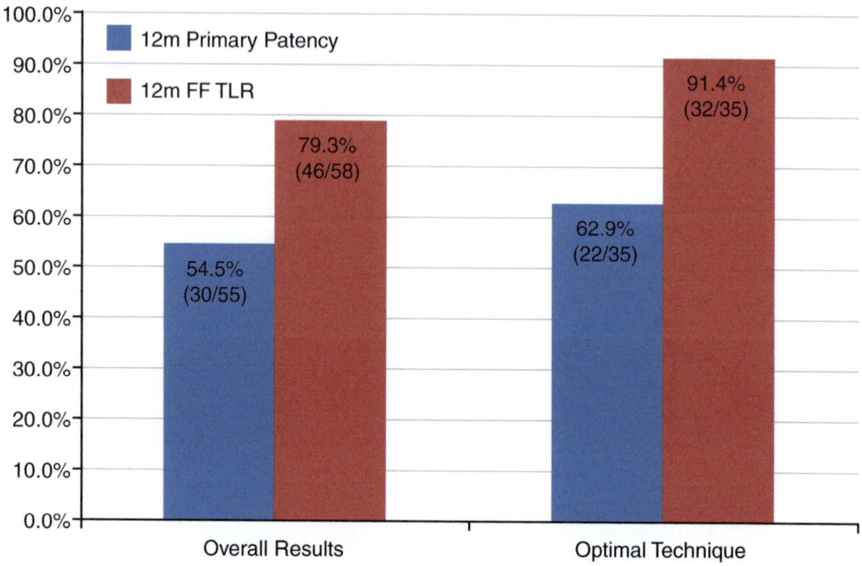

Fig. 9.2 12-month primary patency and freedom from target lesion revascularization (FF-TLR)

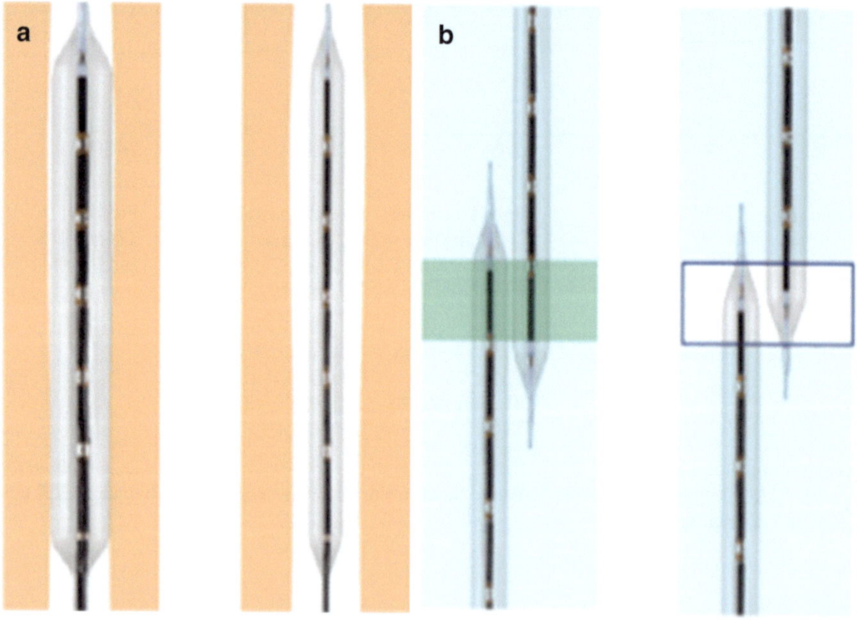

Fig. 9.3 Optimal technique. (**a**) Balloon sizing 1.1:1 balloon-to-reference vessel ratio. (**b**) At least 1 cm emitter overlap

Effect of Calcium on Drug Elution

The use of drug-coated balloons (DCB) as adjunctive therapy in peripheral angioplasty has been tested as a means to overcome the shortcomings of traditional angioplasty. Studies have shown excellent vessel patency and low rates of both target lesion revascularization (TLR) and complications [21–23]. Drug-eluting technologies have lower efficacy rates in severe calcific disease, likely a result of reduced drug penetration into the vessel wall [24]. As a result, combination therapy utilizing specialty balloons and atherectomy devices prior to DCB has shown promising results; however, long-term efficacy remains unproven.

The recently presented DISRUPT PAD III trial was designed to compare the use of combination IVL and DCB versus combination PTA and DCB [25]. DISRUPT PAD III provides the first level I evidence comparing the effect of calcific disease on drug elution. 306 patients were randomized in a 1:1 fashion to receiving IVL + DCB/stent versus PTA + DCB/stent with primary endpoint being procedural success, defined as residual stenosis of <30% without flow-limiting dissection. Powered secondary endpoints included primary patency and clinically driven target lesion revascularization (CD-TLR) at 12 months of 80.5% and 95.7% in the IVL + DCB group, vs. 68.0% and 98.3% in the PTA + IVL group, respectively; P= 0.94 for FF TLR and P= 0.017 for primary patency [26]. Lower maximum inflation pressures were seen in the IVL group (6.3 atm vs. 11.3 atm) which resulted in a 75% relative risk reduction in bailout stenting. DISRUPT PAD III also included 2% below-the-knee, 15% iliac, and 13% common femoral artery target lesions vs. only femoropopliteal lesions in DISRUPT PAD I/II. Moreover, DISRUPT PAD III lesion characteristics were more challenging- longer lesion lengths, greater calcification, higher percentages of CTO, and CLI patients. These encouraging results suggest that lesion preparation and calcium modification with IVL prior to drug-eluting devices are more effective, and safe, than PTA in the management of moderate to severe calcific peripheral artery disease. Although more evidence is needed, it can be surmised that calcium modification prior to DCB provides better milieu for drug elution.

IVL-Facilitated Large-Bore Vascular Access

With the increasing use of minimally invasive strategies for the management of aortic and cardiac valvular disease, large-bore vascular access is frequently required. Randomized trials in the investigation of TAVR included transfemoral as well as other alternative access sites in the approach to valve delivery [27]. Transfemoral access has become the access site of choice as studies have shown it to be the only superior access site when compared to traditional surgical aortic valve replacement [28]. Unfortunately, given concurrent peripheral artery disease with calcified aorto-iliac bifurcations, up to 15–20% of TAVR candidates may be deemed ineligible for transfemoral access due to the inability to successfully and safely advance the required large-bore delivery sheaths resulting in more invasive methods such as trans-axillary, trans-aortic, trans-apical, trans-carotid, trans-septal, and trans-caval [29]. Initial case reports suggested the feasibility of IVL technology to aid in the delivery of large-bore access [30, 31]. In a prospective registry of 40 patients with peripheral artery disease who were deemed ineligible for transfemoral access, IVL facilitated successful placement of the delivery sheaths in >90% with no iliofemoral perforations or dissections observed [32]. Numerous case reports have highlighted the efficacy of IVL in the facilitation of other large-bore vascular access including percutaneous LV assist devices, TEVAR, and EVAR [33, 34]. IVL therefore provides a useful tool in the management of this complex patient population.

Indications for IVL in Specific Vascular Beds with Case Examples

Brachiocephalic Lesions in Patient with Symptomatic Arm Claudication or TIA

Endovascular treatment of brachiocephalic arteries is challenging due to their larger diameter, short length, and proximity to the intracranial vasculature [35]. The presence of calcific disease adds to procedural complexity and increases risks of complications due to perforation, dissection, embolization, and stent underexpansion. Case 9.1 demonstrates the use of IVL to treat symptomatic concomitant innominate and subclavian calcific disease.

Carotid In-Stent Restenosis (ISR) Due to Stent Underexpansion

Dense calcification of carotid bifurcation stenoses is a frequent exclusion for enrollment in studies of carotid artery stenting (CAS). In cases of CAS ISR due to stent underexpansion, IVL may be used to allow for further stent expansion *(off-label use)* as illustrated in Case 9.2. There are very limited options for treating underexpanded stents. High-pressure inflations may be ineffective or induce dissections or rupture. This is the first reported use of IVL for CAS ISR and was included in a first published review of IVL for use in calcified carotid lesions [36].

Mesenteric Ischemia Due to Calcific Stenosis of the Superior Mesenteric Artery (SMA)

The feasibility of IVL both for the treatment of symptomatic mesenteric ischemia for native de novo calcific stenosis and for the treatment of managing ISR due to stent underexpansion was recently reported by Khan et al. [37]. Case 9.3 illustrates the ability to treat severe circumferential underlying calcified stenosis with IVL, allowing for full stent expansion.

Treatment of Aorto-Iliac Calcific Disease

IVL disrupts both intimal and deep wall calcification improving vessel compliance, allowing for the introduction of large-bore devices, and may offer an alternative for high-pressure dilation (with associated risk of dissection or rupture) or expandable sheaths and may obviate the need for open exposure with conduit placement ("pave and crack" technique). A recent report from a subset of the Disrupt PAD III study confirms the safety and efficacy of IVL for the treatment of calcified stenotic iliac arteries [38]. Case 9.4 demonstrates a case of severe aorto-iliac calcific occlusive disease in a patient deemed high risk for open repair treated with IVL and stenting, performed as an outpatient. Case 9.5 illustrates the off-label use of IVL for acute iliac stent suboptimal stent expansion.

Treatment of Calcific Common Femoral Artery (CFA) Stenosis

Endarterectomy has been an established treatment for CFA disease but is associated with extended length of stay and higher 15% composite rate of morbidity and mortality than endovascular techniques [39]. Brodmann evaluated 21 patients with calcified CFA stenoses treated with IVL with an acute lumen gain of 3.1 ± 1.3 mm, few non-flow-limiting dissections, and no perforations, distal embolization, thrombus, and no-reflow or abrupt closure [40]. IVL is an effective treatment for calcific common femoral disease as stand-alone therapy, or in combination with atherectomy and/or drug-coated balloon angioplasty, as seen in Case 9.6.

Calcified Femoropopliteal Lesions in Patients with Symptomatic Claudication or Critical Limb Ischemia

Calcified femoropopliteal lesions are often long occlusions, and traversal is often subintimal where use of atherectomy may result in a higher incidence of dissection or perforation. IVL, by virtue of its ability to penetrate transmural calcification, is uniquely suited to the treatment of subintimal calcification. As described earlier, in DISRUPT PAD III, IVL demonstrated a significant reduction in dissections and provisional stenting and less need for bailout stenting in the largest randomized clinical trial of severely calcified femoropopliteal lesions. Case 9.7 is an example of the utility of IVL to achieve an excellent result without the need for a stent in "no-stent zones" such as the CFA and popliteal arteries.

Calcified Below-the-Knee (BTK) Lesions in Patients with Symptomatic Claudication or Critical Limb Ischemia (CLI)

Medial calcification is more prevalent in BTK arteries and is a marker for amputation in patients with PAD [41]. This is particularly true for patients with diabetes mellitus, chronic kidney disease, and CLI, where diffuse calcific disease with infrapopliteal occlusions is common. Stents are limited to short lesions in proximal locations, and balloon angioplasty is burdened by a high rate of recoil and restenosis [42]. Atherectomy devices are problematic in these patients due to the risks of perforation with possible resultant compartment syndrome. Distal embolization after atherectomy may have catastrophic consequences and transform the CLI patient into an acute limb ischemia patient, with high risk of amputation. IVL has been shown to have a high procedural success and excellent safety profile.

Future Applications

As the population ages, calcified vascular disease is a growing challenge for the cardiovascular interventionist. Since its foray in the cardiovascular space, IVL has shown significant utility in the safe and effective treatment of moderate to severe calcified stenosis. Future applications will extend into other vascular beds. Already being evaluated is the use of IVL in the coronary arteries as has been adjudicated in the DISRUPT CAD studies, with recent FDA approval in the USA [11, 12, 43]. IVL has been used off-label in the treatment of aortic arch vessel angioplasty as well as to aid in the treatment of carotid artery revascularization, both transfemoral and trans-carotid [44, 45]. Increasing clinical experience supports the utility of combination atherectomy to create a pilot channel followed by IVL as the mechanism for enhanced luminal gain. Future improvements of IVL will include larger vessel diameters and longer balloon lengths. Currently, research and development are underway for the evaluation of IVL for the management of calcific cardiac valvular disease; however, no evidence currently exists to support its use. IVL has shown promising potential in many aspects of cardiovascular intervention, with its ceiling yet to be defined.

Case 9.1 Brachiocephalic

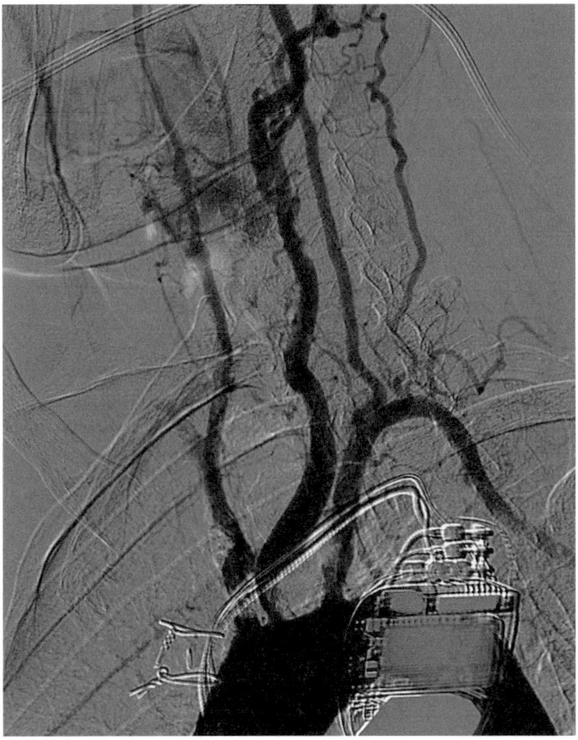

Baseline aortogram showing densely calcified innominate stenosis

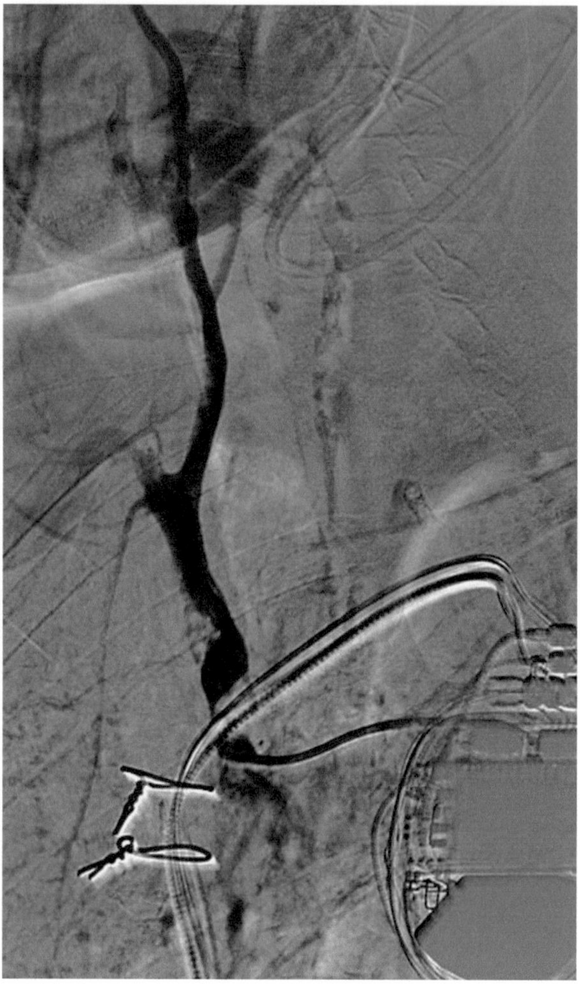

Selective innominate angiogram demonstrating eccentric densely calcified high-grade innominate artery stenosis and proximal right subclavian stenosis, left anterior oblique view (LAO)

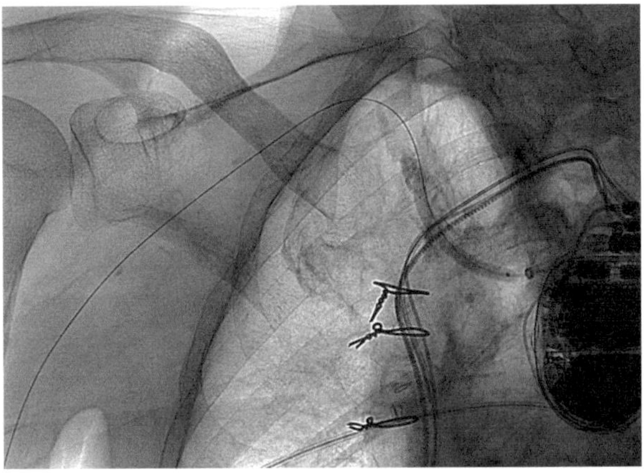

PTA of the innominate artery stenosis with a 4 mm balloon after delivery of a 7F sheath from the left common femoral access

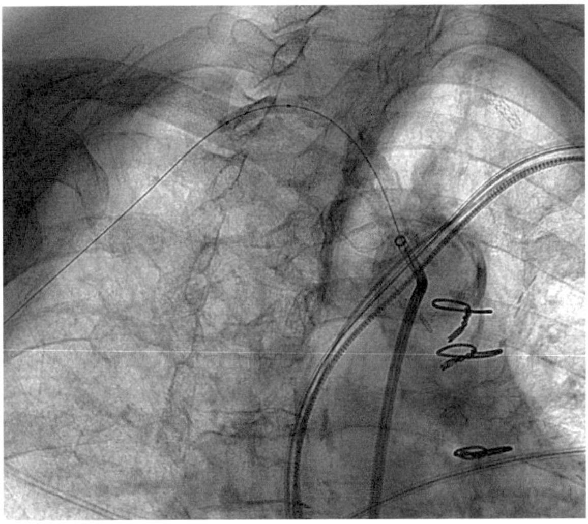

IVL of right subclavian artery with a 7 mm × 60 mm Shockwave Medical balloon

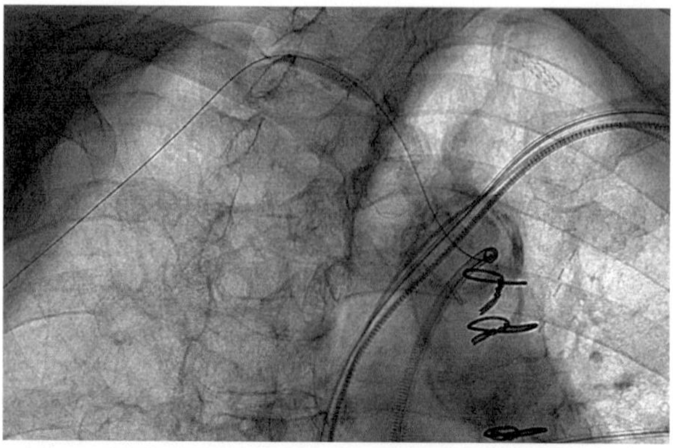

IVL of right subclavian artery with a 7 mm × 60 mm Shockwave Medical balloon

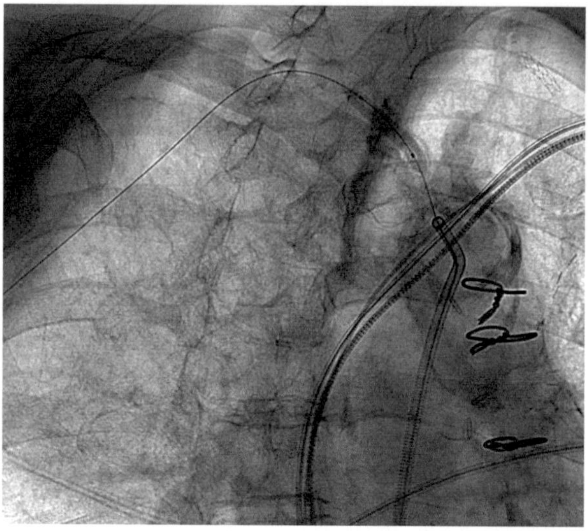

IVL of right subclavian artery with a 7 mm × 60 mm Shockwave Medical balloon

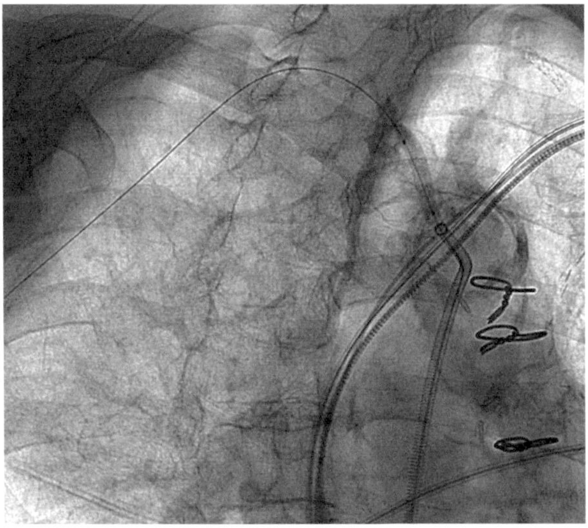

IVL of innominate artery with a 7 mm × 60 mm Shockwave Medical balloon

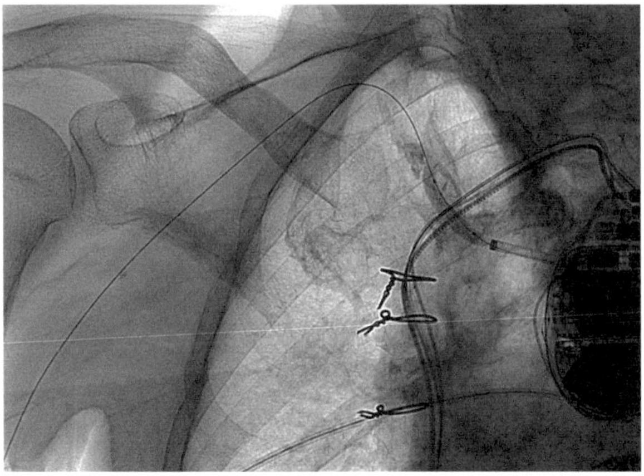

IVL of innominate artery with a 7 mm × 60 mm Shockwave Medical balloon

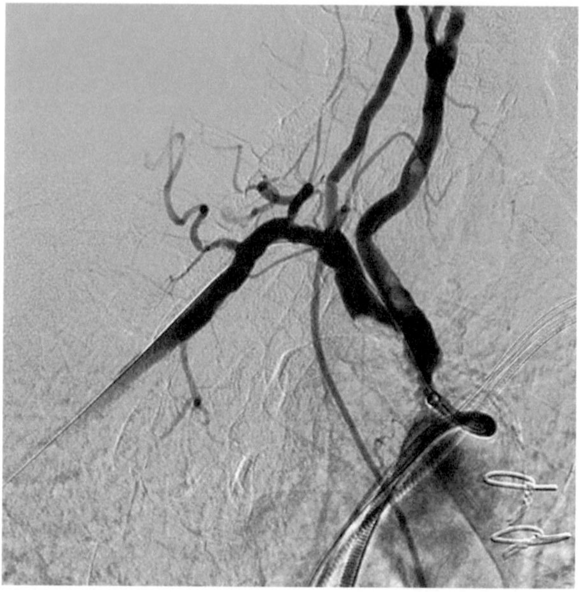

Post-IVL angiogram

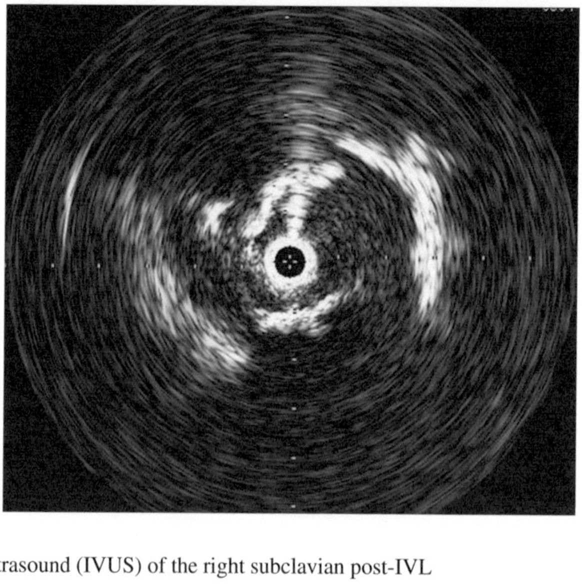

Intravascular ultrasound (IVUS) of the right subclavian post-IVL

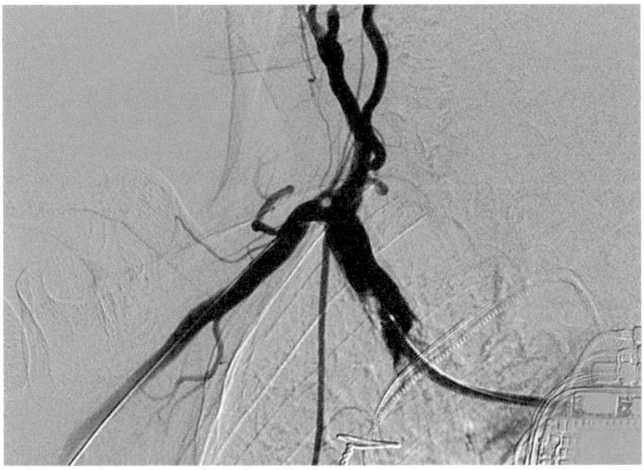

Post-subclavian and innominate IVL, LAO

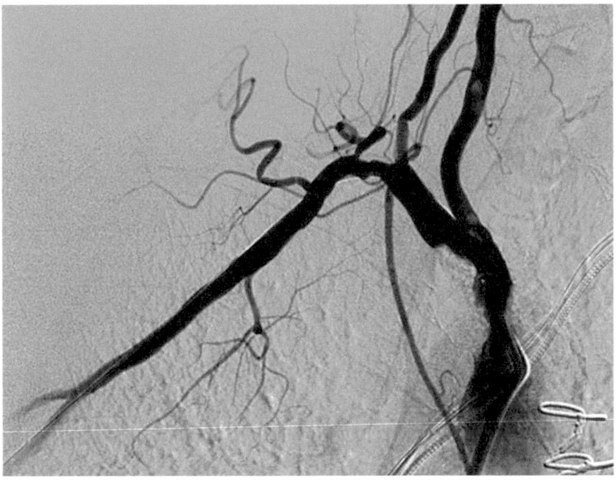

Post-subclavian and innominate IVL, RAO

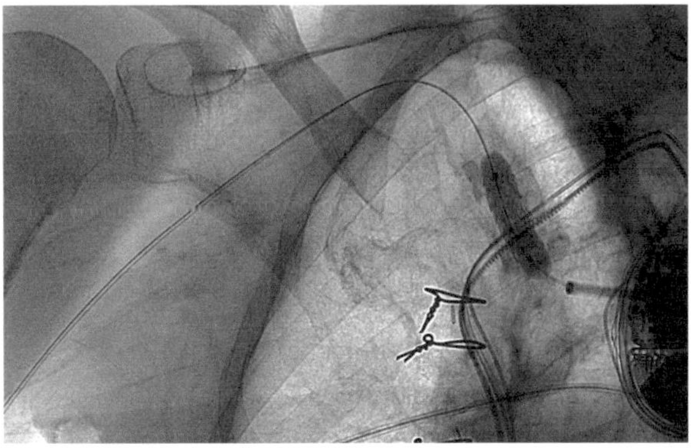

Deployment of 8 mm × 24 mm Cordis Genesis balloon-expandable stent

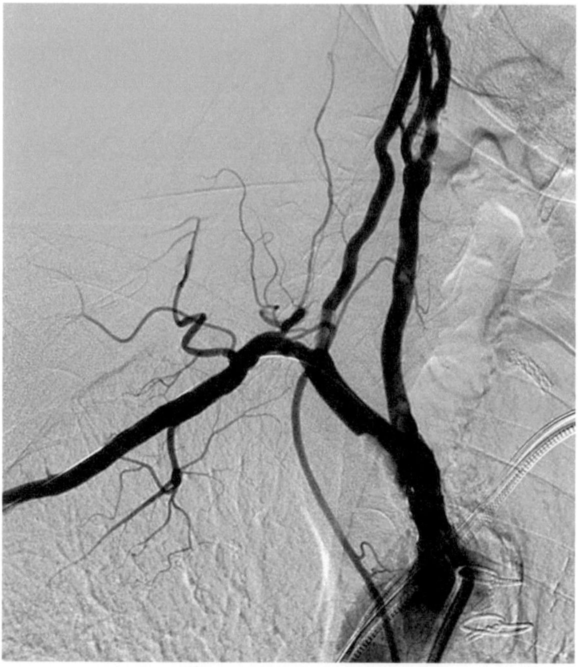

Final angiogram after post-dilation of stent with a 9 mm × 20 mm balloon

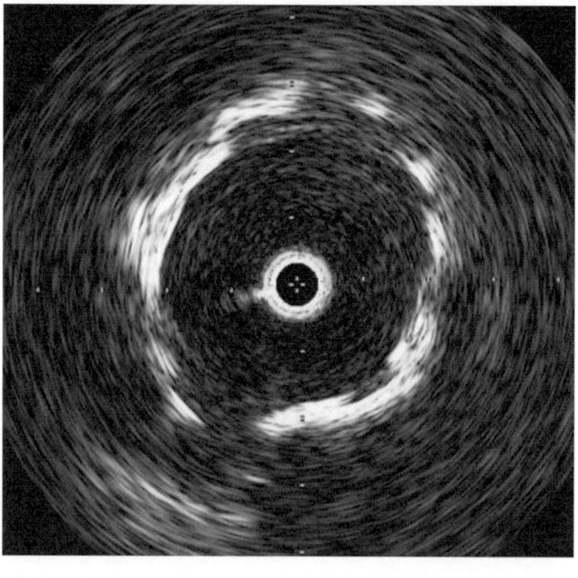

IVUS of innominate artery post-IVL/stenting

Case 9.2 Carotid In-Stent Restenosis (ISR): Off-Label Indication!

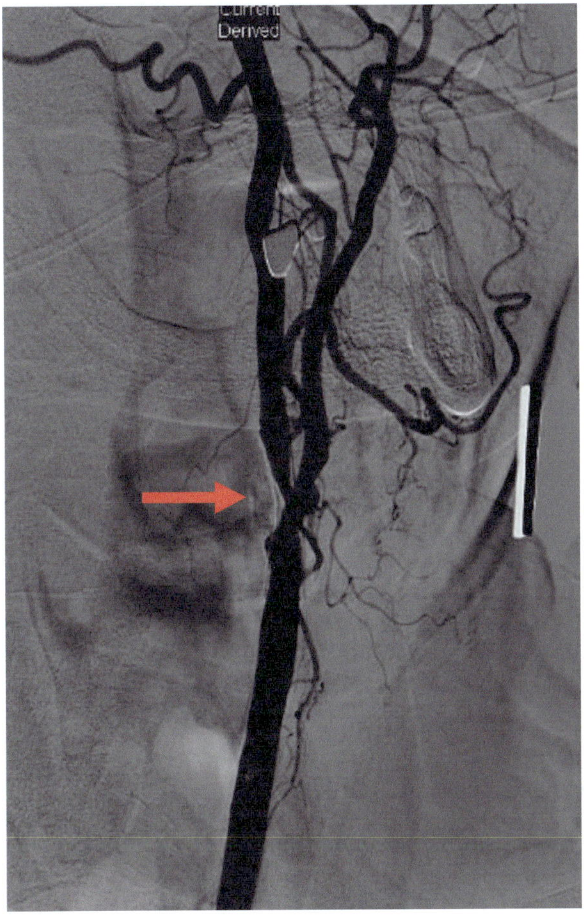

Baseline angiogram demonstrating calcific stenosis of CCA bifurcation with 80% stenosis within the stent, arrow

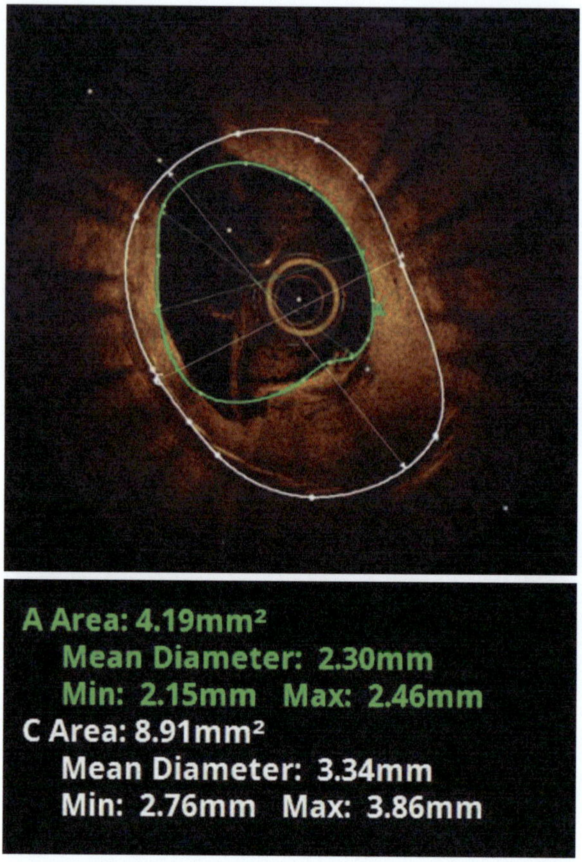

Baseline optical coherence tomography (OCT) image showing circumferential vessel wall calcification with reduced stent diameters and cross-sectional area

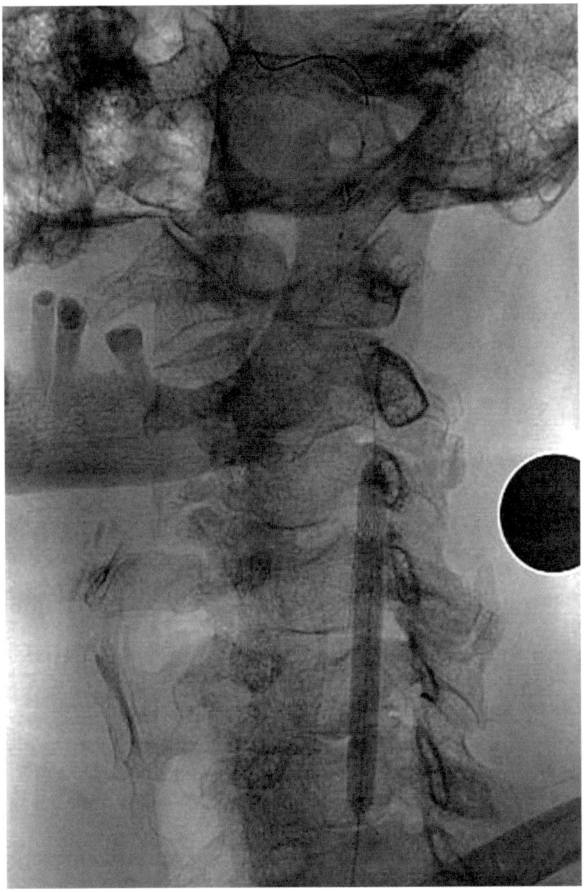

IVL of the carotid artery with 6 mm × 60 mm Shockwave balloon

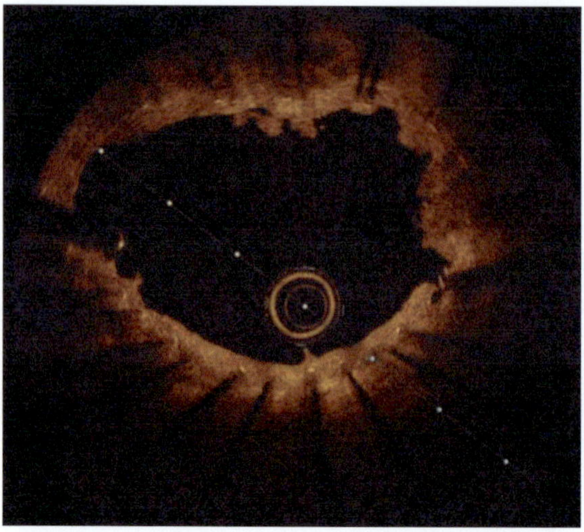

OCT post-IVL showing doubling of stent lumen cross-sectional area

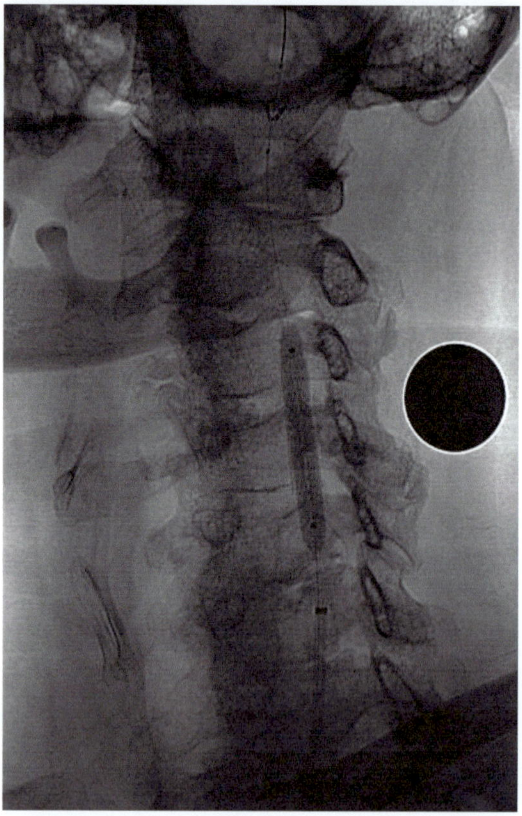

Post-IVL dilation with a 6 mm × 40 mm Bard Lutonix drug-coated balloon (DCB)

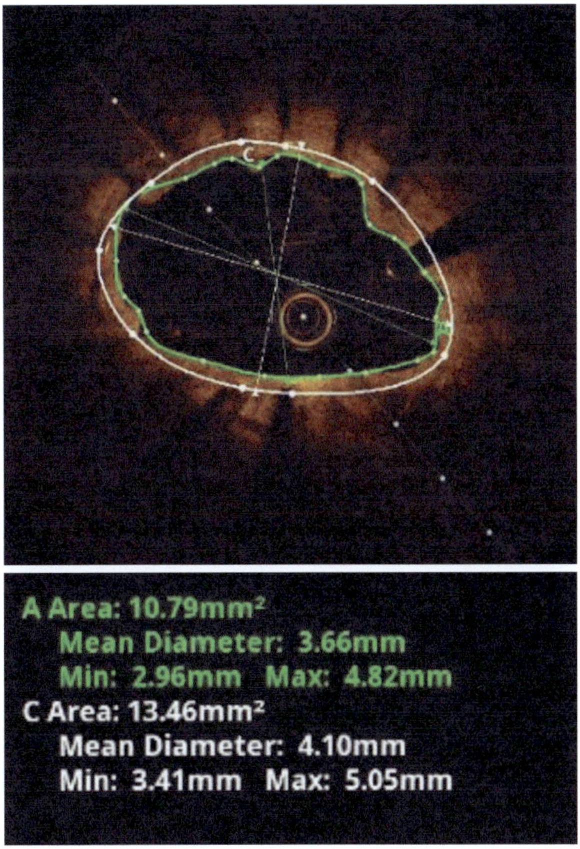

OCT post IVL/DCB showing minimal additional lumen gain and stent expansion post DCB—most gain from IVL

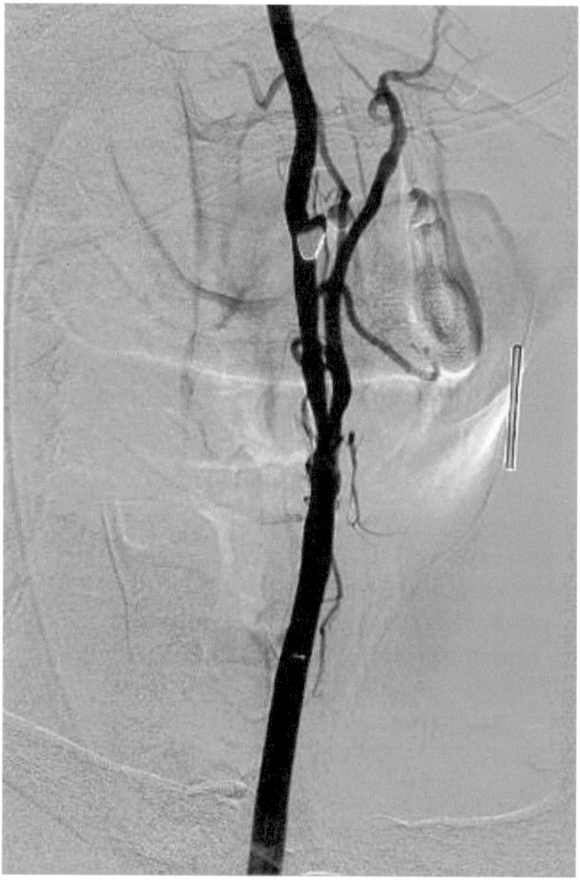

Final angiogram post-IVL/DCB demonstrating excellent stent expansion after IVL/DCB

Case 9.3 Calcified Superior Mesenteric Artery Stenosis

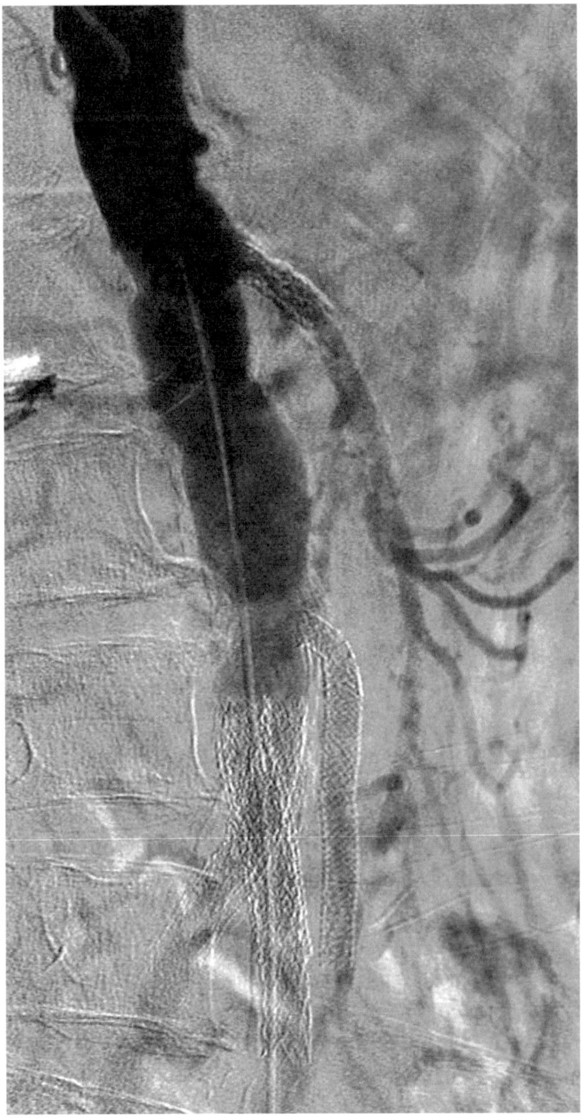

Baseline angiogram showing celiac occlusion, patent iliac, IMA stents, and patent ostial SMA stent with proximal SMA calcified stenosis

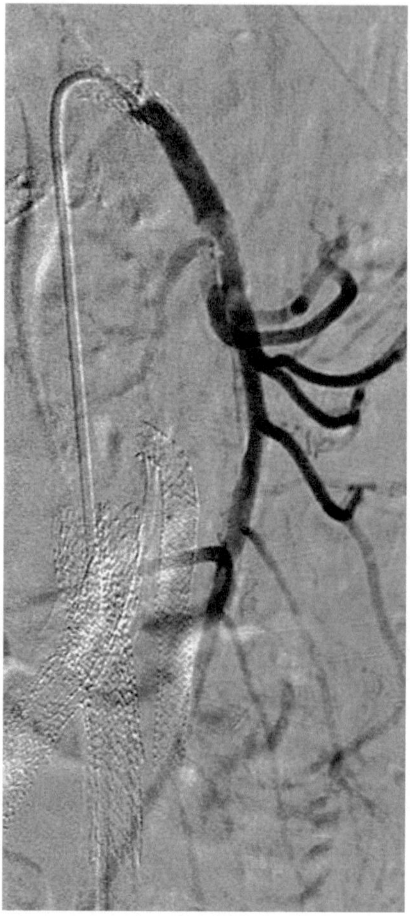

Selective SMA angiogram demonstrating patent ostial SMA stent with calcified proximal stenosis

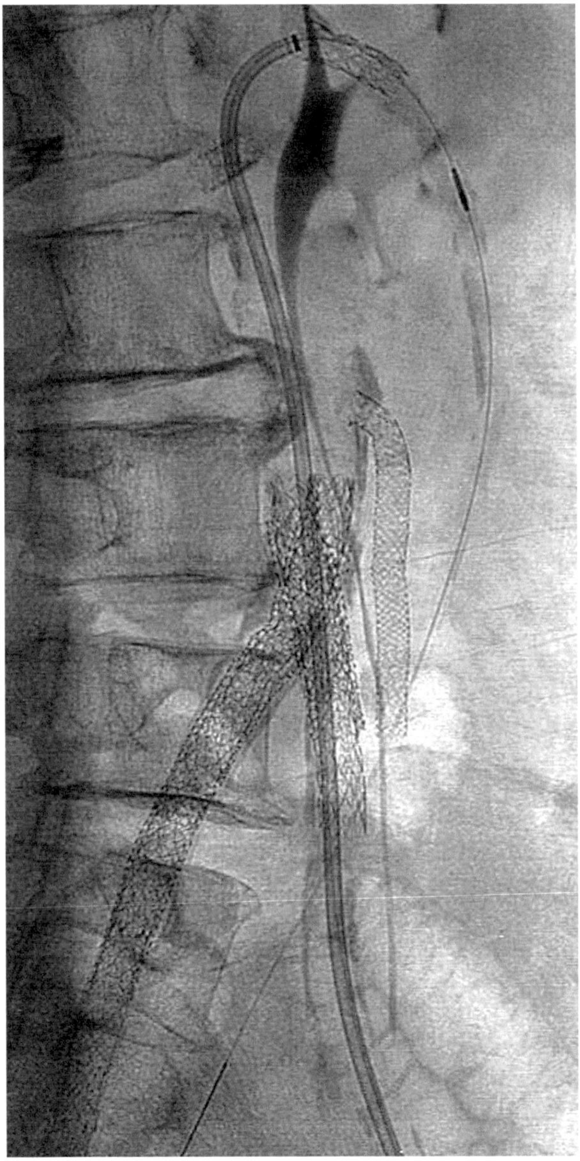

Intravascular ultrasound of the SMA

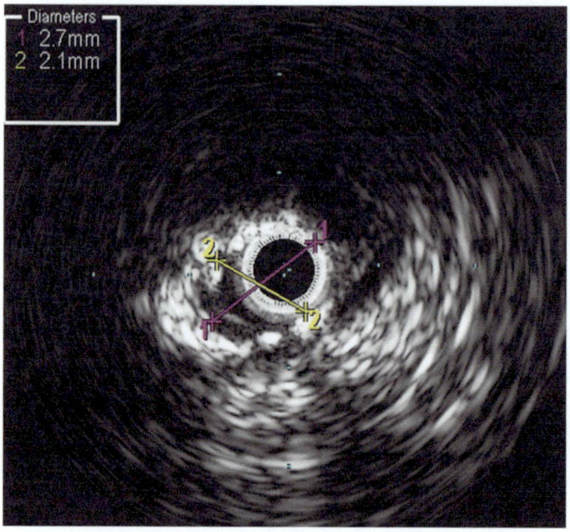

IVUS image showing circumferential severe calcification with high grade cross sectional stenosis

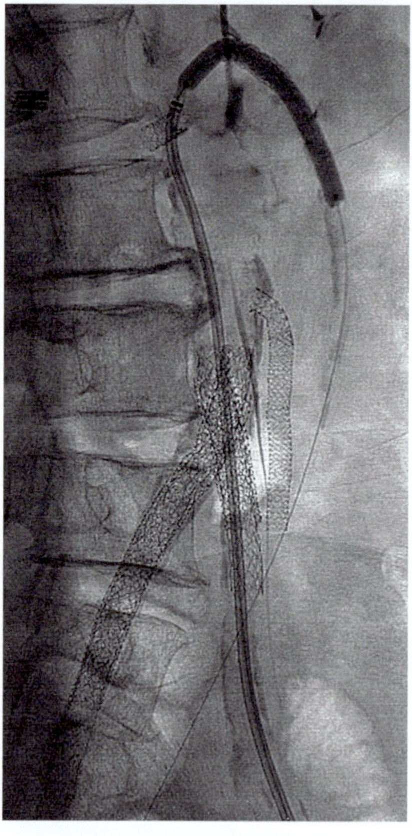

IVL SMA 5.0 mm × 60 mm balloon

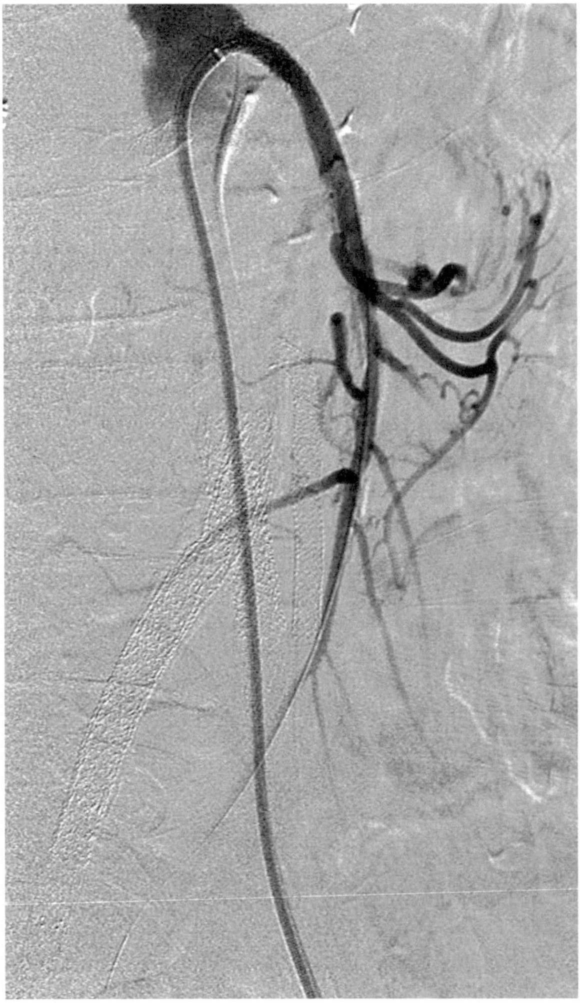

Angiogram post-IVL showing good lumen expansion

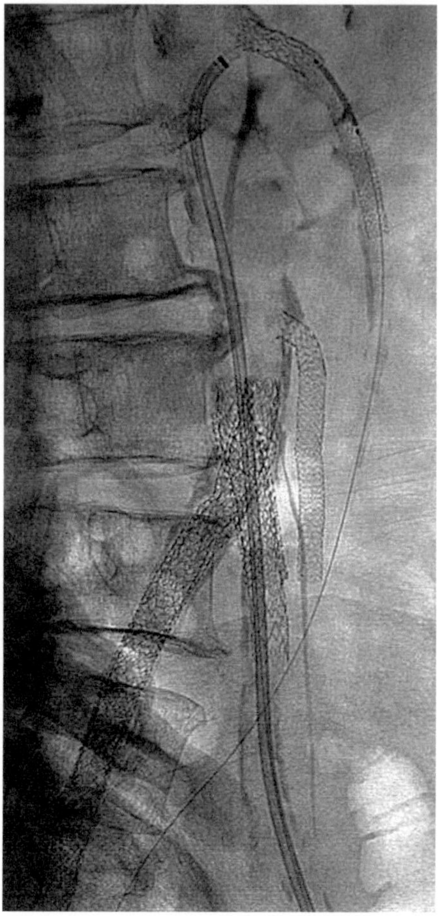

4.5 mm × 30, 5.0 mm × 15 mm Onyx drug-eluting stents after IVL

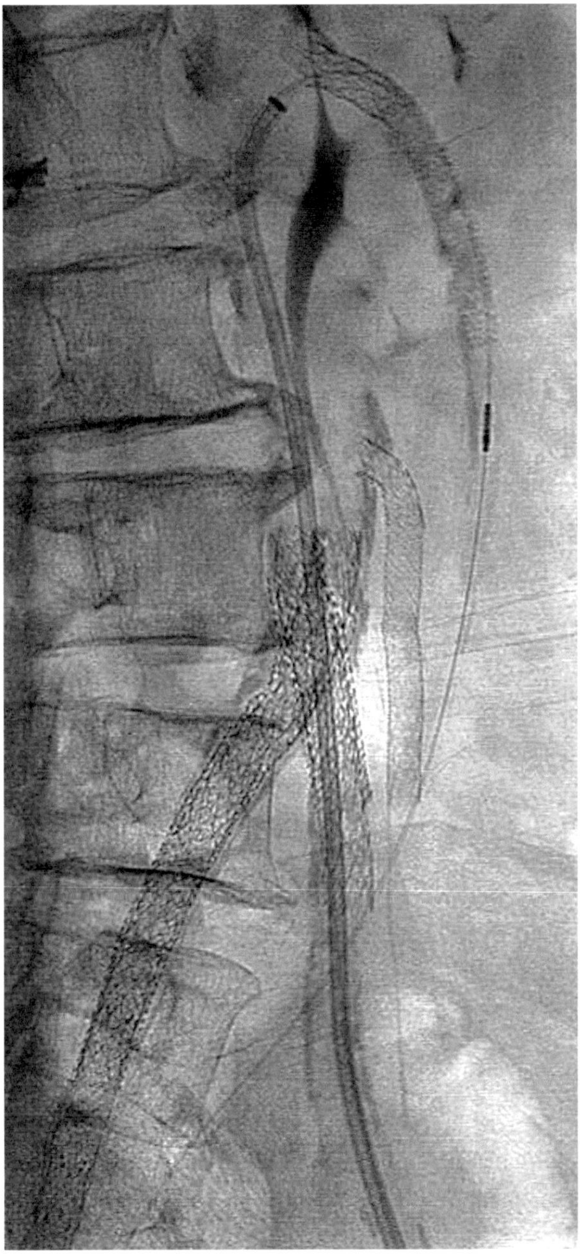

IVUS post-stenting

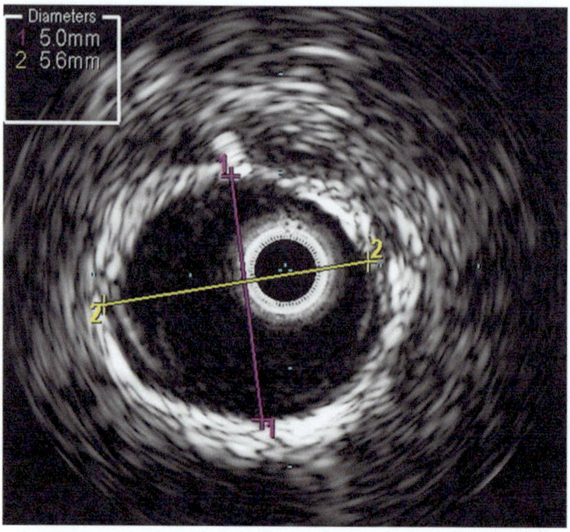

IVUS image post-IVL/stenting showing full stent apposition and expansion

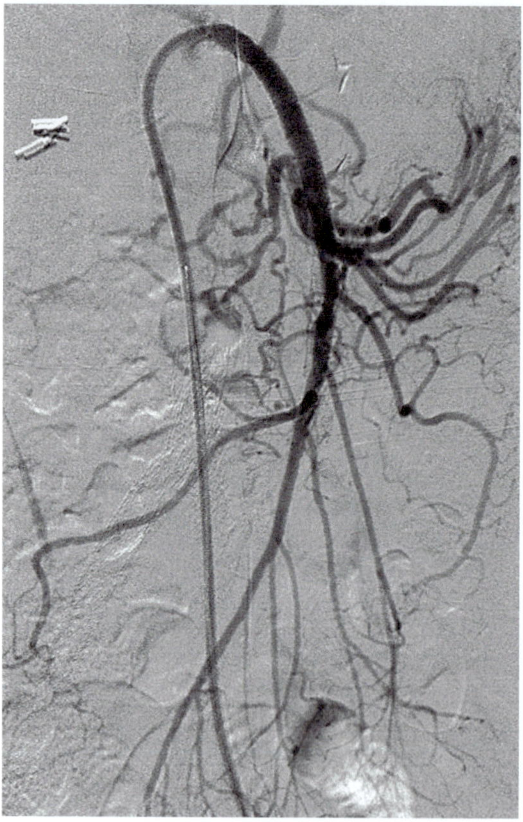

Final angiogram post-IVL/stenting

Case 9.4 Calcified Aorto-Iliac Occlusions

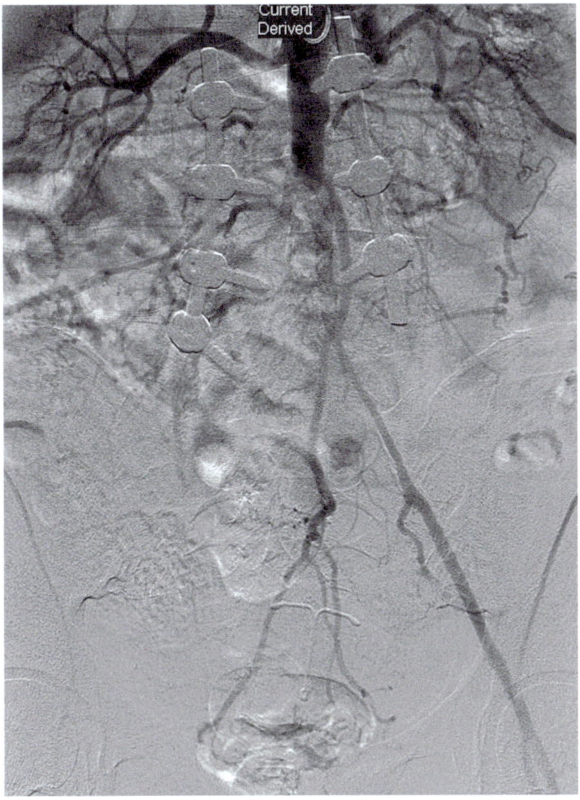

Baseline angiogram showing distal aortic occlusion with dense calcified common iliac artery occlusions

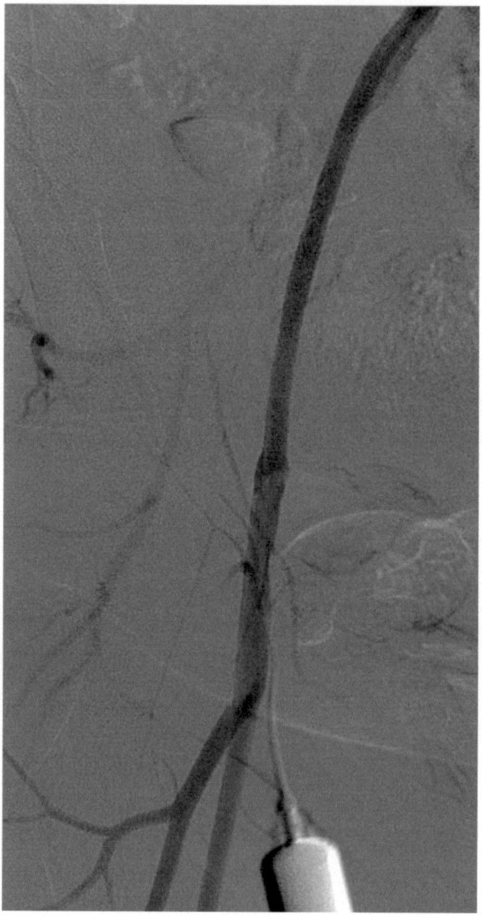

Angiography after obtaining retrograde right CFA access

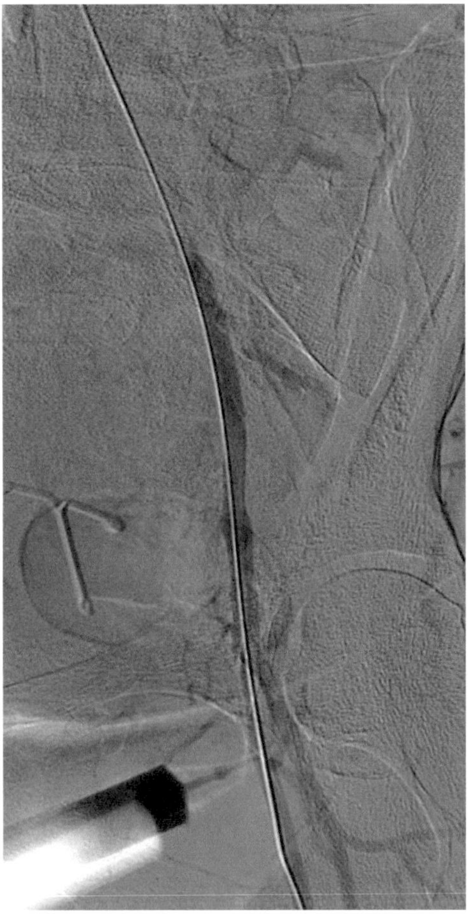

Angiography after obtaining retrograde left CFA access

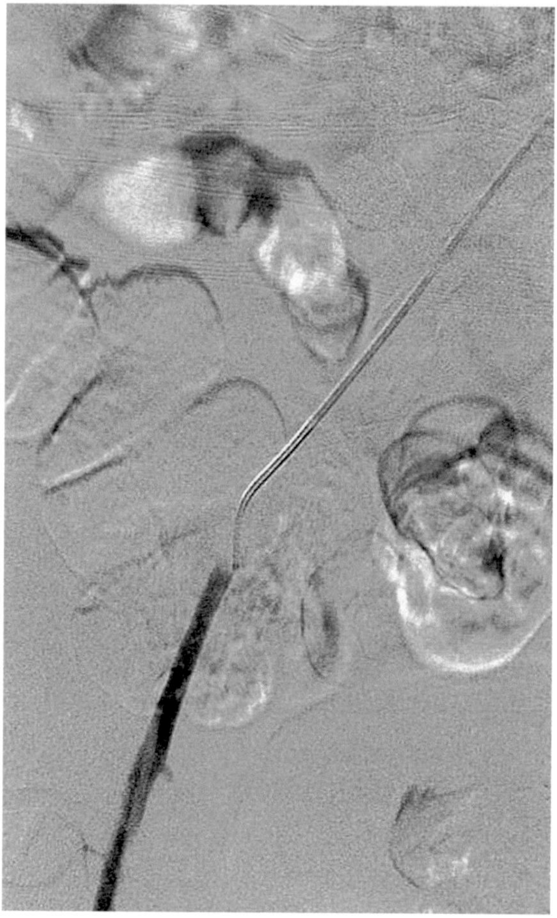

Right iliac occlusion crossed antegrade, wire then exteriorized

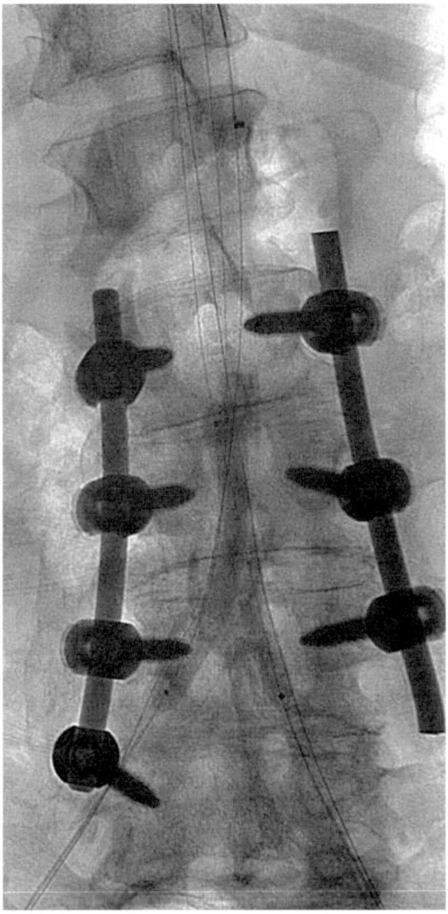

Upsized to 7F sheaths, pre-dilated with 5 mm balloons

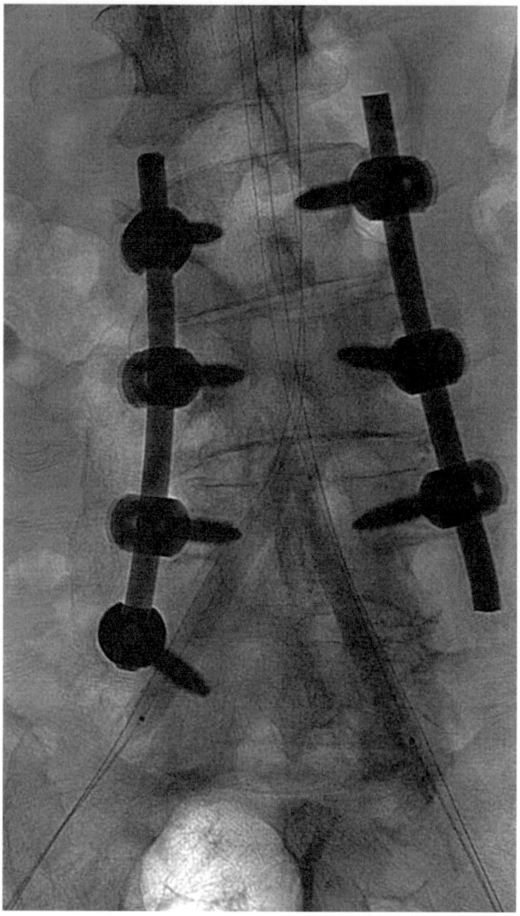

Kissing inflations of distal aorta with two 7 mm × 60 mm Shockwave balloons

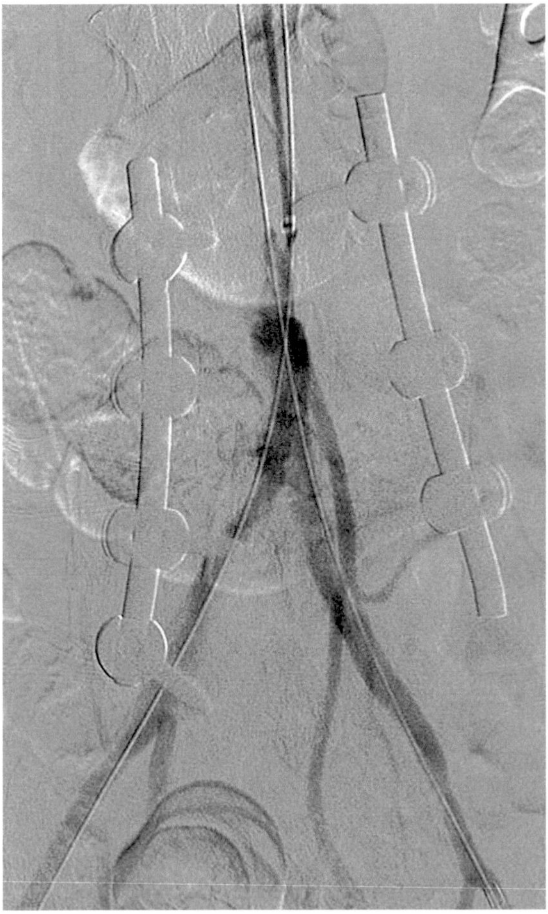

Kissing inflations of proximal common iliac arteries with two 7 mm × 60 mm Shockwave balloons

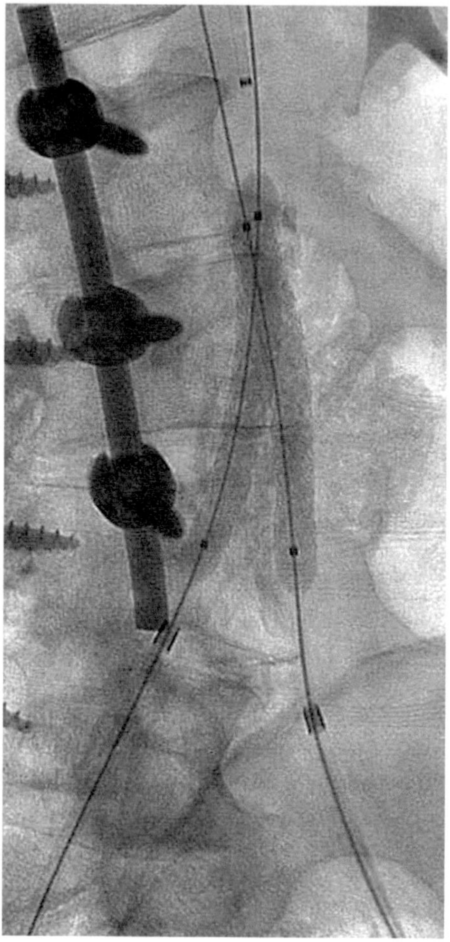

Angiogram post-IVL showing restoration of antegrade flow

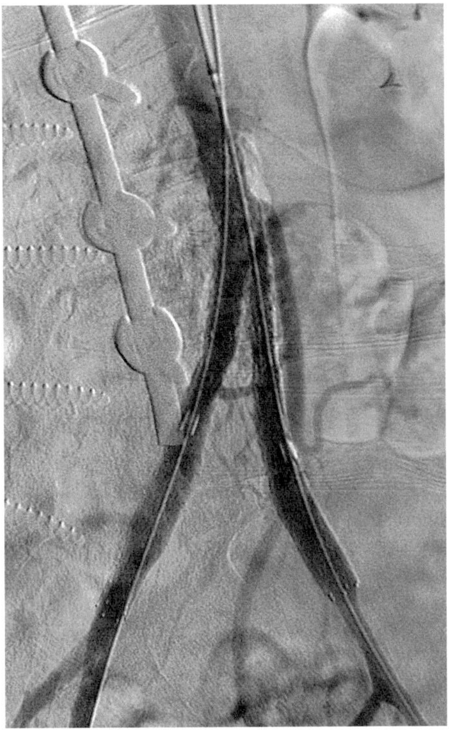

Final angiogram after post-dilation with 8 mm balloons

Case 9.5 IVL to Treat Stent Underexpansion

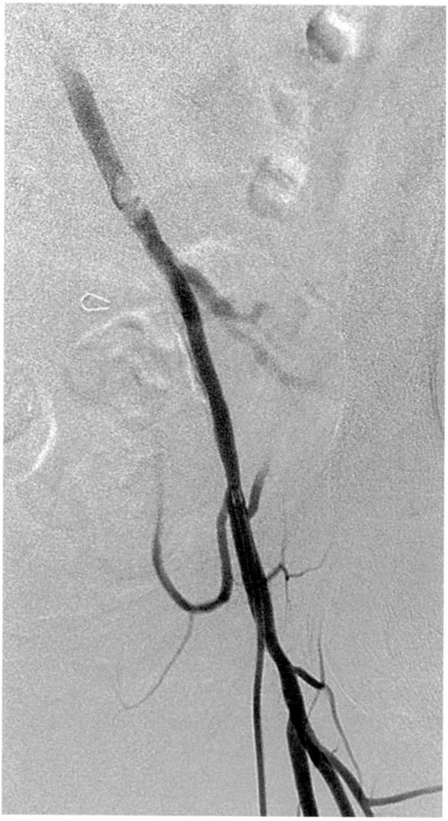

Baseline angiogram showing eccentric calcified iliac stenosis

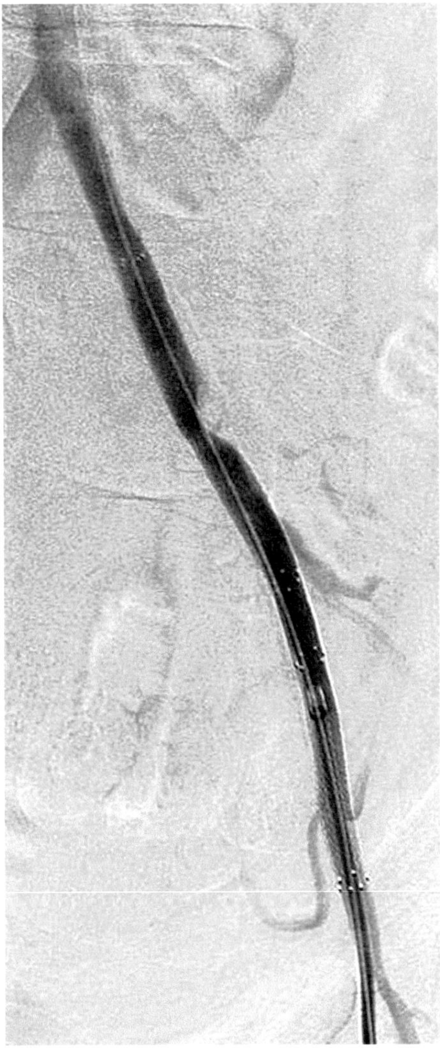

Significant residual stenosis post-stenting

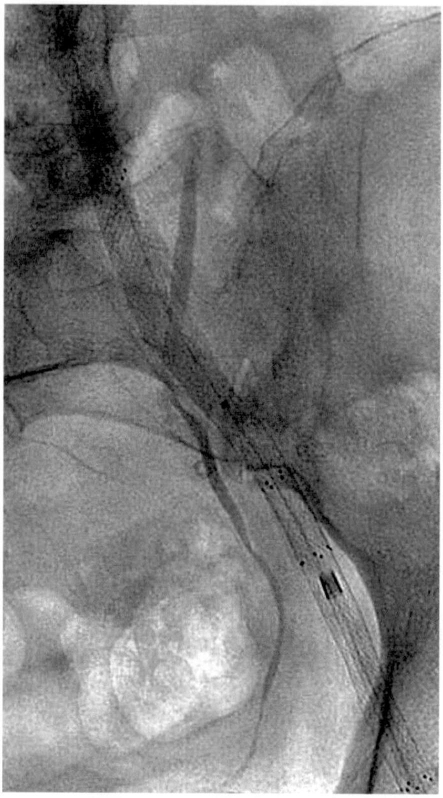

IVL of iliac ISR with 7 mm × 60 mm Shockwave balloon

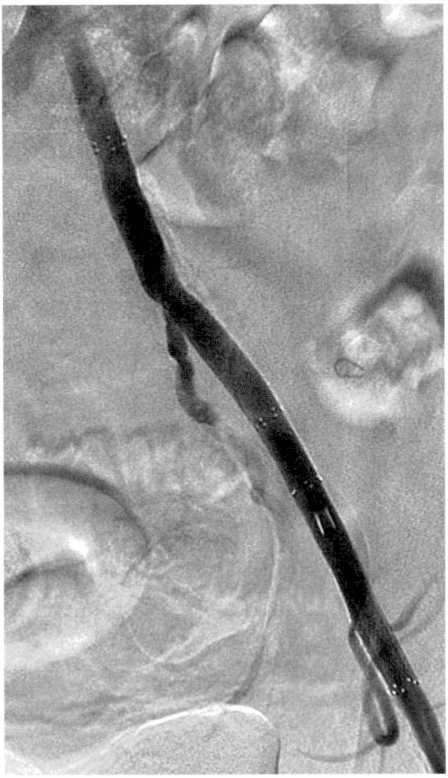

Successful stent expansion post-IVL

Case 9.6 IVL to Treat Stent Underexpansion

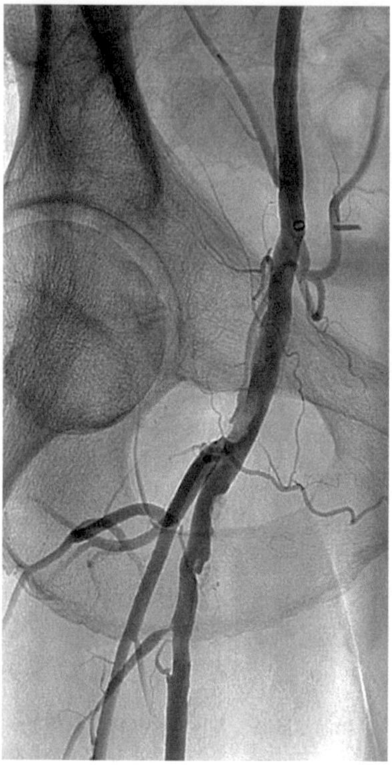

Baseline angiogram showing high-grade calcified CFA stenosis

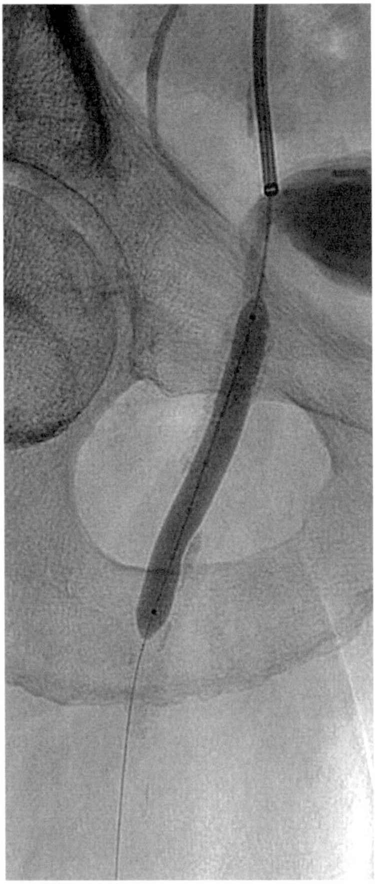

IVL CFA with 7 mm × 60 mm Shockwave Medical balloon

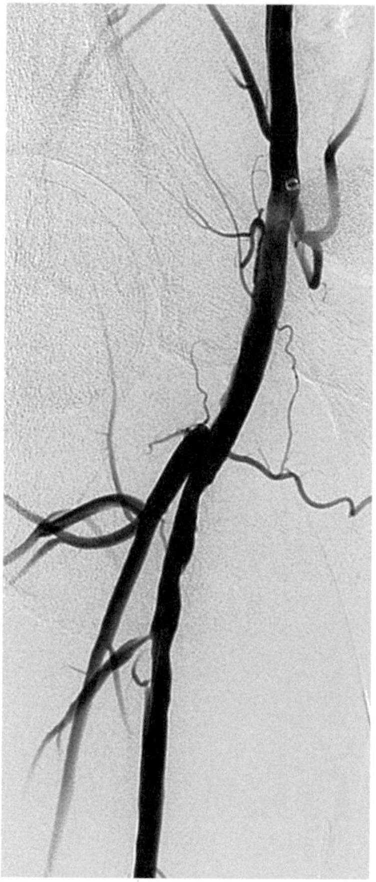

Angiogram after IVL shows full vessel expansion

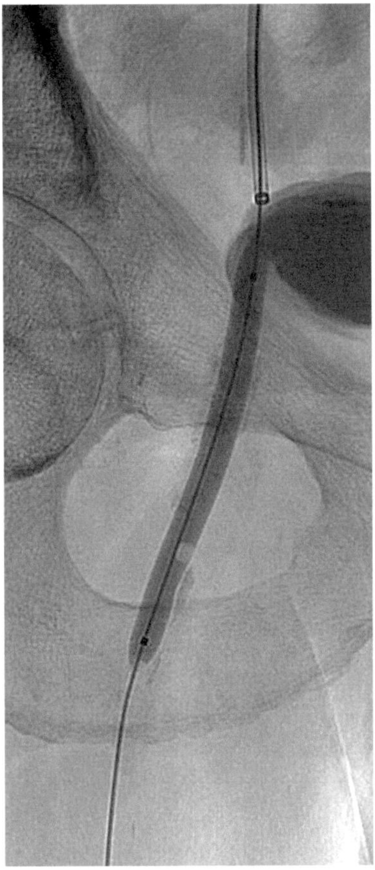

DCB CFA with 7 mm × 60 mm

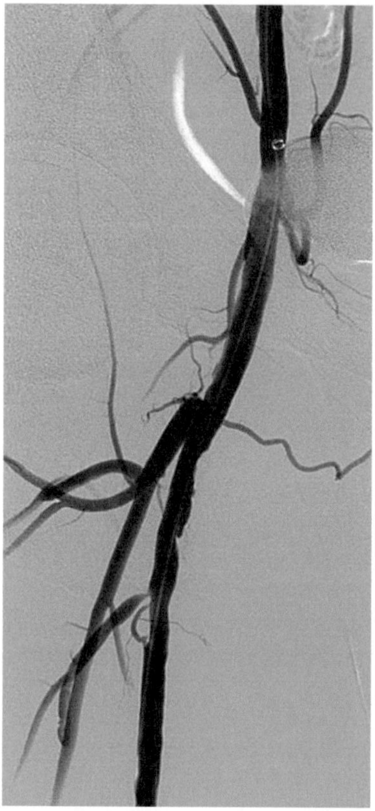

Final angiogram post-IVL/DCB

Case 9.7 IVL to Treat a Heavily Calcified Popliteal Artery "No-Stent Zone" Stenosis

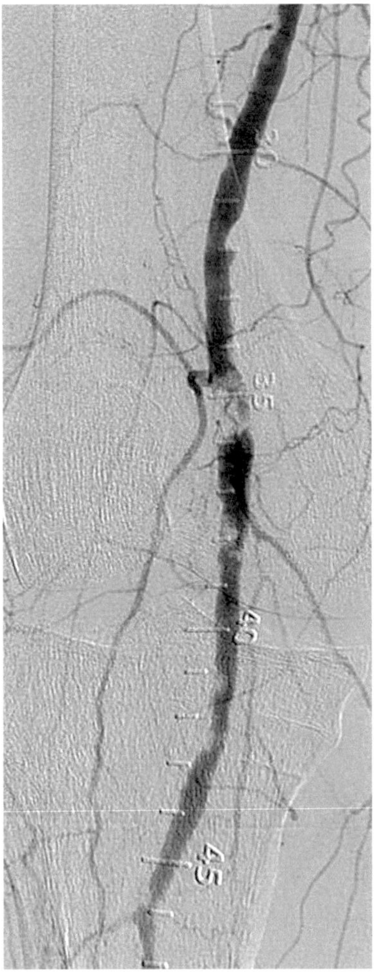

Baseline angiogram showing heavily calcified popliteal artery stenosis

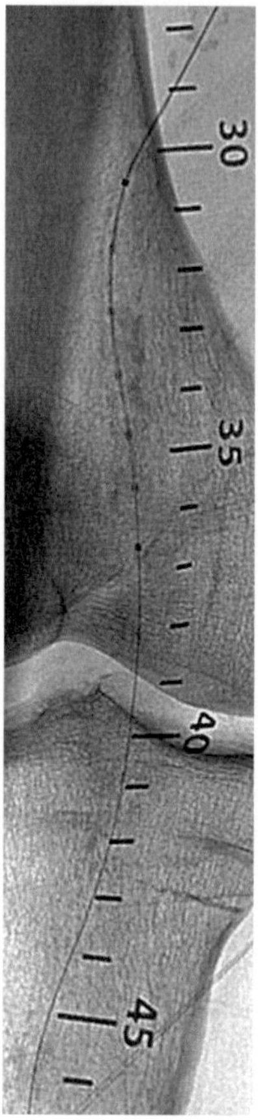

Fluoroscopy demonstrating severe calcification pre-inflation of IVL balloon

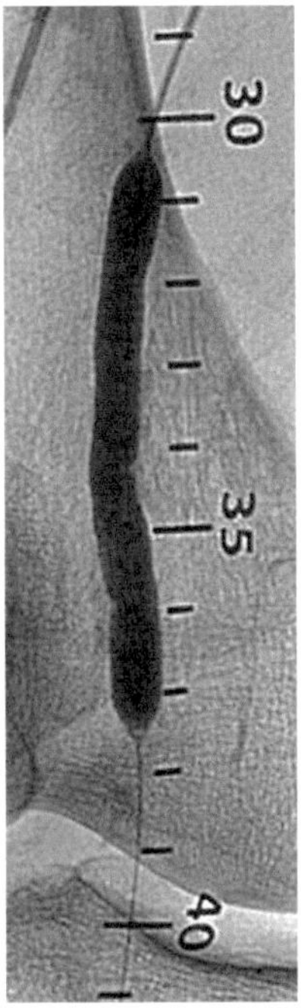

IVL of proximal popliteal stenosis with 6 mm × 60 mm Shockwave balloon

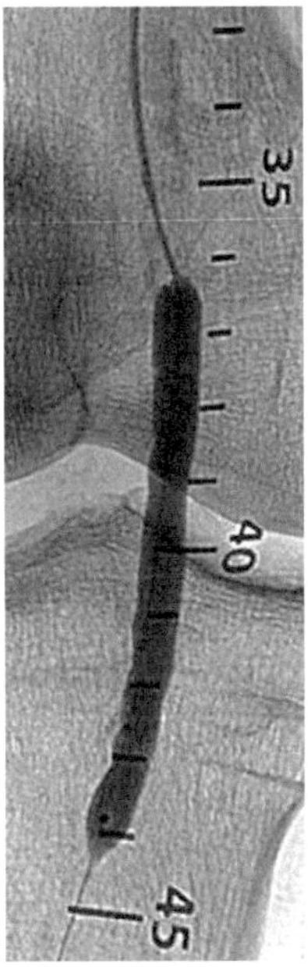

IVL of behind knee popliteal with same balloon

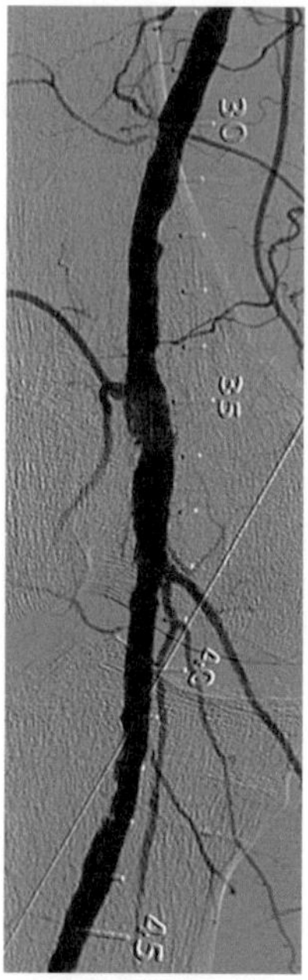

Angiogram post-IVL

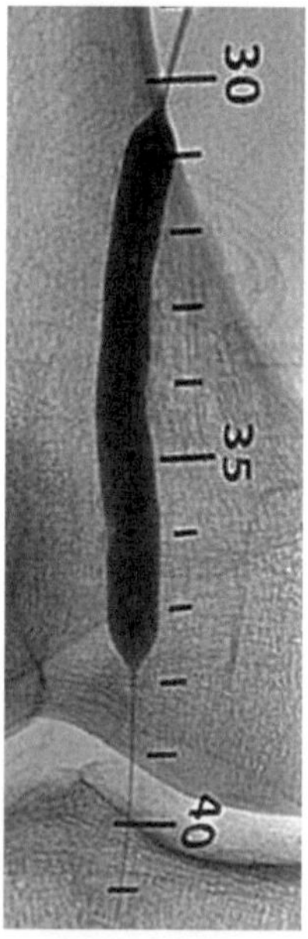

IVL popliteal artery with 6.5 mm × 60 mm Shockwave balloon

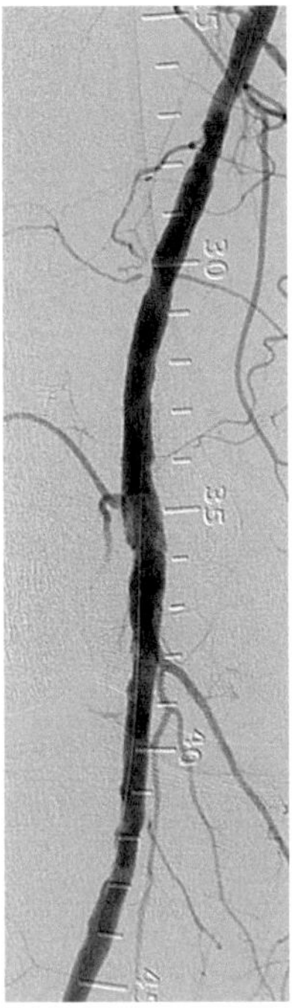

Angiogram post-IVL showing excellent vessel expansion

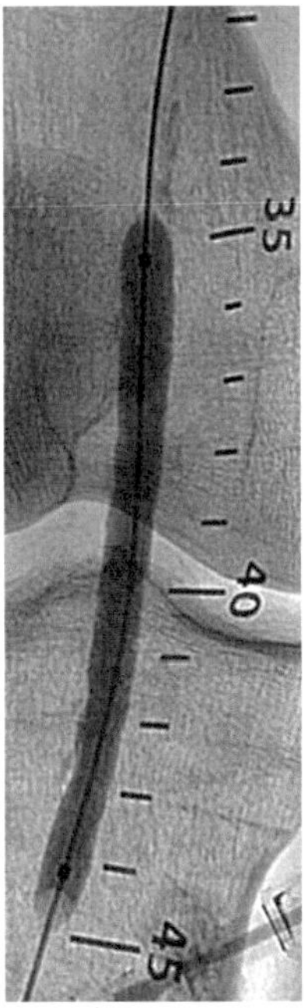

DCB of the popliteal artery with 7 mm × 80 mm IN.PACT balloon

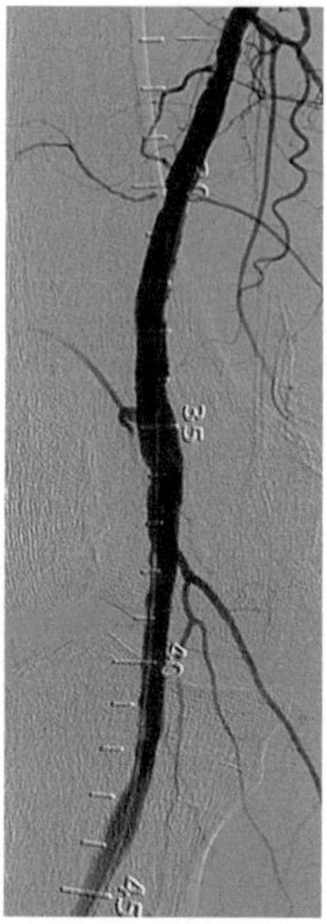

Final angiogram showing excellent expansion without dissection

References

1. Généreux P, Madhavan MV, Mintz GS, et al. Ischemic outcomes after coronary intervention of calcified vessels in acute coronary syndromes. Pooled analysis from the HORIZONS-AMI (harmonizing outcomes with revascularization and stents in acute myocardial infarction) and ACUITY (acute catheterization and urgent intervention triage strategy) TRIALS. J Am Coll Cardiol. 2014;63:1845–54.
2. Soor GS, Vukin I, Leong SW, Oreopoulos G, Butany J. Peripheral vascular disease: who gets it and why? A histomorphological analysis of 261 arterial segments from 58 cases. Pathology. 2008;40:385–91.
3. Frink RJ, Achor RW, Brown AL Jr, Kincaid OW, Brandenburg RO. Significance of calcification of the coronary arteries. Am J Cardiol. 1970;26:241–7.
4. Tan K, Sulke N, Taub N, Sowton E. Clinical and lesion morphologic determinants of coronary angioplasty success and complications: current experience. J Am Coll Cardiol. 1995;25:855–65.
5. Noble S, Roffi M. Overcoming the challenges of the transfemoral approach in transcatheter aortic valve implantation. Interv Cardiol. 2013;8(2):131–4.
6. Walker KL, Nolan BW, Columbo JA, et al. Lesion complexity drives the cost of superficial femoral artery endovascular interventions. J Vasc Surg. 2015;62:998–1002.
7. Fitzgerald PJ, Ports TA, Yock PG. Contribution of localized calcium deposits to dissection after angioplasty. An observational study using intravascular ultrasound. Circulation. 1992;86:64–70.
8. McAteer JA, Bailey MR, Williams JC Jr, et al. Strategies for improved shock wave lithotripsy. Minerva Urol Nefrol. 2005;57(4):271–87.
9. Davros WJ, Garra BS, Zeman RK. Gallstone lithotripsy: relevant physical principles and technical issues. Radiology. 1991;178:397–408.

10. Ali ZA, Brinton TJ, Hill JM, et al. Optical coherence tomography characterization of coronary lithoplasty for treatment of calcified lesions: first description. JACC Cardiovasc Imaging. 2017;10(8):897–906.
11. Brinton TJ, Ali ZA, et al. Feasibility of shockwave coronary intravascular lithotripsy for the treatment of calcified coronary stenoses. Circulation. 2019;139:834–6.
12. Ali ZA, Nef H, et al. Safety and effectiveness of coronary intravascular lithotripsy for treatment of severely calcified coronary stenoses; the disrupt CAD II study. Circ Cardiovasc Interv. 2019;12:e008434.
13. Feldman DN, Armstrong EJ, Aronow HD, et al. SCAI consensus guidelines for device selection in femoral-popliteal arterial interventions. Catheter Cardiovasc Interv. 2018;92(1):124–40.
14. Patel MR, Conte MS, Cutlip DE, et al. Evaluation and treatment of patients with lower extremity peripheral artery disease: consensus definitions from peripheral academic research consortium (PARC). J Am Coll Cardiol. 2015;65(9):931–41.
15. Rocha-Singh KJ, Zeller T, Jaff MR. Peripheral arterial calcification: prevalence, mechanism, detection, and clinical implications. Catheter Cardiovasc Interv. 2014;83(6):E212–20.
16. Thukkani AK, Kinlay S. Endovascular intervention for peripheral artery disease. Circ Res. 2015;116(9):1599–613.
17. Dini CS, Tomberli B, Mattesini A, et al. Intravascular lithotripsy for calcific coronary and peripheral artery stenoses. EuroIntervention. 2019;15:714–21.
18. Brodmann M, Werner M, Brinton TJ, et al. Safety and performance of lithoplasty for treatment of calcified peripheral artery lesions. J Am Coll Cardiol. 2017;70(7):908–10.
19. Brodmann M, Werner M, Holden A, et al. Primary outcomes and mechanism of action of intravascular lithotripsy in calcified, femoropopliteal lesions: result of disrupt PAD II. Catheter Cardiovasc Interv. 2019;93(2):335–42.
20. Brodmann M, Holden A, Zeller T. Safety and feasibility of intravascular lithotripsy for treatment of below-the-knee arterial stenoses. J Endovasc Ther. 2018;25(4):499–503.
21. Schneider PA, Laird JR, Tepe G, et al. Treatment effect of drug-coated balloons is durable to 3 years in the femoro-popliteal arteries: long-term results of the IN.PACT SFA randomized trial. Circ Cardiovasc Interv. 2018;11(1):e005891.
22. Lugenbiel I, Grebner M, Zhou Q, et al. Treatment of femoropopliteal lesions with the AngioSculpt scoring balloon—results from the Heidelberg PANTHER registry. Vasa. 2018;47(1):49–55.
23. Zeller T, Langhoff R, Rocha-Singh KJ, et al. Directional atherectomy followed by a paclitaxel-coated balloon to inhibit restenosis and maintain vessel patency: twelve-month results of the DEFINITIVE AR study. Circ Cardiovasc Interv. 2017;10(9):e004848.
24. Fanelli F, Cannavale A, Gazzetti M, et al. Calcium burden assessment and impact on drug-eluting balloons in peripheral arterial disease. Cardiovasc Intervent Radiol. 2014;37(4):898–907.
25. Adams G, Shammas N, Mangalmurti S, et al. Intravascular lithotripsy for treatment of calcified lower extremity arterial stenosis: initial analysis of the disrupt PAD III study. J Endovasc Ther. 2020;27(3):473–80.
26. Tepe G, Brodmann M, Bachincky W, Holden A, Zeller T, Mangalmurti S, Nolte-Ernsting C, Virmani R, Parikh S, Gray W, for the Disrupt PAD III Investigators. Intravascular lithotripsy for peripheral artery calcification: mid-term outcomes from the randomized disrupt PAD III trial. JSCAI. 2022. https://doi.org/10.1016/j.jscai.2022.100341.
27. Bavaria JE, Tommaso CL, Brindis RG, et al. 2018 AATS/ACC/SCAI/STS expert consensus systems of care document: operator and institutional recommendations and requirements for transcatheter aortic valve replacement: a joint report of the American Association for Thoracic Surgery, the American College of Cardiology, the Society for Cardiovascular Angiography and Interventions, and the Society of Thoracic Surgeons. J Am Coll Cardiol. 2019;73:340–74.
28. Holmes DR, Nishimura RA, Grover FL, et al. Annual outcomes with transcatheter valve therapy: from the STS/ACC TVT registry. J Am Coll Cardiol. 2015;66:2813–23.
29. Biasco L, Ferrari E, et al. Access sites for TAVI: patient selection criteria, technical aspects, and outcomes. Front Cardiovasc Med. 2018;5:88.

30. Di Mario C, Chiriatti N, et al. Lithoplasty-assisted transfemoral aortic valve implantation. Eur Heart J. 2018;41(8):942.
31. Gorla R, Cannone GS, et al. Transfemoral aortic valve implantation following lithoplasty of iliac artery in a patient with poor vascular access. Catheter Cardiovasc Interv. 2019;93:E140–2.
32. Di Mario C, Goodwin M, et al. A prospective registry of intravascular lithotripsy-enabled vascular access for transfemoral transcatheter aortic valve replacement. JACC Cardiovasc Interv. 2019;12(5):502–4.
33. Rosseel L, De Backer O, Søndergaard L, Bieliauskas G. Intravascular iliac artery lithotripsy to enable transfemoral thoracic endovascular aortic repair. Catheter Cardiovasc Interv. 2020;95:E96–9.
34. Riley RF, Corl JD, Kereiakes DJ. Intravascular lithotripsy-assisted Impella insertion: a case report. Catheter Cardiovasc Interv. 2019;93(7):1317–9. https://doi.org/10.1002/ccd.28168.
35. Mordasini P, Gralla J, Do DD, Schmidli, Keseru B, Arnold M, Fischer U, Schmidli G, Brekenfeld C. Percutaneous and open retrograde endovascular stenting of symptomatic high-grade innominate artery stenosis: technique and follow-up. AJNR Am J Neuroradiol. 2011;32(9):1726–31.
36. Giannopoulos S, Speziale F, Vadal G, Soukas PA, Kuhn BA, Stolz CL, Foteh MI, Mena-Hurtado C, Armstrong EJ. Intravascular lithotripsy for treatment of calcified lesions during carotid artery stenting. J Endovasc Ther. 2021;28(1):93–9. https://doi.org/10.1177/1526602820954244. Epub 2020 Sep 1. PMID: 32869718.
37. Khan MS, Baig M, Hyder ON, Aronow HD, Soukas PA. Intravascular lithotripsy for the treatment of severely calcified mesenteric stenosis. JACC Case Rep. 2020;2(6):956–60.
38. Armstrong EJ, Soukas PA, Shammas N, Chamberlain J, Pop A, Adams G, de Freitas D, Valle J, Woo E, Bernardo NL. Intravascular lithotripsy for the treatment of calcified, stenotic iliac arteries: a cohort analysis from the disrupt PAD III study. Cardiovasc Revasc Med. 2020;21(10):1262–8. https://doi.org/10.1016/j.carrev.2020.02.026. Epub 2020 Mar 2. PMID: 32147133.
39. Nguyen BN, Amdur RL, Abugideiri M, et al. Postoperative complications after common femoral endarterectomy. J Vasc Surg. 2015;61(6):1489–1494.e1.
40. Brodmann M, Schwindt A, Argyrios A, Gammon R. Safety and feasibility of intravascular lithotripsy for treatment of common femoral artery stenoses. J Endovasc Ther. 2019;26(3):283–7.
41. Guzman RJ, Brinkley DM, Schumacher PM, et al. Tibial artery calcification as a marker of amputation risk in patients with peripheral artery disease. J Am Coll Cardiol. 2008;51(2):1967–74.
42. Bauman F, Fust J, Engelberger RP, et al. Early recoil after balloon angioplasty of tibial artery obstructions in patients with critical limb ischemia. J Endovasc Ther. 2014;21(1):44–51.
43. Hill JM, Kereiakes DJ, et al. Intravascular lithotripsy for treatment of severely calcified coronary artery disease. J Am Coll Cardiol. 2020;76(22):2635–46.
44. Case B, Yurasi C, Waxman R, et al. Intravascular lithotripsy facilitated percutaneous endovascular intervention of the aortic arch: a single-center experience. Cardiovasc Revasc Med. 2020;21(8):1006–15.
45. Henry CL, Hansen SK, et al. Intravascular lithotripsy during trans-carotid arterial revascularization for highly calcified lesions in high- risk patients. J Vasc Surg Cases Innov Tech. 2020;7(1):68–73. https://doi.org/10.1016/j.jvscit.2020.10.018.

Chapter 10
Preserving Vessel Integrity and Reducing Vascular Recoil with Focal Force Balloons

Effie K. Lambrinos, Edward D. Tubberville, Vinayak Subramanian, and George L. Adams

Introduction

Percutaneous angioplasty (PTA) has been the trailblazer in the management of vascular disease for many years. More innovative tools have been created to treat various types of arterial lesions as the understanding of peripheral arterial disease has advanced. Scoring balloons and focal force balloon technologies have become an essential part of the interventionalist's equipment. The "leave nothing behind" strategy has gained traction over the years due to the prevalence of in-stent restenosis and vessel recoil following peripheral vascular interventions (PVI). This method intends to diminish the development of permanent vascular prosthesis, which can likely allow for future restenosis [1, 2]. Furthermore, recent developments in drug technology have allowed for even more strides in the individualization of patient care. In the following chapter, we will review the techniques utilizing focal force and scoring balloons for vessel preparation and further evaluate the literature for the use of such devices.

E. K. Lambrinos · E. D. Tubberville
Campbell University School of Osteopathic Medicine, Raleigh, NC, USA
e-mail: e_lambrinos1012@email.campbell.edu; edtubbervill0919@email.campbell.edu

V. Subramanian
Department of Internal Medicine, UT Southwestern Medical Center, Dallas, TX, USA
e-mail: Vinayak.subramanian@utsouthwestern.edu

G. L. Adams (✉)
UNC -Medical Center, Chapel Hill, NC, USA
e-mail: george.adams@unchealth.unc.edu

N. W. Shammas (ed.), *Peripheral Arterial Interventions*, Contemporary Cardiology, https://doi.org/10.1007/978-3-031-09741-6_10

The idea of vessel preparation has become mainstreamed among endovascular specialists specifically aiming to treat patients with infrainguinal arterial disease [3, 4]. Focal force balloons are used mainly for two vessel preparatory purposes, the first one being to decrease vessel elastic recoil [5] and the second, to reduce the risk of perforation and/or dissection [6].

The acknowledgement of the role of plaque characteristics can aid in differentiating between which device is most appropriate for preparing the vessel. Plaque characteristics span a vast range of features, from including calcific, heterogenous, and homogenous plaque [7]. Homogenous plaque is linked with thrombus development, typically seen in chronic total occlusions (CTO) and acute occlusions, and also contains fibrocalcific or fibroelastic matter which is often seen in lesions of chronic stenosis [8, 9]. In contrast, heterogenous plaque is associated with an increased amount of calcification and cerebrovascular symptoms along with a predominance in carotid artery stenosis when compared to homogenous plaque [10, 11]. Calcified plaque is made of predominantly calcific deposits with a large variety in presentation and is typically observed as deposits within intimal and medial layer of the vessel [12]; they are mostly found in diabetic patients or those with chronic renal insufficiency and are commonly found in the blood vessels inferior to the knee. The evaluation of the various plaque characteristics can be performed by considering the patient risk factors, the angiographic pattern, and the intraprocedural intravascular ultrasound (IVUS) which allows the angiologist to personalize care improving outcomes and reducing complications.

Functionalities of Balloon Angioplasty and Focal Force Balloons

The functionalities of balloon angioplasty are intricate and can be found in other literature. In summary, a radial circumferential force is administered on the walls of the individual vessel following the distention of the balloon, thereby causing the size of the lumen to increase.

The greatest force from the balloon is focused primarily on the disease-free portions of the artery. A large force is also focused on the area between the disease-free portions and the plaque causing the stenosis [13], followed by an elastic recoil that presents whenever these over-expanded portions are returned to their normal size. A potential poor outcome involves an arterial wall dissection that may occur when the stress produced by the PTA is distributed through a fragile portion of either the plaque or the vessel itself and is spread down the vessel. In the worst-case scenario, this stress can produce an arterial perforation.

The purpose of the scoring balloons and focal force is to allow for a progressive expansion of the vessel by focusing the pressure strictly on the plaque as opposed to the vessel. A number of different designs have been manufactured to utilize this strategy (Table 10.1).

Table 10.1 Summary of focal force balloon types and sizes

Focal force balloons	
Device name	Size range
Peripheral cutting balloon	5–8 mm diameter, 15–20 mm lengths
Chocolate balloon	2.5–6 mm diameter, 40–120 mm lengths
Angiosculpt	2–8 mm diameter, 10–40 mm lengths
VascuTrack	2.0–7.0 mm diameter, 20–300 mm lengths
FLEX scoring catheter	Variable diameter, 40–120 cm working length

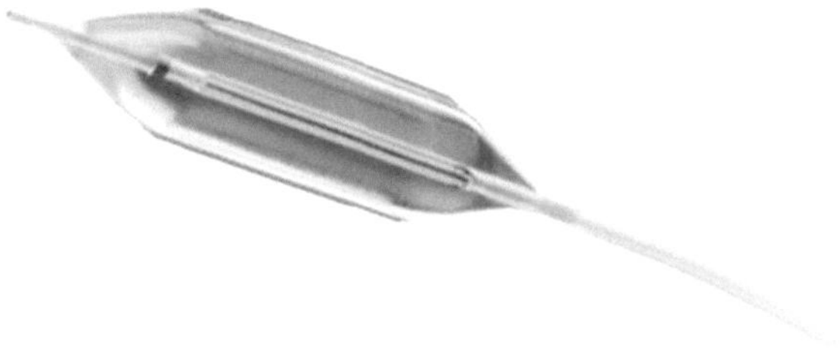

Fig. 10.1 Peripheral Cutting Balloon device by Boston Scientific

Peripheral Cutting Balloon (Boston Scientific) (Fig. 10.1)

Device Mechanism

The peripheral cutting balloons are standard balloons that include four blades of microsurgical precision found along the balloon surface, whose function is to make distinct longitudinal cuts within the plaque. Initially, inflation of the balloon occurs to a pressure of 2 atm to set the blades into position, which are then followed by an inflation to nominal pressures of 6 atm once in contact with the plaque in order to cut into the plaque.

Specifications

There are two accessible forms of the peripheral cutting balloon: a monorail rapid exchange (RX) catheter system and an over the wire (OTW). The two balloon lengths that are currently marketed are 15 and 20 mm, with available balloon diameters that span from 5.0 to 8.0 mm. Catheter lengths range from 50 to 137 cm (OTW) and 142 cm (RX).

Evidence and Use

Current evidence pertaining to the complexity of cutting balloons (CB) is limited. RESCUT, the largest randomized controlled trial, analyzed the use of cutting balloons in the coronary arteries for in-stent restenosis [14]. The conclusion of this study stated that the occurrence of in-stent restenosis did not decrease with the use of cutting balloon angioplasty. However, it did in fact decrease the quantity of balloons that were required for each intervention and pointed toward a decrease in a need for the use of stenting. Within the femoropopliteal arteries, studies have indicated safety in the treatment of these lesions. The use of cutting balloons in contrast to plain old balloon angioplasty (POBA) in small (defined as <5 cm) focal femoropopliteal lesions was analyzed in a randomized controlled trial [15, 16]. The study concluded that POBA was superior to cutting balloon angioplasty and that cutting balloon angioplasty, at 6 months, has greater rates of restenosis. Furthermore, PTA use was weighed against CB-PTA use in a prospective study involving 83 patients with femoropopliteal lesions of short calcified occlusive nature (<3 cm). This study concluded that elastic recoil, arterial perforations, and dissections requiring stenting were not experienced by lesions treated with CB-PTA, along with rates of both primary and secondary patency improving with the use of cutting balloon angioplasty [17].

There is inadequate proof that supports the use of CB as the first-line treatment of femoropopliteal lesions. An appreciation of plaque characteristics can allow for better understanding of the use of this device. Additionally, the CB may be used for hemodialysis fistula site lesions, but further analysis shows that the CB has primarily been used and studied only within the treatment of in-stent stenosis and femoropopliteal stenosis, although the use of these balloons to treat these issues may be considered an off-label use for this equipment. Care should be taken when stationing this balloon during the treatment of in-stent restenosis due to the possibility of fracturing the stent from the microsurgical blades.

Chocolate PTA Balloon (Medtronic) (Fig. 10.2)

Device Mechanism

The Chocolate PTA balloon incorporates a semi-compliant balloon surrounded by a cage made of nitinol. Enlargement of the balloon allows for the balloon to expand through the open spaces of the cage. At the locations where the balloon does not expand, on the frame of the cage, it creates a network that places increased forces on the plaque which gives rise to limited breaks within the plaque. The capacity to focus the force from the balloon onto a smaller location allows for angioplasty to be performed under lower pressures with lower rates of flow-limiting dissection.

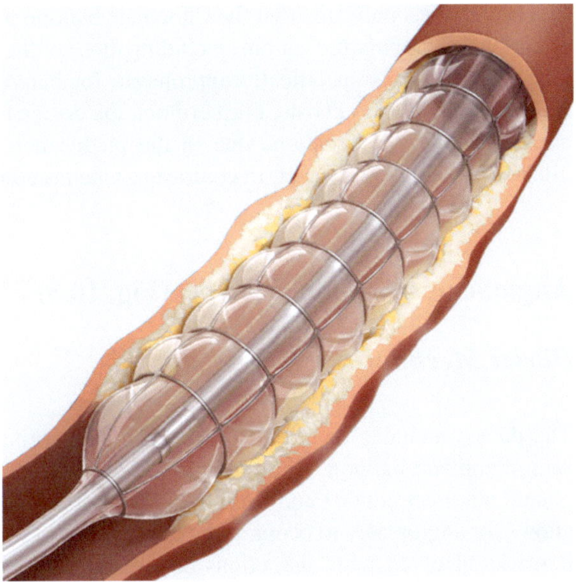

Fig. 10.2 CHOCOLATE PTA device by Medtronic

Device Specifications

The Chocolate balloon can be currently found in diameters of 2.5–6.0 mm and with balloon lengths of 40–120 mm and a working length of 120–150 cm. Compatibility with a 0.014″ and 0.018″ guidewire is possible with its over-the-wire design. Another version, with paclitaxel coating, is available and being assessed for effectiveness and safety in the USA.

Evidence and Use

The majority of evidence for the use of the Chocolate balloon can be found in the Chocolate BAR registry, a prospective multicenter study used to examine the Chocolate balloon when treating patients with peripheral artery disease [18]. The study consisted of 262 patients totaling 290 femoropopliteal lesions with most of the patients having moderate to severe peripheral artery disease (PAD, including Rutherford 3–6). The average length of each lesion among those evaluated in the study was 83.5 mm, and 63.5% had calcific disease. In 85.1% of the cases, success in the procedure was attained, with the dissection rate at 22.6%. Additionally, no flow-limiting dissections were noted. Only 1.6% of cases necessitated bail-out stenting. A drug-coated adaptation of the Chocolate balloon is being assessed for effectiveness and safety.

The FDA has indicated that the Chocolate balloon may be used for the treatment of peripheral vasculature lesions, including those of the iliac and infrainguinal arteries. The balloon is specifically appropriate for heterogenous calcific plaque and lesions of in-stent restenosis. Furthermore, the device is appropriate for lesions that are located near bifurcations due to the plaque not typically shifting when the inflated balloon is in contact, in contrast to when used in conventional angioplasty.

AngioSculpt Balloon (Philips) (Fig. 10.3)

Device Mechanism

The device includes two helical nitinol struts (scoring elements) that surround a semi-compliant balloon. Upon inflation of the balloon, the helical struts pierce the plaque on direct contact and limit the balloon force onto these struts. This method allows for angioplasty to occur at lower pressures of inflation and overall decreases the risks involved with dissections of uncontrolled nature. Originally, the device was created to treat coronary lesions but has more recently been utilized for the treatment of patients with peripheral arterial disease.

Device Specifications

The AngioSculpt balloon can be currently found in diameters of 2.0–8.0 mm and with balloon lengths of 10–40 mm, with a working length of 90–155 cm. Compatibility is with a 0.014 and 0.018 guidewire along with 5–6 F sheaths.

Evidence and Use

A multicenter prospective study researched the technique of the AngioSculpt balloon for the treatment of infrapopliteal disease. The study included 42 patients (with a total of 56 lesions). Most patients had a severe case of PAD, with Rutherford class ≥4 (90.5%). A total of 73% of lesions that were treated had moderate to severe

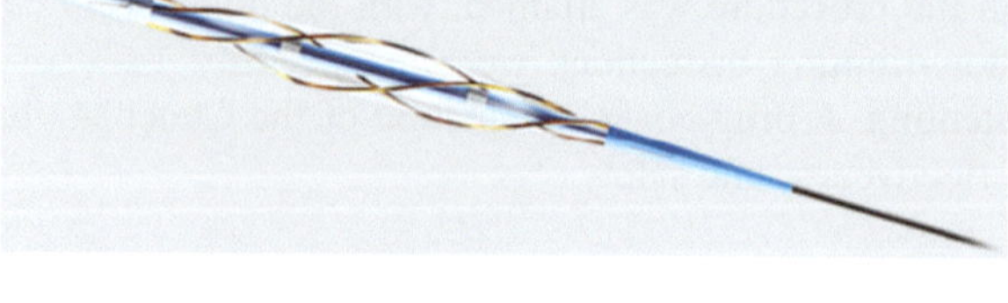

Fig. 10.3 Agniosculpt PTA device by Phillips

calcific disease with an average lesion length of 33.9 ± 42.2 mm. Procedural success was achieved in 98.2% of all cases. Dissections that occurred following the angioplasty were present in 10.7% of lesions [19]. Another prospective study evaluated 31 patients (with a total of 36 lesions) with severe infrapopliteal disease to gauge the effectiveness and safety of the device, with its successful use in all cases. A rate of 35.5% was evaluated for the stenting rate performed after device use due to a dissection of sub-optimal therapy. The survival rate after 1 month without complications was 96.8%, and the primary patency after 1 year was 61% [20].

The AngioSculpt may be used for lesion dilation in peripheral vasculature—more specifically the femoropopliteal, iliac, and infrapopliteal arteries.

VascuTrak (Bard) (Fig. 10.4)

Device Mechanism

The device includes two wires attached to a semi-compliant balloon. After the balloon expands, the stress from the balloon is transferred through the wires to produce contained breaks within the plaque. This equipment has not been studied systematically but is similar in action to other focal force balloons.

Specifications

The VascuTrak can be found with diameter of 2–7 mm and with balloon lengths of 20–300 mm. The working length ranges from 80 to 140 cm and is compatible with a guidewire of 0.014 and 0.018.

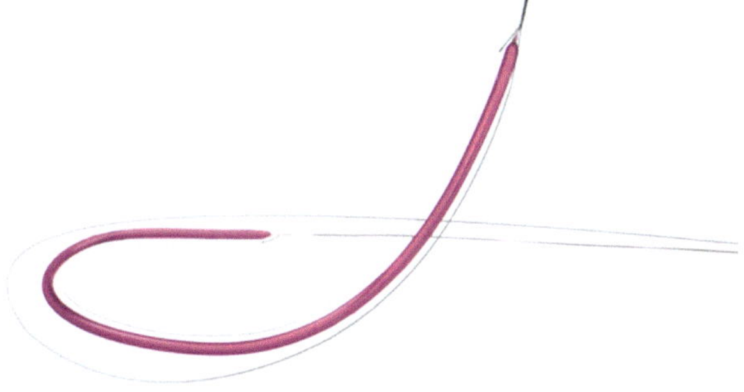

Fig. 10.4 VascuTrack Device by BARD

Evidence and Use

There is little evidence assessing the use of the VascuTrak balloon. Indications for use of the VascuTrak include treatment of peripheral vessel lesions. The device may also be used to treat fibrocalcific disease. The device's simplistic design allows for a vast selection of balloon lengths and sizes. Traditionally, a second wire was used alongside an inflated balloon to attain the same result in most coronary interventions.

Shockwave Intravascular Lithotripsy (IVL) (Shockwave) (Fig. 10.5)

Device Mechanism

Shockwave intravascular lithotripsy (IVL) comprises of a traditional angioplasty balloon mounted with ultrasound emitters capable of emitting pulsatile ultrasound waves which mechanically modify the hard, typically calcific, plaque in the lesion without damaging the elastic components of the healthy artery. The balloon is first inserted into the occluded artery and inflated to a pressure of 4 atm, and 30 shock-wave impulses followed by 60 more are delivered after dilation to nominal pressure has been achieved. The impulses function to break the calcified lesions into small particles while preserving vessel integrity.

Specifications

The Shockwave IVL device is available in two configurations: the Shockwave M5 used for treating peripheral arteries above the knee and the Shockwave S4 used to target arteries below the knee (BTK). The M5 series ranges from 3.5 to 7.0 mm in

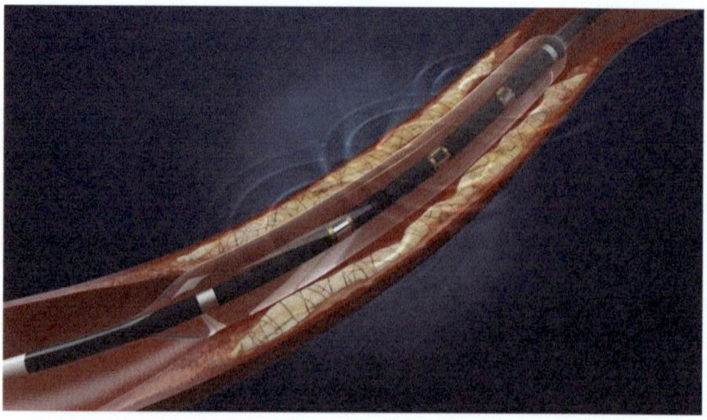

Fig. 10.5 Shockwave intravascular lithotripsy by Shockwave Medical

diameter, has a length of 60 mm and a working length of 110 cm, and can deliver up to 300 pulses maximally. The S4 series ranges from 2.5 to 4.0 mm in diameter, is 40 mm in length, has a 135 cm working length, and can deliver up to 160 maximum impulses.

Evidence and Use

Research on the use of Shockwave IVL has shown its effectiveness in treating lesioned vessels resulting in better outcomes compared to traditional PTA. In a study conducted by Marianne et al., 35 individuals presented with femoropopliteal lesions that were on average 76.3% stenotic with an average lesion length of 61.5 mm [21]. These lesions were heavily calcified in 64.1% of the patients with an average calcified lesion length of 80.3 mm. The study concluded with all patients having procedural success with an average residual stenosis of 23.4% and a 2.9 mm acute gain. There were no implanted stents or vascular complications during the procedure. The patients also showed 100% vessel patency as defined as <50% restenosis and 100% freedom from target lesion revascularization (TLR) at a 30-day follow-up and 82.1% patency and 100% freedom from TLR at a 6-month follow-up.

Further studies demonstrated the increased efficacy of intravascular lithotripsy (IVL) compared to traditional PTA [22, 23]. The largest randomized clinical trial of IVL vs. PTA demonstrated that IVL was superior in most aspects. IVL demonstrated higher procedural success by 15.5%, higher lesions with residual stenosis <30% by 14.5%, fewer flow-limiting dissections by 5.4%, fewer post-dilatations by 14.8%, and fewer stent placements by 13.7%. The main shortcoming of IVL was that it was on par with PTA in TLR and major adverse events, although minimal in both techniques.

Although IVL has had more extensive research in above-the-knee vessels, further evidence is still being collected for use in BTK treatment. Currently, there is 1 available study, conducted on a cohort of 20 patients with 100% calcification in BTK vessels that resulted in 100% success in residual stenosis being <50% at 30 days [24]. Overall, IVL is useful in a multitude of scenarios including where stenting is contraindicated and in high-risk locations such as bifurcating lesions.

FLEX Scoring Catheter (VentureMed) (Fig. 10.6)

Device Mechanism

The FLEX scoring catheter functions by preparing the lesion for balloon angioplasty by way of three microblades attached to three flexible struts located along the end of the catheter. FLEX focuses on improving vessel compliance, leading to lower balloon pressures, leading to less vessel trauma. The catheter is mounted on a

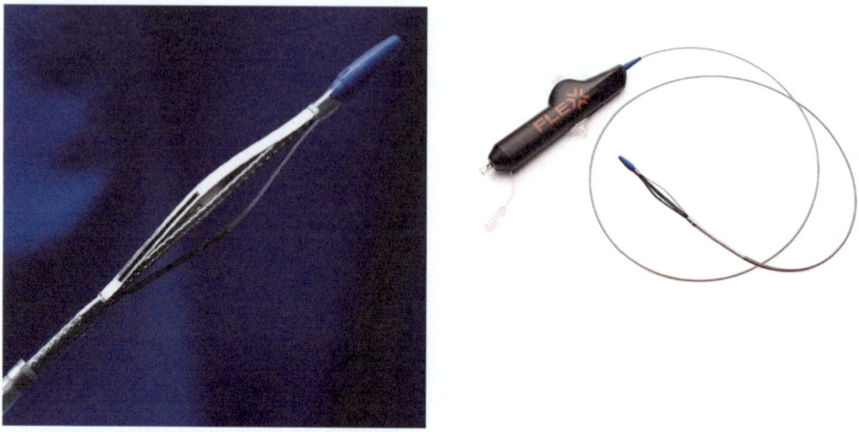

Fig. 10.6 Flex Scoring Catheter by Venturemed

guidewire, and the section with three microblades is directed to the distal end of the lesion. The operator can then engage the scoring elements of the catheter and pull retrograde across the lesions within vessel. The unique aspect of the FLEX catheter is that it will maintain 1 atm of pressure on the blades as the operator pulls the catheter retrograde through the vessel. This dynamic scoring technology allows for precise parallel cuts along the treated vessel segment. Once proximal to the lesion, the catheter blades can be disengaged, sent distal to the lesion, and rotated 30° or 90°, and the process repeated for maximal plaque modification.

Specifications

The FLEX catheter comes in one design. It is 6F compatible and can be used with both 0.014″ and 0.018″ guidewire platforms and has working lengths of 40 or 120 cm.

Evidence and Use

Studies using the FLEX scoring catheter have produced evidence supporting the use in vessel preparation prior to angioplasty. In particular, the International Symposium on Endovascular Therapy in 2018 referenced compiled data from multiple hospitals and operators on the FLEX catheter prior to angioplasty [25]. From the symposium, the study titled "Early Clinical Results Using the FLEX Scoring Catheter in 100 Femoropopliteal Chronic Total Occlusions" showed that of 100 patients with femoropopliteal chronic total occlusions, FLEX catheter prep was successful in 99% of the cases with only 4% having minimal dissections, and stents were provisionally used in 19% of cases. Efficacy of FLEX prep was seen when less than nominal balloon opening pressures averaged at 4.1 atm with maximum pressures of 9.4 atm. Another abstract, "Use of the FLEX Scoring Catheter as a New Arteriovenous Access Management Device," presented data on 59 patients treated with FLEX before balloon angioplasty and demonstrated balloon opening pressures averaging 6.5 atm and maximal balloon pressures averaging 12.1 atm.

The FLEX scoring catheter's main advantage is that there is no need for constant inflation and deflation as with other scoring elements. With its dynamic scoring technology, lesion preparation can be achieved in much less time, and risk of vessel dissection is minimal. Current research suggests that optimal use of the FLEX scoring catheter should be used as preparation for drug-coated balloon angioplasty. However, further evidence is needed to demonstrate if the device assists in lowering restenosis with adequate treatment as other scoring elements do.

Conclusions

Peripheral arterial disease includes a diverse patient population with a multitude of disease presentations. Acknowledgement of various plaque characteristics can aid in providing individualized care to patients presenting with varying lesion features. The use of focal force balloons in conjunction with other therapies can minimize elastic recoil and dissections, ultimately decreasing the necessity of a scaffold.

The principal objective of using focal force balloons is to not only decrease the necessity of supplementary stenting but also eliminate elastic recoil after therapeutic intervention by using a mechanical advantage when attempting to treat stenotic plaque. High procedural success rates have been observed in prospective studies of the devices described in this chapter. However, some patients still develop arterial wall dissections and require bail-out stents.

As drug-coated balloons (DCBs) have emerged in the treatment algorithm for PAD, the adjunctive use of focal force technologies may aid in improved outcomes as a result of more thorough vessel preparation. Known evidence of restenosis along with increased awareness of financial responsibility should be considered when adding these devices, especially in multilevel disease where numerous devices may need to be used. With these factors considered, new technologies such as the XO Score (Transit Scientific) are being developed. The XO Score catheter allows operators to use a single catheter designed device with multiple balloon sizes making it well suited for multilevel disease. Also, the ability to use one specialized device multiple times with balloons widely available to practitioners will reduce overall cost. Along with development of new device designs, the addition of biologics to current focal force technologies may provide the next generation of this treatment.

References

1. Alfonso F, Cuesta J, Pérez-Vizcayno MJ, del Blanco BG, Rumoroso JR, Bosa F, et al. Bioresorbable vascular scaffolds for patients with in-stent restenosis: the RIBS VI study. JACC Cardiovasc Interv. 2017;10(18):1841–51.
2. Giannopoulos S, Armstrong EJ. Newly approved devices for endovascular treatment of femoropopliteal disease: a review of clinical evidence. Expert Rev Cardiovasc Ther. 2019;17(10):729–40.
3. Tzafriri AR, Garcia-Polite F, Zani B, Stanley J, Muraj B, Knutson J, et al. Calcified plaque modification alters local drug delivery in the treatment of peripheral atherosclerosis. J Control Release. 2017;264:203–10.
4. Rocha-Singh KJ, Zeller T, Jaff MR. Peripheral arterial calcification: prevalence, mechanism, detection, and clinical implications. Catheter Cardiovasc Interv. 2014;83(6):E212–20.
5. Dick P, Barth B, Mlekusch W, Sabeti S, Amighi J, Schlager O, et al. Complications after peripheral vascular interventions in octogenarians. J Endovasc Ther. 2008;15(4):383–9.
6. Fiehrlein C, Zimmerman M, Pill J, Metz J, KüBLER W, von Hodenberg E. The role of elastic recoil after balloon angioplasty of rabbit arteries and its prevention by stent implantation. Eur Heart J. 1994;15(2):277–80.
7. Brevetti G, Giugliano G, Brevetti L, Hiatt WR. Inflammation in peripheral artery disease. Circulation. 2010;122(18):1862–75.
8. Guo J, Maehara A, Mintz GS, Ashida K, Pu J, Shang Y, et al. A virtual histology intravascular ultrasound analysis of coronary chronic total occlusions. Catheter Cardiovasc Interv. 2013;81(3):464–70.
9. Gonzalo N, Serruys PW, Okamura T, van Beusekom HM, Garcia-Garcia HM, van Soest G, et al. Optical coherence tomography patterns of stent restenosis. Am Heart J. 2009;158(2):284–93.
10. European Carotid Plaque Study Group. Carotid artery plaque composition—relationship to clinical presentation and ultrasound B-mode imaging. Eur J Vasc Endovasc Surg. 1995;10:23–30.
11. Meskauskiene A, Barkauskas E, Gaigalaite V. Carotid artery atherosclerotic stenosis, plaque structure and stroke. Medicina (Kaunas). 2005;41:335–42.
12. Meissner OA, Rieber J, Babaryka G, Oswald M, Reim S, Siebert U, et al. Intravascular optical coherence tomography: comparison with histopathology in atherosclerotic peripheral artery specimens. J Vasc Interv Radiol. 2006;17(2):343–9.
13. Holzapfel GA, Schulze-Bauer CA, Stadler M. Mechanics of angioplasty: wall, balloon and stent, vol. 242. New York: ASME Applied Mechanics Division-Publications-AMD; 2000. p. 141–56.
14. Albiero R, Silber S, Di Mario C, Cernigliaro C, Battaglia S, Reimers B, et al. Cutting balloon versus conventional balloon angioplasty for the treatment of in-stent restenosis: results of the restenosis cutting balloon evaluation trial (RESCUT). J Am Coll Cardiol. 2004;43(6):943–9.
15. Dick P, Sabeti S, Mlekusch W, Schlager O, Amighi J, Haumer M, et al. Conventional balloon angioplasty versus peripheral cutting balloon angioplasty for treatment of femoropopliteal artery in-stent restenosis: initial experience. Radiology. 2008;248(1):297–302.
16. Amighi J, Schillinger M, Dick P, Schlager O, Sabeti S, Mlekusch W, et al. De novo superficial femoropopliteal artery lesions: peripheral cutting balloon angioplasty and restenosis rates—randomized controlled trial. Radiology. 2008;247(1):267–72.
17. Rabbi JF, Kiran RP, Gersten G, Dudrick SJ, Dardik A. Early results with infrainguinal cutting balloon angioplasty limits distal dissection. Ann Vasc Surg. 2004;18(6):640–3.
18. Mustapha JA, Lansky A, Shishehbor M, Miles McClure J, Johnson S, Davis T, et al. A prospective, multi-center study of the chocolate balloon in femoropopliteal peripheral artery disease: the chocolate BAR registry. Catheter Cardiovasc Interv. 2018;91(6):1144–8.
19. Scheinert D, Peeters P, Bosiers M, O'Sullivan G, Sultan S, Gershony G. Results of the multicenter first-in-man study of a novel scoring balloon catheter for the treatment of infra-popliteal peripheral arterial disease. Catheter Cardiovasc Interv. 2007;70(7):1034–9.

20. Bosiers M, Deloose K, Cagiannos C, Verbist J, Peeters P. Use of the AngioSculpt scoring balloon for infrapopliteal lesions in patients with critical limb ischemia: 1-year outcome. Vascular. 2009;17(1):29–35.
21. Marianne B, Martin W, Brinton Todd J, Uday I, Alexandra L, Jaff Michael R, Andrew H. Safety and performance of lithoplasty for treatment of calcified peripheral artery lesions. J Am Coll Cardiol. 2017;70:908–10.
22. Brodmann M, Werner M, Holden A, Tepe G, Scheinert D, Schwindt A, Wolf F, Jaff M, Lansky A, Zeller T. Primary outcomes and mechanism of action of intravascular lithotripsy in calcified, femoropopliteal lesions: results of disrupt PAD II. Catheter Cardiovasc Interv. 2019;93:335–42.
23. Tepe G, Brodmann M, Werner M, Bachinsky W, Holden A, Zeller T, Mangalmurti S, Nolte-Ernsting C, Bertolet B, Scheinert D, Gray WA. Intravascular lithotripsy for peripheral artery calcification: 30-day outcomes from the randomized disrupt PAD III trial. JACC Cardiovasc Interv. 2021;14:1352–61.
24. Brodmann M, Holden A, Zeller T. Safety and feasibility of intravascular lithotripsy for treatment of below-the-knee arterial Stenoses. J Endovasc Ther. 2018;25:499–503.
25. Abstracts from the International Symposium on Endovascular Therapy (ISET) 2018. J Vasc Interv Radiol. 29:1180.

Chapter 11
Reducing the Metal Burden in the Infrainguinal Arteries: Tack Endovascular System

Marianne Brodmann

Intentional dissection is a key mechanism for luminal gain post-balloon angioplasty (PTA). Balloon angioplasty functions by both mechanically stretching the atherosclerotic artery and inducing dissection, resulting in acute vascular injury [1] (Fig. 11.1).

Angiographic evidence of dissections is frequent, reported in up to 84% of femoropopliteal angioplasties [2]. Acutely, dissection can reduce or obstruct flow, requiring additional therapeutic intervention, and over the long term, lesions with dissections have 3.5 times the rate of repeat target lesion revascularization (TLR) than lesions without [3–5].

Controlling the severity of dissections has been the subject of many adjunctive technologies prior to PTA including debulking with atherectomy [6–8] or treatment with scoring or focal force balloons [9–11].

Data show that despite debulking of plaque, atherectomy is not superior to PTA in achieving better patency and target lesion revascularization [12, 13], which may partly be explained by the occurrence of deep and wide dissections, which can be seen if IVUS is used in addition to angiography.

In the drug-coated balloon (DCB) era, the negative impact of dissections on outcomes appears to have been partially mitigated, as seen in the Thunder trial [4], but with increasing lesion complexity, the stent rate is increasing even after DCB treatment, mainly due to visible dissections.

Dissections are mostly treated with stent placement. By scaffolding the vessel wall with high radial outward force, stents treat the dissections but can present additional challenges, especially with longer lesions. Stents have been shown to improve

M. Brodmann (✉)
Division of Angiology, Medical University Graz, Graz, Austria
e-mail: Marianne.brodmann@medunigraz.at

N. W. Shammas (ed.), *Peripheral Arterial Interventions*, Contemporary Cardiology, https://doi.org/10.1007/978-3-031-09741-6_11

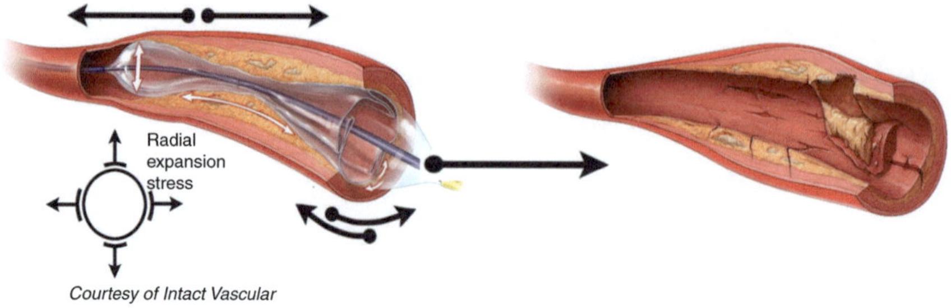

Fig. 11.1 Mechanism of angioplasty: dissection. (*Courtesy of Intact Vascular*)

procedural outcomes, but beyond the acute treatment phase, the aggressive radial force combined with an extensive amount of nitinol can cause inflammation and lead to intimal hyperplasia formation, in-stent restenosis, and high rates (20–37%) of restenosis 1 year posttreatment [14–17]. The dynamic forces exerted in the femoropopliteal segment can lead to additional shear stress, inflammation, and occasional stent fracture [18, 19].

Given the inherent limitations of stent placement, limiting the metal footprint for dissection treatment represents an alternative solution.

The Tack Endovascular System (Intact Vascular, Wayne, Pennsylvania) is a novel device specifically designed to address the limitations of stents while providing durable repair of post-PTA dissections in the superficial femoral artery (SFA) and infrapopliteal arteries. To reduce the metal surface area in contact with the luminal wall, Tack implants are short (4–6 mm), also for BTK, with an open-cell design resulting in lower chronic outward force compared with similar-sized stents (Fig. 11.2). This allows focal dissection treatment and scaffolding with less metal implant (Fig. 11.3).

A large data set for this technique has been created and presented for above- and below-the-knee treatment.

The first trial, the TOBA trial, which was a prospective, single-arm study, evaluated 130 patients with Rutherford clinical category 2–4 and lesions of the superficial femoral and popliteal arteries. Patients were treated with standard balloon angioplasty, and post- PTA dissections were treated with Tacks. The primary endpoints were core laboratory-adjudicated device technical success, defined as the ability of the Tack implants to resolve post-PTA dissection, and device safety, defined as the absence of new onset major adverse events. Patients were followed up to 12 months after implantation.

Tacks were used in 130 patients with post-PTA dissections (74.0% ≥ grade C). Technical success was achieved in 128 (98.5%) patients with no major adverse events at 30 days. The 12-month patency was 76.4%, and freedom from target lesion revascularization was 89.5%. Significant improvement from baseline was observed in Rutherford clinical category (82.8% with grade ≤1) and ankle-brachial index (0.68 6 0.18 to 0.94 6 0.15; $p < 0.0001$) [20].

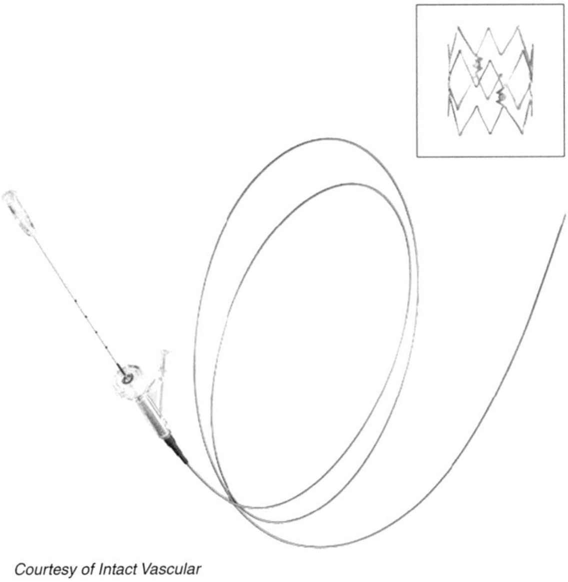

Fig. 11.2 Mode of dissection repair by Tack. (*Courtesy of Intact Vascular*)

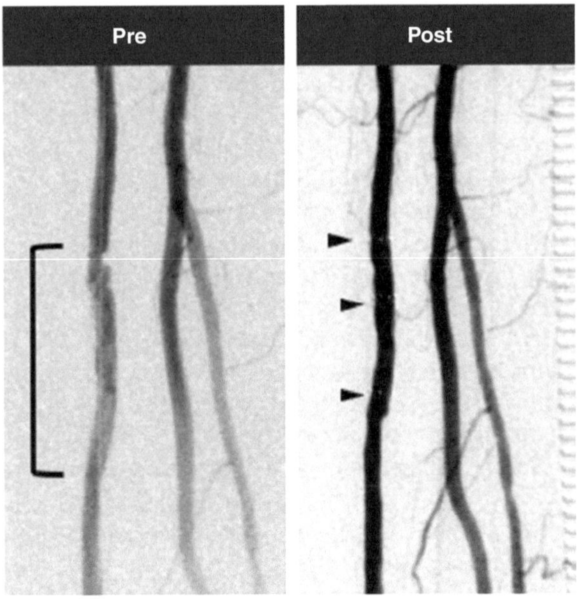

Fig. 11.3 Mode of dissection repair by Tack

The authors concluded that Tack implant treatment of post-PTA dissection was safe, produced reasonable patency and resulted in low rates of target lesion revascularization, and represents a new, minimal metal paradigm for dissection repair that can safely improve the clinical results associated with PTA.

This study was followed by TOBA II which is a prospective, single-arm, multicenter study enrolling 213 patients, all with dissection following angioplasty [21]. Eligibility included Rutherford classification 2–4 with a de novo or nonstented restenotic lesion in the superficial femoral artery or proximal popliteal artery. The study allowed the use of plain balloon angioplasty (POBA) or Lutonix drug-coated balloons (DCBs) for treatment of the SFA or PPA. Balloon choice was at the discretion of the operator. Training in dissection identification and the use of the study device was provided to each operator prior to the index procedure. For the first time, the additional benefit of minimal metal as a concept of dissection treatment after DCB angioplasty was evaluated. Following dilation, lesions with <30% residual stenosis and the presence of ≥1 dissection were enrolled.

The 12-month efficacy endpoint was primary patency (freedom from duplex-derived binary restenosis and clinically driven target lesion revascularization).

Patients' mean age was 68 ± 9 years, and 43.2% had diabetes. Twenty-three percent of lesions were chronic total occlusions, and around 60% had moderate to severe calcium. The mean lesion length was 74.3 ± 40.6 mm. Severe dissections (grade ≥C) were present in 69.4%. By operator choice, 57.7% of patients underwent DCB angioplasty. Most (92.1%) dissections resolved completely, and only 1 bailout stent was required. There were no 30-day major adverse events. The 12-month efficacy endpoint was met, with Kaplan-Meier primary patency and freedom from clinically driven target lesion revascularization of 79.3% and 86.5%, respectively. At 12 months, there were no device fractures or clinically significant migrations, and significant improvements were noted in Rutherford category, ankle-brachial index, and quality of life.

The TOBA II study results support the use of the Tack Endovascular System as a therapeutic option that is both safe and effective for focal dissection repair following standard and DCB angioplasty of the SFA and PPA.

TOBA III addressed the issue of dissection repair in a purely DCB-treated cohort in the femoropopliteal arterial segment to show the effect of minimal metal repair after drug-coated technology [22].

The Tack Optimized Balloon Angioplasty III (TOBA III) study is a prospective, multicenter, single-arm study in which patients who underwent percutaneous transluminal angioplasty with the Medtronic IN.PACT™ Admiral™ drug-coated balloon and experienced post-angioplasty dissection(s) were treated with Tack implants. The primary endpoints were freedom from major adverse events at 30 days and primary patency at 12 months. Within this study also, the additional benefit of minimal metal as a treatment concept for patients with complex long lesions and dissections after DCB treatment was evaluated.

A total of 201 patients were enrolled in the trial, 169 with standard length lesions (≥20 mm and ≤150 mm) and 32 with long-length lesions (>150 mm and ≤250 mm). Safety and effectiveness results were favorable compared with historical benchmarks at 12 months in the standard lesion cohort. Notably, patients in the standard lesion length cohort experienced 95.0% primary patency, 97.5% freedom from clinically driven target lesion revascularization, 100% freedom from amputation, and 100% survival at 12 months ($p < 0.0001$). Primary patency in long lesion patients was 89.3%, freedom from clinically driven target lesion revascularization was 96.8%, and freedom from amputation was 100% at 12 months. Device success was achieved in 95.8% (182/190) and 97.7% (43/44) of devices deployed into standard and long lesion patients, respectively. Procedural success was 99.4% (168/169) and 100% (44/44) in the standard and long lesion cohorts, respectively, with only 1 bailout stent placed in the entire population.

These data show that the Tack Endovascular System is a safe and effective treatment option for patients with post-angioplasty dissections in the superficial femoral and proximal popliteal arteries, with a high patency, low rates of secondary intervention, and a low incidence of bailout stenting when used in combination with drug-coated balloon angioplasty, even in a long and complex lesion cohort.

In infrapopliteal arteries, there is even more discussions with regard to the adequate treatment for mechanical issues after angioplasty. No final solution so far can be proposed for this vessel area. Drug eluting stents in short lesions have shown some benefit, but there is still reluctance with regard to broader acceptance [23].

In a prospective, single-arm study, the concept of minimal metal for dissection repair in BTK arteries after POBA treatment was evaluated in patients with CLI and BTK lesions [24]. 11.4% were Rutherford category (RC) 4 and 88.6% were RC 5. BTK occlusive disease was treated with standard PTA, and post-PTA dissections were treated with Tack placement. The primary safety endpoint was a composite of major adverse limb events (MALE) and perioperative death (POD) at 30 days. Other endpoints included device success, procedure success (vessel patency in the absence of MALE), freedom from clinically driven target lesion revascularization (CD-TLR), primary patency, and changes in RC. Data through 12 months are presented.

Thirty-two of 35 (91.4%) patients had post-PTA dissection and successful deployment of Tacks. Procedural success was achieved in 34/35 (97.1%) patients with no MALEs at 30 days. The 12-month patency rate was 78.4% by vessel, 77.4% by patient, and freedom from CD-TLR was 93.5%. Significant ($p < 0.0001$) improvement from baseline was observed in RC (75% of patients improved four or five steps).

Tack implant treatment of post-PTA dissection was safe and effective for treatment of BTK dissections and resulted in reasonable 12-month patency and low rates of CD-TLR.

The concept proving TOBA BTK trial was followed by the TOBA II BTK study, which is a prospective, single-arm pivotal IDE study, including 233 patients with CLI and angiographic evidence of a dissection post-PTA requiring repair in the mid-popliteal/distal popliteal, tibial, and/or peroneal arteries at 41 US international sites [25]. Device success was achieved in 96.5% (303/314) of patients, bailout stent rate was low with 1.3% (3/233), and only 1 stent 0.4% (1/233) had to be placed within the tacked segment. The mean dissection length was 24 ± 18 mm, and a mean of 4.0 ± 2.8 tacks was placed per patient. The primary efficacy endpoint (freedom from MALE at 6 m + POD at 30 days) was achieved in 95.6% (196/205). Primary target lesion patency was 87.3%, freedom from CD-TLR was 92.0%, and this resulted in target limb salvage of 98.6% at 6 months. 6-month amputation-free survival was 95.7%. With regard to the clinical aspect of wound healing or improving in a CLI cohort, this could be achieved in 73.8% of wounds at 6 months.

References

1. Schneider PA, Giasolli R, Ebner A, Virmani R, Granada JF. Early experimental and clinical experience with a focal implant for lower extremity post-angioplasty dissection. JACC Cardiovasc Interv. 2015;8:347–54.
2. Fujihara M, Takahara M, Sasaki S, et al. Angiographic dissection patterns and patency outcomes after balloon angioplasty for superficial femoral artery disease. J Endovasc Ther. 2017;24:367–75.
3. Tepe G, Zeller T, Albrecht T, et al. Local delivery of paclitaxel to inhibit restenosis during angioplasty of the leg. N Engl J Med. 2008;358:689–99.
4. Tepe G, Zeller T, Schnorr B, et al. High-grade, non-flow-limiting dissections do not negatively impact long-term outcome after paclitaxel-coated balloon angioplasty? An additional analysis from the THUNDER study. J Endovasc Ther. 2013;20:792–800.
5. Kokkinidis DG, Armstrong EJ. Emerging and future therapeutic options for femoropopliteal and infrapopliteal endovascular intervention. Interv Cardiol Clin. 2017;6:279–95.
6. Dattilo R, Himmelstein SI, Cuff RF. The COMPLIANCE 360° trial: a randomized, prospective, multicenter, pilot study comparing acute and long-term results of orbital atherectomy to balloon angioplasty for calcified femoropopliteal disease. J Invasive Cardiol. 2014;26:355–60.
7. McKinsey JF, Zeller T, Rocha-Singh KJ, Jaff MR, Garcia LA, DEFINITIVE LE Investigators. Lower extremity revascularization using directional atherectomy: 12-month prospective results of the DEFINITIVE LE study. JACC Cardiovasc Interv. 2014;7:923–33.
8. Shammas NW, Lam R, Mustapha J, et al. Comparison of orbital atherectomy plus balloon angioplasty vs balloon angioplasty alone in patients with critical limb ischemia: results of the CALCIUM 360 randomized pilot trial. J Endovasc Ther. 2012;19:480–8.
9. Scheinert D, Peeters P, Bosiers M, et al. Results of the multicenter first-in-man study of a novel scoring balloon catheter for the treatment of infra-popliteal peripheral arterial disease. Catheter Cardiovasc Interv. 2007;70:1034–9.
10. Dick P, Sabeti S, Mlekusch W, et al. Conventional balloon angioplasty versus peripheral cutting balloon angioplasty for treatment of femoropopliteal artery in-stent restenosis: initial experience. Radiology. 2008;248:297–302.
11. Bosiers M, Deloose K, Cagiannos C, et al. Use of the AngioSculpt scoring balloon for infrapopliteal lesions in patients with critical limb ischemia: 1-year outcome. Vascular. 2009;17:29–35.
12. Shammas NW, Coiner D, Shammas GA, et al. Percutaneous lower-extremity arterial interventions with primary balloon angioplasty versus Silverhawk atherectomy and adjunctive balloon angioplasty: randomized trial. J Vasc Interv Radiol. 2011;22:1223–8.
13. Diamantopoulos A, Katsanos K. Atherectomy of the femoropopliteal artery: a systematic review and meta-analysis of randomized controlled trials. J Cardiovasc Surg. 2014;55:655–65.
14. Schillinger M, Sabeti S, Loewe C, et al. Balloon angioplasty versus implantation of nitinol stents in the superficial femoral artery. N Engl J Med. 2006;354:1879–88.
15. Krankenberg H, Schlüter M, Steinkamp HJ, et al. Transluminal angioplasty in superficial femoral artery lesions up to 10 cm in length: the femoral artery stenting trial (FAST). Circulation. 2007;116:285–92.
16. Bosiers M, Torsello G, Gissler H-M, et al. Nitinol stent implantation in long superficial femoral artery lesions: 12-month results of the DURABILITY I study. J Endovasc Ther. 2009;16:261–9.
17. Laird JR, Katzen BT, Scheinert D, et al. Nitinol stent implantation versus balloon angioplasty for lesions in the superficial femoral artery and proximal popliteal artery: twelve-month results from the RESILIENT randomized trial. Circ Cardiovasc Interv. 2010;3:267–76.
18. Klein AJ, Chen SJ, Messenger JC, et al. Quantitative assessment of the conformational change in the femoropopliteal artery with leg movement. Catheter Cardiovasc Interv. 2009;74:787–98.
19. Scheinert D, Scheinert S, Sax J, et al. Prevalence and clinical impact of stent fractures after femoropopliteal stenting. J Am Coll Cardiol. 2005;45:312–5.

20. Bosiers M, Scheinert D, Hendriks JM, Wissgott C, Peeters P, Zeller T, Brodmann M, Staffa R, TOBA Investigators. Results from the Tack Optimized Balloon Angioplasty (TOBA) study demonstrate the benefits of minimal metal implants for dissection repair after angioplasty. J Vasc Surg. 2016;64(1):109–16. https://doi.org/10.1016/j.jvs.2016.02.043. Epub 2016 Apr 29. Erratum in: J Vasc Surg. 2016 Nov;64(5):1552.
21. Gray WA, Cardenas JA, Brodmann M, Werner M, Bernardo NI, George JC, Lansky A. Treating post-angioplasty dissection in the femoropopliteal arteries using the tack endovascular system: 12-month results from the TOBA II study. JACC Cardiovasc Interv. 2019;12(23):2375–84. https://doi.org/10.1016/j.jcin.2019.08.005.
22. Brodmann M, Wissgott C, Brechtel K, Nikol S, Zeller T, Lichtenberg M, Blessing E, Gray W, TOBA III Investigators. Optimized drug-coated balloon angioplasty of the superficial femoral and proximal popliteal arteries using the tack endovascular system: TOBA III 12-month results. J Vasc Surg. 2020;72(5):1636–1647.e1. https://doi.org/10.1016/j.jvs.2020.01.078. Epub 2020 May 12.
23. Varcoe RL, Paravastu SC, Thomas SD, Bennett MH. The use of drug-eluting stents in infrapopliteal arteries: an updated systematic review and meta-analysis of randomized trials. Int Angiol. 2019;38(2):121–35. https://doi.org/10.23736/S0392-9590.19.04049-5. Epub 2019 Jan 16.
24. Brodmann M, Wissgott C, Holden A, Staffa R, Zeller T, Vasudevan T, Schneider P. Treatment of infrapopliteal post-PTA dissection with tack implants: 12-month results from the TOBA-BTK study. Catheter Cardiovasc Interv. 2018;92(1):96–105. https://doi.org/10.1002/ccd.27568. Epub 2018 Mar 24.
25. Geraghty PJ, Adams G, Schmidt A, TOBA II BTK Investigators. Six-month pivotal results of tack optimized balloon angioplasty using the Tack Endovascular System in below-the-knee arteries. J Vasc Surg. 2021;73(3):918–929.e5. https://doi.org/10.1016/j.jvs.2020.08.135. S0741–5214(20)32060–7. Online ahead of print.

Chapter 12
Drug-Coated Balloons in Infrainguinal Arteries

Sriya A. Avadhani, Serdar Farhan, and Prakash Krishnan

Background

Peripheral arterial disease (PAD) affects >200 million people worldwide and contributes to significant lifestyle-limiting claudication and to significant morbidity and mortality [1]. It involves some of the largest conduits in the body and is associated with significant atherosclerotic disease burden. Advances in endovascular therapies offer a minimally invasive approach to revascularization as an alternative to surgery with equal efficacy and lower periprocedural risk and complications [2, 3]. However, these therapies have limited long-term durability and have a high risk of restenosis.

The discovery of balloon angioplasty in 1977 by Andreas Gruentzig revolutionized the field of interventional cardiology as it offered a minimally invasive therapy for the treatment of coronary artery disease [4]. This was followed by the use of bare metal stents (BMS), which were initially developed to treat complications such as dissections and acute vessel closure; however, these were also limited by high rates of in-stent restenosis that affected nearly 30–40% of percutaneous coronary interventions (PCIs) [5]. This led to the discovery of drugs that inhibit smooth muscle proliferation and neointimal hyperplasia, processes which underlie the pathophysiology of restenosis.

S. A. Avadhani · S. Farhan · P. Krishnan (✉)
Zena and Michael A. Wiener Cardiovascular Institute, Mount Sinai Heart, Icahn School of Medicine at Mount Sinai Medical Center, New York, NY, USA
e-mail: sriya.avadhani@mountsinai.org; serdar.farhan@mountsinai.org; prakash.krishnan@mountsinai.org

N. W. Shammas (ed.), *Peripheral Arterial Interventions*, Contemporary Cardiology, https://doi.org/10.1007/978-3-031-09741-6_12

Drug-coated balloons (DCBs) were developed as a therapy to address restenosis by the delivery of antiproliferative drugs to the arterial wall upon balloon inflation. DCBs were first described in human use in 1995 by Camenzind et al. with the use of a coil-based dispatch balloon in 22 patients in the coronary arteries [6]. The porous balloon was designed to elute intracoronary heparin (known inhibitor of smooth muscle cells) under low-pressure inflation while maintaining distal perfusion for targeted therapy in an area of restenosis. This was fallen out of favor by the lack of significant inhibition of neointimal proliferation by the low molecular weight heparin, reviparin [7]. Other antiproliferative drugs such as colchicine and methotrexate were tested, however unsuccessful due to high washout rates and inadequate retention [8, 9]. Scheller et al. first described paclitaxel use in coronary arteries as a treatment for in-stent restenosis [10]. In a small study of 52 patients, 1 out of 22 (5%) patients treated with DCB had restenosis as compared to 10/23 (43%) in the uncoated balloon angioplasty group [10]. Subsequent studies also demonstrated efficacy of paclitaxel in the inhibition of coronary artery restenosis [11, 12]. The evolution and subsequent success of drug-coated therapies in the coronary arteries led to their extension into the treatment of peripheral artery disease.

Patency rates in femoropopliteal disease are limited by long lesions (which can sometimes measure between 200 and 300 mm) that are often accompanied by severe calcifications and chronic total occlusions (CTOs). Patency rates also vary depending on the therapy used. Percutaneous transluminal angioplasty (PTA) in focal lesions has patency rates of about 87% at 6 months and 78% at 3 years [13]. However, in longer lesions, this can be as low as 20–33% at 1 year [14, 15]. Data for the use of atherectomy in addition to PTA is limited to small single-center or registry data which demonstrate improved luminal gain and less bailout stenting; however, patency rates still remain around 60–80% at 1 year [16–18]. Although stents improve initial patency compared with PTA alone [18], the sustained benefit remains suboptimal, in particular for longer SFA lesions, with 1-year patency rates of 63–81% [19, 20]. Patency rates of contemporary drug-eluting stents (DES) remain at 79–86% and 77–83% at 12 and 24 months, respectively [21, 22], and drop to 72.4% at 5 years [23]. Challenges for stenting in the femoropopliteal space might include the length and calcification of arteries that can contribute to stent underexpansion and other factors including external compression and torsional forces from hip flexion/extension which can contribute to stent deformation and fractures and thereby lower patency.

Drug-coated balloons (DCBs) were developed to offer an attractive alternative therapy for femoropopliteal disease. With the delivery of sustained, localized anti-restenotic therapy upon balloon inflation, these devices avoid residual scaffold and polymer effects that might contribute to inflammatory or hypersensitivity reactions and thereby restenosis. DCBs are semi-compliant balloons covered in an antineoplastic drug, designed to locally deliver the drug upon contact with the vessel wall. At the time of writing of this chapter, DCB technology contains three main components which include currently approved cytostatic therapeutic agent, coating, and an excipient designed for efficient drug delivery to the vessel wall.

Technical and Pharmacologic Considerations of DCBs

The three components of the DCB—drug, coating, and excipient—play a crucial role in ensuring adequate drug uptake and retention, efficient transfer of the drug to the vessel wall, and minimal systemic loss and toxicity. Paclitaxel and sirolimus have been tested for use in DCBs. While both demonstrate rapid uptake and binding, paclitaxel achieves greater tissue concentrations, especially in the presence of contrast agents [24]. Paclitaxel's lipophilicity, which ensures drug uptake and retention by the vessel wall, wide therapeutic window, and lack of systemic toxicity at the doses adequate to inhibit restenosis, make it a drug of choice for DCBs.

Paclitaxel, a taxane, is an antineoplastic agent that induces the polymerization of elastin and tubulin leading to the formation of nonfunctional microtubules, thereby impairing intracellular signaling, protein secretion, and cell migration [25]. The inhibition of smooth muscle cell migration and endothelial cells occurs at much lower doses compared to those needed to achieve its antineoplastic effects. The lower doses seemingly affect the microtubule assembly leading to inhibition of cell structure, secretory processes, and motility; however, higher doses are necessary for cell apoptosis [26]. The local antiproliferative effects on vascular smooth muscle and extracellular matrix and inhibition of neointimal proliferation and hyperplasia make it an attractive agent for the treatment of de novo and restenotic atherosclerotic lesions. Early studies revealed inhibition of smooth muscle proliferation up to 14 days after a single-dose exposure to paclitaxel [26].

Current DCBs contain paclitaxel doses ranging from 1.3 to 3.5 μg/mm^2 with doses as low as 1 μg/mm^2 showing effective inhibition of neointimal hyperplasia [27]. Porcine studies have demonstrated that about 10% of the drug dosage is lost before it reaches target site and about 80% is released during balloon inflation [28]. However, only 20% is retained at the target site, while the remainder is lost into the distal circulation. While drug concentration may decline for a few days after delivery, up to 80% in 24 h [29], there is persistent drug concentration at the site even 6 months after therapy [30]. Additionally, studies show persistent inhibition of smooth muscle cells and collagen accumulation up to 90 days after DCB therapy [31]. Freyhardt et al. studied the bioavailability of paclitaxel in the plasma among 14 patients with SFA disease who underwent paclitaxel DCB therapy [32]. A maximum paclitaxel plasma concentration of 40.1 ± 76.6 ng/mL was found immediately after intervention, and within 24 h, the paclitaxel plasma level was below detectable levels in all patients [32]. In an FDA analysis, paclitaxel dose during treatment with current drug-coated balloons and stents corresponded to a dose range of 0.167–3.5 μg/mm^2 (maximum total drug load of 0.1–17 mg), while cytotoxic effects were noted to occur when drug concentrations exceeded 135–175 mg/m^2 over 3 to 24-h period [33].

There are several forms of paclitaxel in current DCB coatings ranging from amorphous, crystalline, hybrid, microcrystalline, and nanoencapsulations. Crystalline and amorphous are the most common forms and affect the amount of drug retention, drug loss, and, thereby, the pharmacokinetic behavior of the coating. While the amorphous paclitaxel provides a more homogenous coating, it results in a shorter duration of drug retention. In contrast, the crystalline form results in a prolonged retention time and, thereby, higher tissue levels and biologic efficacy, however at the expense of more drug loss. The crystalline formulation was found to have a lower washout rate (88.6% vs. 99.9% with amorphous at 7 days) and thereby higher concentration in the vessel wall at 7 and 28 days after treatment [34].

However, lipophilic substances are not necessarily soluble, a property required for quick release from the balloon and efficient delivery of the drug to the arterial wall. This was circumvented by the use of excipients or substances that prevent paclitaxel washout and enhance its transfer to the vessel wall. Paclitaxel in a contrast agent resulted in a higher local tissue concentration indicating the need for additional compounds to ensure drug transfer [28]. Early studies use iopromide, a contrast agent to enhance drug delivery, retention, and bioavailability by increasing the solubility of paclitaxel [28]. Preclinical data by Albrecht et al. investigated inhibition of restenosis in varying paclitaxel doses and coating with or without contrast medium [35]. Compared to a rate of in-stent restenosis close to 38% in the control group of uncoated balloons, there was a reduction of restenosis to about 18% in all subgroups treated with paclitaxel doses of 330 μg, 480 μg, and 6.4 mg dissolved in iopromide [35]. Polymer-based carriers, resorbable polymers, or non-polymeric agents such as urea, fatty acids, and contrast agents are also used to enhance efficient drug delivery.

Several other compounds have been used in various DCB platforms—including urea, shellac, BTHC (n-butyryl tri-n-hexyl citrate), polyethylene glycol (PEG), and ATEC (acetyl triethyl citrate). BTHC, a hydrophobic excipient used in the Passeo-18 Lux DCB (Biotronik), enhances paclitaxel retention in tissue to nearly 28 days after exposure [36]. Studies [37, 38] have suggested that there is heterogeneity in drug uptake with the use of various excipients. In a study of 45 patients [39], the IN.PACT Falcon DCB (urea-based) was associated with lower late lumen loss (LLL) and diameter stenosis at 6 months compared to the shellac-based DIOR DCB (Eurocor). The urea-based DCB was also associated with a higher in-stent fractional flow reserve (FFR) and lower decrease in neointimal volume at follow-up by optical coherence tomography (OCT) suggesting variations in the inhibition of neointimal hyperplasia and restenosis [39]. Interestingly, the Lutonix 035 and Stellarex excipient were noted to bind very strongly to the drug causing a slower dissolution rate and minimal drug release upon inflation [40]. Current DCBs that are approved for use in the United States along with their properties are summarized in Table 12.1.

Other important characteristics that play a role in drug delivery to the vessel wall include properties of the balloon catheter and vessel wall characteristics. Homogenous drug coating over the balloon catheter is essential to ensure uniformity in vessel wall coverage. Drug delivery catheters have gone through a series of evolution from hydrogel coated to double balloons and iontophoretic balloon catheters. Contemporary DCBs use balloons in which the drug is stored within pleats and folds to minimize drug loss during transfer. Vessel wall and plaque characteristics are also critical determinants of drug absorption. Calcium presents a barrier to paclitaxel absorption as shown by Fanelli et al. In lesions with significant calcium burden, the effect of paclitaxel was significantly lower [41]. In lesions treated with DCB, those with greater than 270 degree arc of calcium on CT angiography had

Table 12.1 Paclitaxel DCBs currently available for treatment of PAD in the United States

DCB	Company	Dose (μg/mm²)	RCT	Dose range in RCT (mg)	Excipient	Length (mm)	Diameter (mm)
IN.PACT	Medtronic	3.5	IN.PACT SFA I, II	1.9–21.7	Urea, THF, pyrogen-free water	40–220	4–7
Stellarex	Phillips	2	ILLUMENATE	1.3–9.4	PEG 8000 and iodine	40–120	4–6
Lutonix	Bard	2	LEVANT 1/2	1.0–11.3	Polysorbate and sorbitol	40–220	4–7
Ranger	Boston scientific	2	RANGER SFA	6.97 (Avg dose)	Acetyltributyl citrate	30–200	2–7

PEG polyethylene glycol, *RCT* randomized controlled trial, *THF* tetrahydrofuran

lower primary patency, ABIs, and higher LLL, TLR, and major adverse events compared to those with less than 90 degree arc of calcium suggesting that the effect of paclitaxel was diminished by the presence of calcium [41].

Lastly, the mechanical effect of balloon inflation not just allows for arterial wall stretch and plaque reduction to achieve an acute luminal gain but also facilitates drug delivery and retention. Drug delivery depends on the duration of balloon inflation, usually 30–60 s, after which drug concentrations plateau. The duration of balloon inflations was evaluated by Cremers et al. who found that balloon inflation times of 10 s were equally efficacious as longer inflations in the treatment of restenosis [42]. The study suggested that the drug (5 μg/mm² coated balloons) was rapidly transferred, within seconds after balloon inflation. In addition, they also demonstrated that doses up to 10 μg/mm² from two consecutive DCB inflations did not necessarily correlate with increased toxicity such as aneurysm formation or thrombosis [42].

Since drugs are mounted on semi-compliant balloons, adequate lesion preparation is also essential prior to DCB therapy. Pre-dilation is not just recommended for its acute mechanical effects; it is also shown to improve drug penetration into the vessel wall. Adequate pre-dilation minimizes drug loss upon balloon delivery and results in a more uniform expansion, hence more homogenous drug delivery to the lesion [43].

Clinical Applications of DCBs in PAD

Drug-Coated Balloons in Native Femoropopliteal Lesions

Current guidelines for the management of femoropopliteal disease after failed guideline-directed medical and exercise therapy support the use of endovascular therapies (Class IIA, LOE A) [44]. Endovascular intervention is recommended for patients with lifestyle-limiting claudication with hemodynamically significant lesions (Class IIA). Most lesions that contribute to intermittent claudication (70%) include femoropopliteal lesions, while the others include aortoiliac disease. Although treatment approaches may vary depending on the location, length, and lesion characteristic and clinical factors, an endovascular-first approach is usually recommended for iliac and femoropopliteal disease [45]. DCB use in native femoropopliteal disease is generally associated with improved patency rates compared to plain balloon angioplasty (PTA) as evaluated in several clinical trials, summarized in Table 12.2.

Drug-coated balloons in PAD were first evaluated in the *Local Taxan with Short Time Contact for Reduction of Restenosis in Distal Arteries* (THUNDER) trial in 2008 which assessed the efficacy of using DCBs in femoropopliteal disease among 154 patients [46]. Sixty six of these patients, followed up to 5 years, demonstrated restenosis rate of 17% (vs. 54% in PTA) and target lesion revascularization (TLR) of 21% in the DCB group (vs. 56% in the uncoated PTA) [46]. There was no evidence of safety concerns in the 5-year data including aneurysm formation and constrictive fibrosis [47]. There was significantly lower late luminal loss (LLL) in the DCB group compared to the balloon angioplasty group. Furthermore, these results were maintained despite the presence of moderate to severe dissections without stent implantation [56].

Similar results were established in the *Femoral Paclitaxel Randomized Pilot* (Fem-Pac) trial of iopromide-paclitaxel DCB vs balloon angioplasty of 87 patients [48]. Significantly lower LLL (0.5 ± 1.1 vs. 1.0 ± 1.1 mm; $p = 0.031$) and TLR

Table 12.2 DCB RCTs in native femoropopliteal lesions

		Treatment groups	Avg. lesion length	Primary EP	Outcome
THUNDER 2015 [46, 47]	Multicenter RCT 1:1:1 $N = 154$	Uncoated balloon PTA vs iopromide-paclitaxel (3 μg/mm^2) vs. paclitaxel diluted in iopromide (0.171 mg/cm^3)	7.5 cm	LLL, TLR at 6 months and 5 years	Iopromide-PCB sig. lower LLL (0.4 mm vs. 1.7 mm vs. 2.2 mm $p < 0.001$) and TLR (4% vs. 29%) for DCB vs. PTA At 5 years: restenosis, 17% DCB vs. 54% PTA TLR of 21% DCB vs. 56% PTA

Table 12.2 (continued)

Fem-Pac 2008 [48]	Multicenter RCT 1:1 $N = 87$	Iopromide-paclitaxel (3 μg/mm²) DCB vs. uncoated PTA	6.0 cm	LLL, TLR at 6 months Sustained at 18 months	Sig. lower LLL (0.5 vs. 1.0 mm, $p = 0.031$) and TLR (6.7% vs. 33% $p = 0.002$) for DCB vs. PTA
PACIFIER 2012 [49]	Multicenter RCT 1:1 $N = 91$	IN.PACT Pacific (3 μg/mm²) vs. uncoated PTA	7.0 cm	LLL, binary restenosis and MAE at 6 months	Sig. lower LLL was −0.01 mm vs. 0.65 mm ($p = 0.001$), binary restenosis (9% vs. 32%) and major adverse events (7% vs. 35%) for DCB vs. control
LEVANT I 2014 [50]	Multicenter RCT 1:1 $N = 101$	PTA vs. bailout stent-assisted strategy-both randomized to Lutonix DCB (2 μg/mm²) vs. uncoated PTA	8.0 cm (42% CTO)	LLL at 6 months	Both PTA and stent groups—better LLL at 6 months with the use of DCB (0.46 mm vs. 1.09, $p = 0.016$)
LEVANT II 2015 [51]	Multicenter RCT 2:1 $N = 543$	Lutonix (2 μg/mm²) DCB ($N = 316$) vs. standard PTA ($n = 160$)	6.27 cm (21% CTO)	Freedom from 1° safety EP and 1° patency at 1 year	65% vs. 52.6% DCB vs. PTA for 1° patency ($p = 0.015$) at 12 months 58.6% patency with DCB at 24 months 84% vs. 79% DCB vs. PTA for freedom from 1° safety EP ($p = 0.005$ for non-inferiority) No diff. in TLR at 1 year

(continued)

Table 12.2 (continued)

		Treatment groups	Avg. lesion length	Primary EP	Outcome
IN.PACT SFA I and II [52, 53]	Multicenter RCT 2:1 *N* = 331	IN.PACT DCB (admiral 3.5 μg/mm²) *N* = 221 vs PTA *N* = 111	8.9 cm (20–25% CTO)	1° patency or freedom from TLR (d/t symptoms or decrease in ABI), 1° safety EP and MACE at 1 year and up to 5 years	At 1 year: 82.2% vs. 52.4% 1° patency DCB vs. PTA ($p < 0.001$) TLR 2.4% vs. 20.6% ($p < 0.001$) Vessel thrombosis 1.4% vs. 3.7% ($p = 0.10$) At 3 years: 1° patency (69% DCB vs. 45% PTA, $p < 0.001$) and freedom from TLR (15.2% vs. 31% $p = 0.02$); not maintained in years 4–5 No sig. safety concerns up to 5 years
ILLUMENATE RCT [54]	Multicenter RCT 3:1 *N* = 294	DCB (Stellarex 2 μg/mm²) vs. PTA with uncoated balloon	7.1–7.2 cm (19% CTO)	1° patency at 12 month 1° safety EP (device-/procedure-related death) at 1 month and freedom from TLR/major amputation at 12 months	Superiority of DCB over POBA for 1° patency (83.9% vs 60.6%) at 12 months $p < 0.001$ Non-inferiority of safety EP (94% freedom from major amputation) and 83% freedom from TLR at 12 months
RANGER SFA [55]	Prospective RCT 2:1 *N* = 105	Ranger DCB (2-μg/mm² hydrophobic paclitaxel with TransPax coating) vs. uncoated balloon	6–6.8 mm (34% CTO)	1° patency Freedom from TLR Time to re-intervention	1° patency 86.4% DCB vs. 56.5% PTA at 12 months $p < 0.001$ freedom from TLR (91.2% DCB vs. 69.9% PTA, $p = 0.01$)

(6.7% vs. 33%; $p = 0.002$) were observed in the DCB cohort compared to uncoated balloon angioplasty [48]. TLR results were maintained up to 18 months of follow-up. The findings of these trials were further confirmed in *the Paclitaxel-coated Balloons in Femoral Indication to Defeat Restenosis* (PACIFIER) trial which assessed the efficacy of IN.PACT Pacific DCBs [49]. In addition to the primary endpoints of LLL and restenosis, there is a significant reduction in TLR and major adverse limb events at 1 year compared to uncoated angioplasty [49].

Lower-dose DCBs were studied in the *Lutonix Paclitaxel-Coated Balloon for the Prevention of Femoropopliteal Restenosis* (LEVANT I and II) trial using Lutonix 2 μg/mm^2 dosing using a sorbitol-based excipient. While the LEVANT I RCT showed promising results of reduced LLL at 6 months, there was no difference in TLR at 24 months [50]. The study was limited by a significant rate of balloon malfunction (due to a manufacturing defect of twisted balloon folds) that resulted in failed deployments [49]. Hence, the LEVANT II trial involving 476 patients with 2:1 randomization to Lutonix DCB vs PTA was conducted with a larger sample size and greater statistical power [51]. While there was a significant improvement in primary patency (defined as a composite freedom from TLR and binary restenosis) at 12 months, DCB was shown to be non-inferior to uncoated balloon angioplasty with respect to safety endpoints such as freedom from limb-related events and perioperative death (83% with DCB vs 79% in control, $p = 0.005$ for non-inferiority) [51]. Notably, there was no significant difference in functional outcomes (including change in Rutherford class, walking impairment score, and quality-of-life measures) and freedom from TLR (87.7% vs 83.2%, $p = 0.21$) which was concerning [51].

Using clinical endpoints such as clinically driven TLR (either due to symptoms or decrease in ABI), the IN.PACT SFA trial demonstrated that primary patency was still significantly higher in the DCB group up to a follow-up duration of 3 years [52]. In the IN.PACT SFA trial, the 3-year patency rate associated with the use of DCB was 69.5% which was significantly higher than PTA (45%) [52]. There was no significant difference between the two groups with respect to functional improvement. Through 5 years of follow-up, the DCB group demonstrated superiority in freedom from clinically driven TLR compared to the PTA group (74.5% DCB vs. 65.3% PTA, $p = 0.02$) [53]. Although there was no difference in the primary safety composite endpoint between the two groups, there was a statistically nonsignificant trend toward higher all-cause death in the DCB arm (15.8% DCB vs 9.6% PTA, $p = 0.156$).

Similar paclitaxel dosing with a polyethylene glycol coating was assessed in the *Randomized Trial of a Novel Paclitaxel-Coated Percutaneous Angioplasty Balloon* (ILLUMENATE) study using the Stellarex DCB (Phillips, Spectranetics). This study met its superiority endpoint over balloon angioplasty with respect to primary patency at 12 months (83.9% DCB vs. 60.6% PTA, $p < 0.001$) [54]. The DCB was found to be non-inferior compared to PTA (94% DCB vs. 83% PTA) for the safety endpoint (defined as freedom from TLR and major amputations) [54].

Recently, the Ranger (Boston Scientific) low-dose paclitaxel DCB with a novel TransPax coating was approved for use. In the pilot RCT of the Ranger DCB which included 105 patients, there was a significant improvement in primary patency (86.4% vs. 56.4% with PTA) and freedom from TLR at 12 months [55]. Subsequently, the Ranger II SFA (presented at Vascular InterVentional Advances, VIVA 2019) of 376 patients aim to randomize 3:1 treatment with the Ranger DCB vs. PTA. The primary patency (defined by ultrasound in the absence of CD-TLR or bypass of the target lesion) was 94.1% in the DCB arm compared to 83.5% wit PTA ($p < 0.01$ for non-inferiority). Significant reduction in CD-TLR (16.5% vs. 5.5%) was seen in the DCB group, and importantly, there was no significant difference in mortality between the two groups.

These proof-of-concept RCTs were supplemented by data from large, multicenter registries. The LEVANT SFA Global was a multicenter, prospective registry that enrolled 691 patients in 38 centers from 10 countries treated with Lutonix DCB for a follow-up period of 24 months [57]. Freedom from TLR, amputation and death was 89.3% overall, 88.2% for long lesions, and 84.6% for in-stent restenosis at 24 months. Site-reported primary patency (defined as the onset of patency failure) was 85.4% and 75.6% at 12 and 24 months, respectively. Seventy-six percent of patients had an improvement in at least 1 Rutherford class [57].

The larger IN.PACT SFA Global Study of 1535 patients and 1773 lesions from 64 sites worldwide and included complex femoropopliteal arterial disease (long lesions (≥150 mm, mean lesion length 12.09 cm), chronic total occlusions (CTOs) (35.5%), calcified lesions (68.7%), and in-stent restenotic (ISR) (18%) lesions) [58]. Procedural and angiographic data were measured by an independent core lab analysis. There was a 92.6% rate of freedom from TLR at 12 months using the IN.PACT Admiral DCB. At 36 months, this dropped to 76.9% and was significantly lower in patients with chronic limb-threatening ischemia (CLTI) vs. intermittent claudication (IC). The composite safety endpoint was met in 75.6% of the study population [58]. Additionally, a multivariate analysis predicted increased lesion length, ISR, bilateral disease, hyperlipidemia, CLTI, and vessel diameter <4.5 mm as predictors of CD-TLR [58].

In the ILLUMENATE Global prospective, multicenter registry of 371 patients treated with the Stellarex DCB, the patency (evaluated by Doppler ultrasound) was 81.4% and freedom from CD-TLR 95% at 12/24 months [59]. This was accompanied by clinical improvement in Rutherford classification to 90.3% and walking impairment questionnaire by 84% [59]. At 2 years, however, the primary patency was lower, at 72.4% [60].

Drug-Coated Balloons in Below-the-Knee Interventions

Endovascular interventions are an emerging tool for the management of below-the-knee critical limb-threatening ischemia (CLTI). Given the increased risk of amputation and major adverse cardiovascular events, the ACC/AHA 2018 guidelines provide an appropriate use indication for both endovascular and surgical approaches to the treatment of below-the-knee vessels [61]. Endovascular therapies to establish direct in-line blood flow to the foot in patients with nonhealing wounds or gangrene (Class I) is recommended. However, strong evidence for the use of DCB in below-the-knee interventions is still lacking.

In a meta-analysis of 6769 patients treated with infrapopliteal disease, primary patency at 1 year was 63%, 15% underwent repeat revascularization, and about the same also underwent amputation and died as a result of all-cause mortality [62]. Possible challenges with tibial artery interventions include extensive calcifications; long, diffusely disease segments; large number of CTOs; inability to estimate true vessel size; and, therefore, appropriate balloon sizing and possible loss of drug from the DCB due to longer delivery time.

Several studies have explored the safety and efficacy of DCBs in infrapopliteal disease. Table 12.3 summarizes the major RCTs that assessed the use of DCBs in major RCTs. Most of these trials are limited by a small sample size. The *Drug-Eluting Balloon Evaluation for Lower Limb Multilevel Treatment* (DEBELLUM) trial [63] which included 50 patients had about 25% below-the-knee lesions. At 6- and 12-month follow-up, the DCB arm had significantly lower LLL (0.5 mm vs 1.6 mm), TLR (6.1% vs. 23.6%), and binary restenosis rates (9.1% vs. 28.9%) compared to PTA. In addition, there was a significant improvement in Fontaine class in the DCB group compared to PTA (80% vs. 56%). The *Drug-Eluting Balloon in Peripheral Intervention for Below-the-Knee Angioplasty Evaluation* (DEBATE-BTK) trial evaluated patients with long lesions below the knee, and a significant proportion of them had occlusions (77–82%). In spite of these high-risk lesions, there was still a superiority benefit with the use of DCBs with respect to TLR and binary restenosis rates at 12 months [64].

These smaller trials which were followed by data from a large, multicenter randomized trial in below-the-knee critical limb ischemia [65] failed to show any significant benefit with the use of DCBs over PTA in the tibial arteries. In the *Randomized IN.PACT Amphirion Drug-Coated Balloon* vs. *Standard Percutaneous Transluminal Angioplasty for the Treatment of Below-the-Knee Critical Limb Ischemia* (IN.PACT DEEP) trial, 358 subjects were randomized 2:1 to DCB angioplasty with the IN.PACT Amphirion balloon or uncoated balloon angioplasty. The study demonstrated no significant benefit of DCB angioplasty over uncoated PTA at 5 years with respect to restenosis and TLR rates. This study also assessed a safety endpoint of all-cause death up to 5 years. While there was no difference in all-cause death, there was a nonsignificant but 2.4-fold increased risk of major amputations compared to the DCB group at 12 months and at 5 years of follow-up [65].

More recently, the IN.PACT BTK study (presented as an LBCT at TCT Connect 2020) evaluated the efficacy of the IN.PACT 0.014 DCB (3.5 μg/mm^2) compared to uncovered balloon angioplasty as a control. The study included patients with critical limb ischemia (CLI) and CTOs of the infrapopliteal arteries and lesions that were severely calcified and long (average length 17.6 cm). The results were promising, as the DCB group was associated with a 53% lower LLL compared to the PTA control group, both in the subsegmental (across the entirety of the lesion) and the classic LLL (at the narrowest segment of the artery) groups. In addition, there was no

Table 12.3 DCB RCTs in infrapopliteal PAD

		Treatment groups	Avg. lesion length	Primary EP	Outcome
DEBELLUM 2014 [63]	RCT 1:1 $N = 50$ patients, $N = 122$ lesions	IN.PACT Amphirion (3.5 μg/mm^2) DCB vs. PTA 75% fem-pop lesions, 25% below-the-knee disease	7.5 cm	LLL, TLR, and restenosis rates at 6 and 12 months	LLL 0.66 DCB vs. 1.69 PTA (0.03) at 6 months BTK TLR 12% vs. 35% Amputation rate 4% vs. 12% ($p = 0.36$) DCB vs. PTA
DEABTE-BTK 2013 [64]	RCT, single center $N = 132$, 158 lesions	IN.PACT Amphirion (3.5 μg/mm^2) DCB vs. PTA	13 cm 77–82% CTO	TLR at 12 months	Superiority of DCB with TLR (18% vs. 43%), binary restenosis rates (27% vs. 74%) and amputation rate (0% vs. 1.5%) DCB vs. PTA
IN.PACT DEEP 2014 [65]	RCT 2:1 $N = 358$	IN.PACT Amphirion ($N = 239$) (3.5 μg/mm^2) DCB vs. PTA ($N = 119$)	10–13 cm	Freedom from TLR at 5 years Safety composite major amputation and all-cause mortality	Freedom from TLR 68.6% vs. 78.4% and from CD-TLR 70.9% vs. 76% DCB vs. PTA Major amputation rate (15.4% DCB vs. 10.6% PTA $p = 0.11$) MAE at 5 years 60.8% vs. 58.4% $p = 0.2$ DCB vs. PTA
IN.PACT BTK 2020 (results to be published)	Prospective multicenter RCT 1:1 $N = 104$	IN.PACT 0.014 DCB (3.5 μg/mm^2) vs. PTA	17.6 cm	LLL (classic and subsegmental), TLR at 9 months Safety EP of device-/procedure-related mortality and freedom from CD-TLR and amputation at 9 months	Subsegmental LLL 0.59 mm vs. 1.26-mm DCB vs. PTA Classic LLL 0.89 mm vs. 1.31-mm DCB vs. PTA No sig. difference in safety EPs

significant difference in the safety endpoints which included device- and procedure-related death, major amputations, and clinically driven TLR at 9 months.

In a network meta-analysis by Katsanos et al., the secondary endpoint of TLR in infrapopliteal arteries demonstrated a significant 40% reduction associated with DCB use. The crude risk of TLR was 11.8% in the DCB group versus 25.6% in the uncoated balloon group. The calculated pooled risk ratio was 0.53 (95% CI 0.35–0.81; $p = 0.004$), with a corresponding number needed to treat eight patients (95% CI 4–25) [66].

DCB Use in Other Lesion Subsets: In-Stent Restenosis, Long Lesions, and Combination Therapy

In-Stent Restenosis (ISR)

Outcomes for the treatment of ISR depends on the type of lesion—focal lesions, classified as <5 cm; diffuse, generally >5 cm; and total occlusions [67]. In-stent lesions that are total occlusions are usually associated with high recurrent ISR than focal lesions in spite of the use of adjunctive therapies such as atherectomy [68].

Early studies from a single-center, Italian registry of 38 patients suggested successful treatment of SFA ISR with PTA followed by DCB post-dilation. This study showed a 2-year patency rate (defined as proximal velocity ratio of <2.4) of 70.3% in those treated with DCB [69]. This was followed by the *Femoropopliteal In-Stent Restenosis Repair: Midterm Outcomes After Paclitaxel-Eluting Balloon Use* (PLAISIR) trial, a small sample size prospective cohort study involving 53 patients with femoropopliteal ISR treated with IN.PACT Admiral DCB, which was found to have a 1-year patency rate of 84% and freedom from TLR of 90.2% [70]. Subsequent studies [71–74] demonstrated the efficacy of DCB in treating ISR lesions; however, these were limited by single-center studies and small study populations. These findings are reviewed in Table 12.4.

A meta-analysis by Cassese et al. included four RCTs which evaluated DCB angioplasty for femoropopliteal ISR [75]. A total of 367 patients were followed for a period of 12 months. The study showed that DCB angioplasty resulted in a lower risk of TLR, recurrent ISR, and sustained improvement in Rutherford class compared to plain balloon angioplasty. The DCB group had a lower risk for TLR (odds ratio 0.20, $p = 0.002$) and recurrent ISR (OR 0.24, $p = 0.003$) and a sustained RC improvement (OR 2.57, $p = 0.002$) compared to PTA [75].

This was also confirmed from a subsequent patient-level meta-analysis (2532 patients and 16 RCTs) which showed superiority of drug-coated therapies in ISR lesions [76]. The analysis compared multiple therapies including bare nitinol stents, covered stents, paclitaxel, or sirolimus stents and paclitaxel balloons with plain balloon angioplasty in femoropopliteal ISR. Restenosis and TLR were the lowest in paclitaxel stents and balloons, respectively, supporting the use of drug-coated therapies in in-stent restenotic lesions [76].

Table 12.4 DCB use in in-stent restenotic lesions

	Trial	Treatment arms	Avg. length	Endpoints	Outcomes
DEBATE-ISR 2014 [71]	RCT $N = 44$ Diabetics + fem-pop ISR	IN.PACT admiral ($N = 44$) (3.5 μg/mm²) DCB vs. PTA ($N = 42$)	137 cm	Recurrent ISR, TLE rate, up to 3 years	Recurrent ISR 19.5% vs. 71.8% DCB vs. POBA TLR 13.6% vs. 31% At 3 years: TLR 40% vs. 43% in DCB vs. PTA
FAIR 2016 [72]	Prospective single-center RCT 1:1 $N = 119$ SFA ISR	IN.PACT admiral (3.5 μg/mm²) DCB vs. PTA (admiral Xtreme)	82.2 mm 29% CTO	Restenosis at 6 months and 1 year Freedom from CD-TLR All-cause mortality at 12 months Thrombosis at 12 months	Restenosis at 1 year 29.5% vs. 62.5% DCB vs. POBA ($p = 0.004$) Freedom from CD-TLR 90.8% vs. 52.6% DCB vs. POBA at 1 year ($p = 0.0001$) All-cause mortality 4.3% vs. 6.8% ($p = 0.59$) at 12 month
PACUBA 2016 [73]	Prospective, dual-center RCT $N = 74$ ISR of fem-pop lesions	Freeway balloon with shellac (3.0 μg/mm²) DCB ($N = 35$) vs. PTA ($N = 39$)	173 mm	1° patency at 12 months (<50% stenosis by duplex or CTA without TLR) Complication rate at 1 month Clinical success (change in Rutherford/ABI, CD-TLR) at 30 days	40.7% vs. 13.4% DCB vs. PTA patency rate at 12 months $p = 0.02$ Freedom from CD-TLR 49% vs. 22% DCB vs. PTA, $p = 0.11$ Change in Rutherford 69% vs. 54.5% DCB vs. PTA

Table 12.4 (continued)

ISAR-PEBIS 2017 [74]	Dual-center RCT 1:1 $N = 70$ SFA ISR	IN.PACT admiral (3.5 μg/mm^2) DCB $N = 36$ vs. PTA $N = 34$	139 mm 36% CTO	% diameter stenosis at 6–8 months Binary restenosis, TLR, amputation/bypass surgery, and all-cause mortality at 24 months	% diameter stenosis 44% vs. 65% at 6–8 months Binary restenosis 30% versus 59% $p = 0.03$ TLE 19% vs. 50% $p = 0.007$ at 24 months

Long Lesions

Long femoropopliteal lesions remain a challenge for endovascular intervention with patency rates of 35–50% and often complicated by restenosis that is difficult to treat [77]. The SFA-Long study specifically addressed the role of DCB therapy in long femoropopliteal lesions [78]. The prospective, multicenter, single-arm study included 105 patients who had lesions greater than 15 cm (average lesion length 251 mm) and followed them for a period of 12 months. At follow-up, the patency rate, defined as freedom from combined endpoints of CD-TLR and by duplex ultrasound, was 83.2% [78]. In addition, at 12 months, there was a significant improvement in the quality of life (measured by walking impairment questionnaire) and in the ankle-brachial indices [78]. There was a 7% risk of adverse events which included death from any cause, thrombosis, or nontarget vessel revascularization [78].

In the single-arm sub-study of 131 patients from the IN.PACT Global study [79] with long and complex native ISR lesions ($N = 149$ lesions, 59% calcified and 34% CTOs), there was an 88% primary patency rate at 12 months treated with DCB. Preliminary data confirmed the safety and efficacy of using DCBs in long and complex ISR lesions in the femoropopliteal arteries [79]. Clinically driven TLR rate was 7.2%, and freedom from device-/procedure-related events was 92.7% at 1 year [79].

Combination Therapies

The increasing prevalence in the use of DCBs was accompanied with the development of several other therapies to address restenosis and improve patency rates in PAD. Most RCTs evaluating the use of DCBs in PAD excluded the use of other adjunctive therapies such as atherectomy, laser atherectomy, scoring balloons, and stents in their trial subjects. Data regarding the use of these adjunctive therapies with drug-coated balloons is limited. Calcium presents a barrier to paclitaxel absorption as shown by Fanelli et al. which showed significantly lower patency rates in calcified lesions treated with DCB [41]. In addition, elastic recoil, incomplete stent expansion, and dissections might affect the patency rates of balloon angioplasty, especially in long and calcified lesions. Atherectomy appears to reduce the risk of dissections and bailout stenting and improve acute procedural results [80, 81].

The *Directional Atherectomy* (HawkOne, Silver Hawk, TurboHawk Medtronic) *Followed by a Paclitaxel-Coated Balloon to Inhibit Restenosis and Maintain Vessel Patency* (DEINITIVE-AR) study first evaluated if vessel preparation with atherectomy prior to drug delivery improved outcomes [82]. It was suggested that plaque modification with directional atherectomy might enable a more homogenous drug delivery and increased penetration into the vessel wall [83]. In this pilot, prospective, multicenter randomized study of 102 patients, subjects were randomized to treatment with DAART (directional atherectomy with anti-restenotic therapy) plus DCB vs. DCB alone (Cotavance paclitaxel balloon with Paccocath coating, 3 μg/mm^2) alone [80]. The mean lesion length was 106 mm, and about 28% of them were occlusions [80]. One-year primary outcome of angiographic percent diameter stenosis was 33.6% in the atherectomy + DCB arm vs. 36.4% in the DCB arm ($p = 0.48$). Primary patency and rates of major adverse events were similar between the two groups demonstrating that the use of directional atherectomy prior to DCB therapy was safe and effective [80]. The rate of flow-limiting dissections was lower in the atherectomy plus DCB arm (2% vs. 19.4%, $p = 0.01$) [82]. In a single-center study of 78 patients, there was a statistically significant difference between primary patencies at 1 year associated with the use of DAART which was 82% compared to 65% with DCB alone [83].

In the recently presented data from the prospective *Directional Atherectomy and DCB to Treat Long Calcified Femoropopliteal Lesions* (REALITY study presented at Vascular InterVentional Advances (VIVA) 2020, November 6–7, 2020) study of 102 subjects evaluated the use of TurboHawk (Medtronic) atherectomy in conjunction with DCB. Preliminary data demonstrated a 12-month primary patency rate (by duplex ultrasound) of 77% and freedom from CD-TLR of 93% with the use of directional atherectomy prior to DCB (IN.PACT Admiral DCB) for long, calcified femoropopliteal lesions. The average lesion length was 17.9 cm, 39% were CTOs, and 86% had moderate-severe calcification.

Other debulking techniques, especially in the setting of in-stent restenosis, have also been gaining traction. The use of laser atherectomy (Philips) to debulk the ISR lesion, prior to the application of DCB, might help reduce restenosis and improve patency. While laser atherectomy has been shown to improve patency rates compared to PTA alone in the treatment of ISR [84], few studies have investigated its application with DCB. A dual-center observational study of 112 patients with Tosaka II–III lesions [67] underwent laser atherectomy plus DCB treatment and compared with laser atherectomy and plain balloon angioplasty. The use of DCB was associated with a significantly higher freedom from reocclusion (86.7% vs. 57.1%) and TLR (72.5% vs. 50.5%) at 1 year [85]. Further data from the currently enrolling Photo-Pac trial by Zeller et al. might add additional information regarding this therapy.

The use of orbital atherectomy (OA, CSI) in ex vivo peripheral arteries demonstrated a 50% increase in radiolabeled paclitaxel uptake and deeper penetration compared to the untreated segment in calcified plaque [86]. OA use was associated with thinner intima and less plaque calcification [86]. OA with the use of DCB was also investigated in a small retrospective study of 113 patients by Kokkinidis et al. [87]. In patients with heavily calcified femoropopliteal lesions, there were similar outcomes at 2 years with the use of OA in addition to DCB treatment compared to DCB alone (p = NS). The 2-year freedom from TLR was 76.1% in the OA plus DCB group vs. 55.5% in the DCB alone group [87]. There was a significantly lower rate of bailout stenting in the OA group; however, other procedural outcomes and complications were similar between the two groups.

More recently, the use of Jetstream atherectomy (JA) device (Boston Scientific), a rotational cutter with aspiration capacity approved for treatment of calcified femoropopliteal disease, was evaluated in adjunction to DCB in the single-center JET-SCE comparative study of 75 patients [88]. At 16 months, there was a significantly higher freedom from TLR associated with JA and DCB use compared with JA plus PTA (94.4% vs. 54%) [88]. The currently enrolling JET-RANGER randomized study will provide additional information.

The use of drug-eluting stents with DCB remains controversial. While the use of two different antineoplastic agents (paclitaxel-based balloons with limus-based stents) might offer a potential option in complex or recurrent ISR lesions, there remains concern about drug toxicity in overlap areas, incomplete endothelialization of stent struts, and the need for longer duration of dual antiplatelet agents [89].

Future Innovations in DCB Technology

A newer-generation, paclitaxel-coated SurVeil® DCB (Surmodics Inc.) was studied in PREVEIL, a prospective, US, multicenter, feasibility trial at three different clinical sites for the treatment of native femoropopliteal arteries. The lower-dose paclitaxel DCB (2 mcg/mm^2 loading dose) uses an excipient that improves efficacy and uniformity of paclitaxel drug transfer and minimizes systemic doses. In total, 13 patients were included with an average lesion length of 56 mm (Vascular InterVentional Advances (VIVA) 2018, Las Vegas, NV). Median paclitaxel plasma concentration peaked immediately post-procedure (Cmax 1.07 ng/mL) and was undetectable at 30 days (Vascular InterVentional Advances (VIVA) 2018, Las Vegas, NV). The plasma concentration achieved was much lower than the currently available DCBs, and there were no adverse events related to the drug or device reported. In addition, there was an improvement in ABI by 0.28, improvement in 6-min walk test by 90.4 m, and improvement in Rutherford class by 69%. Primary patency was achieved in all patients, LLL was 0.27 mm, and there were no reported TLR at 6 months (Vascular InterVentional Advances (VIVA) 2018, Las Vegas, NV). Although not available for clinical use in the United States, further larger trials including TRANSCEND RCT that compares the SurVeil DCB to IN.PACT DCB are still pending.

While sirolimus- and everolimus-coated stents have demonstrated safety and efficacy in the treatment of femoropopliteal disease [90, 91], limus-coated balloons offer a new alternative therapy for de novo and restenotic lesions. Given that limus-based, coronary stents have been shown to have more antiproliferative effect than paclitaxel-based stents [92] and are the cornerstone of interventional therapies for coronary artery disease, limus-based DCBs might offer the same benefit. Sirolimus is a cytostatic molecule that binds to the FKBP-12 molecule blocking cell cycle progression from G1/S phase [93]. However, given short tissue retention time and slow absorption, delivery of sirolimus for several weeks might be necessary for effective inhibition or neointimal proliferation [94]. The physical properties of the drug have made it difficult to be applied in DCB technology. Three sirolimus-coated balloons have been developed for intracoronary use—Magic Touch (Concept Medical) with a phospholipid excipient and carrier, the Virtue balloon (Orchestra BioMed), and SELUTION (MedAlliance). These balloons are also being applied in the peripheral vasculature.

The pilot SELUTION trial was a prospective, multicenter, single-arm trial that assessed 6-month safety and efficacy outcomes of the SELUTION SLR DCB in femoropopliteal arteries [95]. In this study of 50 subjects, outcomes including angiographic late lumen loss (LLL), binary restenosis, improvement in Rutherford class, ankle-brachial index, and patency by duplex ultrasound were all in favor of DCB over plain balloon angioplasty. The patency rate, measured by duplex ultrasound, was 88.4%, and freedom from binary restenosis was 91.2% at 6 months with the use of DCB [95]. Longer-term data pertaining to the use of this DCB remains to be seen. The ongoing XTOSI study by Edward Choke aims to study the application of the Magic Touch, a sirolimus-coated DCB in femoropopliteal arteries in critical limb ischemia.

Paclitaxel scoring balloons also offer an exciting new frontier in the treatment of PAD. With the ability for simultaneous plaque modification and drug delivery, these devices might offer better patency and restenosis rates compared to standard therapy. The recently approved Chocolate Touch DCB balloon was evaluated in the ENDURE trial which included 67 patients, majority with Rutherford class III. The 6-month patency rate was 90% by Duplex ultrasound and LLL of 0.16 mm, which was improved compared to the Lutonix and Stellarex DCBs [90]. Final results remain to be seen.

Mortality and Paclitaxel

In December 2018, a study-level meta-analysis by Katsanos et al. [96], which pooled data from 28 RCTs and included 4432 patients, found an increase in mortality associated with DCB use. While there was no statistically significant difference in 1-year mortality in the 28 RCTs, an increase in 2-year all-cause mortality was reported based on 12 RCTs which persisted at 5 years in 3 studies.

Of the three RCTs (THUNDER, ZILVER-PTX, and IN.PACT SFA) with 5-year follow-up, there was a 14.7% risk of death in the paclitaxel-treated arm vs. 8.1% in the non-paclitaxel arm (6.6% absolute risk) [96]. The authors reported a dose-related increase in mortality postulated to be due to downstream embolization and toxicity. However, the analysis was limited by study-level pooled data and the absence of patient-level data including individual cause of deaths to establish a causal relationship. The study was also limited by several RCTs that were under-powered to detect a mortality difference between the two groups, missing data beyond 2 years, crossover of treatment, and patients lost to follow-up. This led to an FDA guidance to healthcare professionals that cautioned against the use of drug-coated balloons due to an increase in long-term mortality [97].

Following this, a 3-year patient-level meta-analysis of the ILLUMENATE trials [98] was performed and failed to show any association of the Stellarex DCB with mortality for up to 3 years. In the meta-analysis, patient-level data from all patients treated with Stellarex DCB from six studies were included. Of the 1906 patients that were included, all-cause mortality was similar among the groups treated with DCB and PTA [98]. All-cause mortality was 2.1% at 1 year and 7.0% at 3 years of follow-up. Also, an independent patient-level meta-analysis of 1980 patients with 5-year follow-up data of the IN.PACT Admiral DCB showed no association of paclitaxel dose exposure and mortality [99].

Subsequently, an independent FDA analysis included the four RCTs (Zilver PTX, LEVANT 2, IN.PACT SFA I and II, and ILLUMENATE) with available 5-year follow-up data and incorporated trials that were not part of the Katsanos meta-analysis. A patient-level analysis by the FDA also found an increase in mortality associated with paclitaxel use, especially between 2 and 5 years (13.7% vs. 18.3% with DCB); however, this was limited by missing data of 14–38% in some trials [100]. At the same time, the Vascular InterVentional Advances (VIVA) physicians group meta-analysis was performed, which included 2185 subjects from 8 paclitaxel trials with 4-year follow-up of patient-level data and recovered missing data that was not included in the original meta-analysis. This study demonstrated a 4.6% absolute increase in all-cause death in patients treated with paclitaxel devices, which was lower than previously reported [101]. In addition, there was no evidence of drug dose-related exposure and mortality risk over 5 years [101]. However, since freedom from TLR and clinical improvement were still maintained, a full discussion of risks and benefits related to paclitaxel devices was recommended by the FDA.

Following this data, several large observational studies including Vascular Quality Initiative (VQI), OPTUM, and SAFE-PAD attempted to elucidate this mortality signal better. In the propensity-matched, Vascular Surgery VQI analysis of 8376 patients undergoing endovascular treatment of femoropopliteal disease, there was no difference in mortality at 1 year between paclitaxel and non-paclitaxel groups (9.6% vs. 12.6%, respectively) [102]. Mortality was lower in the paclitaxel subgroup of patients with intermittent claudication; however, this was not significant in the CLTI group [102]. A multicenter cohort of 16,560 patients from the Centers for Medicare and Medicaid Services, by contrary, found a lower cumulative incidence of all-cause mortality among those treated with paclitaxel therapies in femoropopliteal arteries (32.5% vs. 34.3%, $p = 0.007$). After multivariate adjustment, there was no difference in all-cause mortality between the two groups including patients with CLI and among those treated with DCB alone or DES with or without DCB [103]. This was also maintained among patients treated with DES compared to BMS in a Medicare cohort of 51,456 patients (51.7% DES vs. 50.1% BMS at 4.1 years, $p = 0.16$) [104]. Further data is awaited in the larger yet SAFE-PAD observational retrospective study by Secemsky et al., which includes all Medicare beneficiaries undergoing lower extremity revascularization.

Additional independent analyses that included large registry data in Germany also failed to show any association of mortality related to paclitaxel devices. In a large, propensity-matched cohort of 14,738 patients, there was no evidence of increase in mortality associated with paclitaxel use [105]. In a propensity-matched model, there was a lower all-cause mortality, amputation, and cardiovascular death in the paclitaxel cohort [105]. Freisinger et al. included all patients with BARMER health insurance who underwent any paclitaxel-based therapy for PAD (64,771 patients) [106]. The study also found no association of paclitaxel-coated devices with mortality for up to 11 years posttreatment [106]. Surprisingly, during the first year of follow-up, there was a decrease in mortality with paclitaxel devices compared to uncoated devices (HR 0.92, $p < 0.001$) which disappeared subsequently [106]. In a retrospective analysis of a similar cohort of 37,914 patients from the BARMER insurance group, a propensity score-matched analysis found an improved overall and amputation-free survival in the paclitaxel-treated CLTI and intermittent claudication (IC) groups [107].

The more recently published results of the SWEDEPAD [108] RCT also support these findings. In this randomized study, 2289 patients were randomized to drug-coated devices vs. uncoated therapies (65% with CLTI) and followed for 2–4 years. The multicenter trial was powered to detect a difference in the primary endpoint of mortality between the two groups. During the follow-up period, there was no difference in all-cause mortality between the two groups. The overall mortality in the DCB group was 10.4%. vs. 9.8% in the uncoated device group [108] which was not significant. The wealth of data since the publication of the meta-analysis by Katsanos et al. continue to support that paclitaxel-coated devices are not associated with an increase in all-cause mortality compared to uncoated devices (Fig. 12.1).

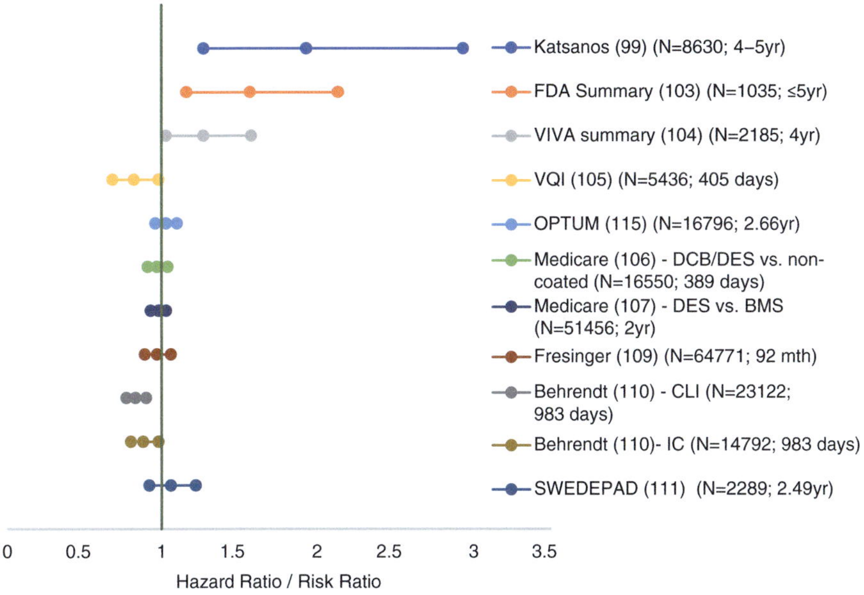

Fig. 12.1 Mortality risk associated with paclitaxel use among various contemporary studies. Hazard ratio greater than one corresponds to an increased risk in mortality. Study population size and duration of follow-up are listed along with the referenced study

Cost-Effectiveness of Drug-Coated Balloons

In addition to the lower rates of TLR and restenosis associated with DCB therapies, there is also evidence for an economic benefit related to these devices. The economic impact of drug-coated therapies was first examined by Pietzch et al. in a systematic economic analysis that included payers and providers in the United States and Germany [109]. Thirteen studies with 2406 subjects were included following BMS, DCB, DES, and plain balloon angioplasty. The 24-month probability for TLR was 14.3% vs. 19.3% vs. 28.1% vs 40.3% in the DCB, DES, BMS, and PTA groups, respectively. This corresponded to a lower economic budget over 24 months in the drug-coated groups compared to uncoated therapies ($10,214 DCB vs. $12,904 DES vs. $13,114 PTA vs. $13,802 BMS) [109].

Following this data, in a prospective randomized economic study of 181 patients from the IN.PACT SFA II trial, Salisbury et al. evaluated resource utilization over 2 years [110]. While the initial costs were $1129 higher in the DCB cohort, at 24 months of follow-up, limb-related costs were $1212 lower in the DCB group compared to uncovered balloon angioplasty (PTA) [110]. This is attributed to a lower number of repeat revascularization procedures in the DCB group including repeat target limb revascularization, amputation, and recurrent hospitalization, thereby contributing to increased costs in the PTA group. Overall, with the offset of costs between the two groups, there was no significant difference between the two groups at 2 years [110]. This data was similar to that derived from the UK National Health Service [111] which also reflected a lower lifetime costs and greater effectiveness associated with drug-coated therapy.

Conclusion

Since their initial discovery and application, drug-coated technology has made major advances and broadened its application in the treatment of infrainguinal peripheral artery disease. From the treatment of native femoropopliteal arteries to their extension into below-the-knee vessels, in-stent restenosis, and in combination therapies, DCBs play a critical role in the prevention of restenosis. The role of DCB in several of these applications remains to be elucidated as long-term data continues to emerge. While earlier concerns regarding the safety of paclitaxel therapies reflected an increase in mortality, several large, multicenter studies since then have failed to reproduce this finding. Sirolimus-coated balloons also offer an emerging therapeutic alternative for this technology. DCBs continue to remain a critical component for the treatment of PAD with their ability to efficiently deliver therapies to inhibit restenosis and improve patency rates in infrainguinal arterial revascularization.

References

1. Fowkes FG, Rudan D, Rudan I, et al. Comparison of global estimates of prevalence and risk factors for peripheral artery disease in 2000 and 2010: a systematic review and analysis. Lancet. 2013;382(9901):1329–40.
2. Antoniou GA, Chalmers N, Georgiadis GS, et al. A meta-analysis of endovascular versus surgical reconstruction of femoropopliteal arterial disease. J Vasc Surg. 2013;57(1):242–53.
3. Jones WS, Dolor RJ, Hasselblad V, et al. Comparative effectiveness of endovascular and surgical revascularization for patients with peripheral artery disease and critical limb ischemia: systematic review of revascularization in critical limb ischemia. Am Heart J. 2014;167:489–98.
4. Gruntzig A. Transluminal dilatation of coronary-artery stenosis. Lancet. 1978;1(8058):263.
5. Byrne RA, Joner M, Kastrati A. Stent thrombosis and restenosis: what have we learned and where are we going? The Andreas Grüntzig lecture ESC 2014. Eur Heart J. 2015;36(47):3320–31.
6. Camenzind E, Kint PP, Di Mario C, et al. Intracoronary heparin delivery in humans. Acute feasibility and long-term results. Circulation. 1995;92(9):2463–72.
7. Baumbach A, Oberhoff M, Bohnet A, et al. Efficacy of low-molecular-weight heparin delivery with the dispatch catheter following balloon angioplasty in the rabbit iliac artery. Catheter Cardiovasc Diagn. 1997;41(3):303–7.
8. Muller DW, Topol EJ, Abrams GD, et al. Intramural methotrexate therapy for the prevention of neointimal thickening after balloon angioplasty. J Am Coll Cardiol. 1992;20(2):460–6.

9. Gradus-Pizlo I, Wilensky RL, March KL, et al. Local delivery of biodegradable microparticles containing colchicine or a colchicine analogue: effects on restenosis and implications for catheter-based drug delivery. J Am Coll Cardiol. 1995;26(6):1549–57.
10. Scheller B, Speck U, Abramjuk C, et al. Paclitaxel balloon coating, a novel method for prevention and therapy of restenosis. Circulation. 2004;110(7):810–4.
11. Gershlick A, De Scheerder I, Chevalier B, et al. Inhibition of restenosis with a paclitaxel-eluting, polymer-free coronary stent: the European evaLUation of pacliTaxel eluting stent (ELUTES) trial. Circulation. 2004;109(4):487–93.
12. Scheller B, Hehrlein C, Bocksch W, et al. Two year follow-up after treatment of coronary in-stent restenosis with a paclitaxel-coated balloon catheter. Clin Res Cardiol. 2008;97(10):773–81.
13. Capek P, McLean GK, Berkowitz HD. Femoropopliteal angioplasty. Factors influencing long-term success. Circulation. 1991;83(2 Suppl):I70–80.
14. Hewes RC, White RI Jr, Murray RR, et al. Long-term results of superficial femoral artery angioplasty. AJR Am J Roentgenol. 1986;146(5):1025–9.
15. Rocha-Singh KJ, Jaff MR, Crabtree TR, et al.; VIVA Physicians, Inc. Performance goals and endpoint assessments for clinical trials of femoropopliteal bare nitinol stents in patients with symptomatic peripheral arterial disease. Catheter Cardiovasc Interv. 2007;69(6):910–919.
16. Dattilo R, Himmelstein SI, Cuff RF. The COMPLIANCE 360° trial: a randomized, prospective, multicenter, pilot study comparing acute and long-term results of orbital atherectomy to balloon angioplasty for calcified femoropopliteal disease. J Invasive Cardiol. 2014;26(8):355–60.
17. Ramaiah V, Gammon R, Kiesz S, et al. Midterm outcomes from the TALON registry: treating peripherals with SilverHawk: outcomes collection. J Endovasc Ther. 2006;13:592–602.
18. Roberts D, Niazi K, Miller W, et al. Effective endovascular treatment of calcified femoropopliteal disease with directional atherectomy and distal embolic protection: final results of the DEFINITIVE Ca++ trial. Catheter Cardiovasc Interv. 2014;84(2):236–44. Epub 2014 Jan 9.
19. Schillinger M, Sabeti S, Loewe C, et al. Balloon angioplasty versus implantation of nitinol stents in the superficial femoral artery. N Engl J Med. 2006;354(18):1879–88.
20. Bosiers M, Torsello G, Gissler HM, et al. Nitinol stent implantation in long superficial femoral artery lesions: 12-month results of the DURABILITY I study. J Endovasc Ther. 2009;16(3):261–9.
21. Garcia L, Jaff MR, Metzger C, et al. Wire-interwoven nitinol stent outcome in the superficial femoral and proximal popliteal arteries: twelve-month results of the SUPERB trial. Circ Cardiovasc Interv. 2015;8(5):e000937.
22. Gray WA, Keirse K, Soga Y, et al. A polymer-coated, paclitaxel-eluting stent (eluvia) versus a polymer-free, paclitaxel-coated stent (Zilver PTX) for endovascular femoropopliteal intervention (IMPERIAL): a randomised, non-inferiority trial. Lancet. 2018;392(10157):1541–51.
23. Dake MD, Ansel GM, Jaff MR, et al. Durable clinical effectiveness with paclitaxel-eluting stents in the femoropopliteal artery: 5-year results of the Zilver PTX randomized trial. Circulation. 2016;133(15):1472–83.
24. Levin AD, Vukmirovic N, Hwang CW, et al. Specific binding to intracellular proteins determines arterial transport properties for rapamycin and paclitaxel. Proc Natl Acad Sci U S A. 2004;101:9463–7.
25. Rowinsky EK, Donehower RC. Paclitaxel (taxol). N Engl J Med. 1995;332(15):1004 14. https://doi.org/10.1056/NEJM199504133321507. Erratum in: N Engl J Med 1995 Jul 6;333(1):75.
26. Axel DI, Kunert W, Göggelmann C, et al. Paclitaxel inhibits arterial smooth muscle cell proliferation and migration in vitro and in vivo using local drug delivery. Circulation. 1997;96(2):636–45.
27. Posa A, Hemetsberger R, Petnehazy O, et al. Attainment of local drug delivery with paclitaxel-eluting balloon in porcine coronary arteries. Coron Artery Dis. 2008;19(4):243–7.

28. Speck U, Scheller B, Abramjuk C, et al. Inhibition of restenosis in stented porcine coronary arteries: uptake of paclitaxel from angiographic contrast media. Invest Radiol. 2004;39(3):182–6.
29. Cremers B, Milewski K, Clever YP, et al. Long-term effects on vascular healing of bare metal stents delivered via paclitaxel-coated balloons in the porcine model of restenosis. Catheter Cardiovasc Interv. 2012;80(4):603–10.
30. Speck U, Cremers B, Kelsch B, et al. Do pharmacokinetics explain persistent restenosis inhibition by a single dose of paclitaxel? Circ Cardiovasc Interv. 2012;5(3):392–400.
31. Yazdani SK, Pacheco E, Nakano M, et al. Vascular, downstream, and pharmacokinetic responses to treatment with a low dose drug-coated balloon in a swine femoral artery model. Catheter Cardiovasc Interv. 2014;83(1):132–40.
32. Freyhardt P, Zeller T, Kröncke TJ, et al. Plasma levels following application of paclitaxel-coated balloon catheters in patients with stenotic or occluded femoropopliteal arteries. Rofo. 2011;183(5):448–55.
33. https://www.accessdata.fda.gov/drugsatfda_docs/label/1998/20262s24lbl.pdf
34. Granada JF, Stenoien M, Buszman PP, et al. Mechanisms of tissue uptake and retention of paclitaxel-coated balloons: impact on neointimal proliferation and healing. Open Heart. 2014;1(1):e000117.
35. Albrecht T, Speck U, Baier C, et al. Reduction of stenosis due to intimal hyperplasia after stent supported angioplasty of peripheral arteries by local administration of paclitaxel in swine. Invest Radiol. 2007;42(8):579–85.
36. Tepe G, Zeller T, Moscovic M, et al. Paclitaxel-coated balloon for the treatment of infrainguinal disease: 12-month outcomes in the all-comers cohort of BIOLUX P-III global registry. J Endovasc Ther. 2020;27(2):304–15.
37. Radke PW, Joner M, Joost A, et al. Vascular effects of paclitaxel following drug-eluting balloon angioplasty in a porcine coronary model: the importance of excipients. EuroIntervention. 2011;7(6):730–7.
38. Kempin W, Kaule S, Reske T, et al. In vitro evaluation of paclitaxel coatings for delivery via drug-coated balloons. Eur J Pharm Biopharm. 2015;96:322–8.
39. Nijhoff F, Stella PR, Troost MS, et al. Comparative assessment of the antirestenotic efficacy of two paclitaxel drug-eluting balloons with different coatings in the treatment of in-stent restenosis. Clin Res Cardiol. 2016;105(5):401–11.
40. Schorn I, Malinoff H, Anderson S, et al. The Lutonix® drug-coated balloon: a novel drug delivery technology for the treatment of vascular disease. Adv Drug Deliv Rev. 2017;112:78–87.
41. Fanelli F, Cannavale A, Gazzetti M, et al. Calcium burden assessment and impact on drug-eluting balloons in peripheral arterial disease. Cardiovasc Intervent Radiol. 2014;37(4):898–907.
42. Cremers B, Speck U, Kaufels N, et al. Drug-eluting balloon: very short-term exposure and overlapping. Thromb Haemost. 2009;101(1):201–6.
43. Tanaka A, Latib A, Jabbour RJ, et al. Impact of angiographic result after predilatation on outcome after drug-coated balloon treatment of in-stent coronary restenosis. Am J Cardiol. 2016;118(10):1460–5.
44. Gerhard-Herman MD, Gornik HL, Barrett C, et al. 2016 AHA/ACC guideline on the management of patients with lower extremity peripheral artery disease: a report of the American College of Cardiology/American Heart Association task force on clinical practice guidelines. Circulation. 2017;135(12):e726–79.
45. Norgren L, Hiatt WR, Dormandy JA, et al. Inter-society consensus for the management of peripheral arterial disease. Int Angiol. 2007;26(2):81–157.
46. Tepe G, Zeller T, Albrecht T, et al. Local delivery of paclitaxel to inhibit restenosis during angioplasty of the leg. N Engl J Med. 2008;358(7):689–99.
47. Tepe G, Schnorr B, Albrecht T, et al. Angioplasty of femoral-popliteal arteries with drug-coated balloons: 5-year follow-up of the THUNDER trial. JACC Cardiovasc Interv. 2015;8(1 Pt A):102–8.

48. Werk M, Langner S, Reinkensmeier B, et al. Inhibition of restenosis in femoropopliteal arteries: paclitaxel-coated versus uncoated balloon: femoral paclitaxel randomized pilot trial. Circulation. 2008;118(13):1358–65.
49. Werk M, Albrecht T, Meyer DR, et al. Paclitaxel-coated balloons reduce restenosis after femoro-popliteal angioplasty: evidence from the randomized PACIFIER trial. Circ Cardiovasc Interv. 2012;5(6):831–40.
50. Scheinert D, Duda S, Zeller T, et al. The LEVANT I (Lutonix paclitaxel-coated balloon for the prevention of femoropopliteal restenosis) trial for femoropopliteal revascularization: first-in-human randomized trial of low-dose drug-coated balloon versus uncoated balloon angioplasty. JACC Cardiovasc Interv. 2014;7(1):10–9.
51. Rosenfield K, Jaff MR, White CJ, et al. Trial of a paclitaxel-coated balloon for femoropopliteal artery disease. N Engl J Med. 2015;373(2):145–53.
52. Laird JR, Schneider PA, Tepe G, et al. Durability of treatment effect using a drug-coated balloon for femoropopliteal lesions: 24-month results of IN.PACT SFA. J Am Coll Cardiol. 2015;66(21):2329–38.
53. Schneider PA, Laird JR, Tepe G, et al. Treatment effect of drug-coated balloons is durable to 3 years in the femoropopliteal arteries: long-term results of the IN.PACT SFA randomized trial. Circ Cardiovasc Interv. 2018;11(1):e005891.
54. Schroeder H, Werner M, Meyer DR, et al. Low-dose paclitaxel-coated versus uncoated percutaneous transluminal balloon angioplasty for Femoropopliteal peripheral artery disease: one-year results of the ILLUMENATE European randomized clinical trial (randomized trial of a novel paclitaxel-coated percutaneous angioplasty balloon). Circulation. 2017;135(23):2227–36.
55. Steiner S, Willfort-Ehringer A, Sievert H, et al. 12-month results from the first-in-human randomized study of the ranger paclitaxel-coated balloon for femoropopliteal treatment. JACC Cardiovasc Interv. 2018;11(10):934–41.
56. Tepe G, Zeller T, Schnorr B, et al. High-grade, non-flow-limiting dissections do not negatively impact long-term outcome after paclitaxel-coated balloon angioplasty: an additional analysis from the THUNDER study. J Endovasc Ther. 2013;20(6):792–800.
57. Thieme M, Von Bilderling P, Paetzel C, et al. The 24-month results of the Lutonix global SFA registry: worldwide experience with Lutonix drug-coated balloon. JACC Cardiovasc Interv. 2017;10(16):1682–90.
58. Torsello G, Stavroulakis K, Brodmann M, et al. Three-year sustained clinical efficacy of drug-coated balloon angioplasty in a real-world femoropopliteal cohort. J Endovasc Ther. 2020;27(5):693–705.
59. Schroë H, Holden AH, Goueffic Y, et al. Stellarex drug-coated balloon for treatment of femoropopliteal arterial disease-the ILLUMENATE global study: 12-month results from a prospective, multicenter, single-arm study. Catheter Cardiovasc Interv. 2018;91(3):497–504.
60. Schroeder H, Meyer DR, Lux B, et al. Two-year results of a low-dose drug-coated balloon for revascularization of the femoropopliteal artery: outcomes from the ILLUMENATE first-in-human study. Catheter Cardiovasc Interv. 2015;86(2):278–86.
61. Bailey SR, Beckman JA, Dao TD, et al. ACC/AHA/SCAI/SIR/SVM 2018 appropriate use criteria for peripheral artery intervention: a report of the American College of Cardiology Appropriate use Criteria Task Force, American Heart Association, Society for Cardiovascular Angiography and Interventions, Society of Interventional Radiology, and Society for Vascular Medicine. J Am Coll Cardiol. 2019;73(2):214–37.
62. Mustapha JA, Finton SM, Diaz-Sandoval LJ, et al. Percutaneous transluminal angioplasty in patients with infrapopliteal arterial disease: systematic review and meta-analysis. Circ Cardiovasc Interv. 2016;9(5):e003468.
63. Fanelli F, Cannavale A, Corona M, et al. The "DEBELLUM"—lower limb multilevel treatment with drug eluting balloon—randomized trial: 1-year results. J Cardiovasc Surg. 2014;55(2):207–16.

64. Liistro F, Porto I, Angioli P, et al. Drug-eluting balloon in peripheral intervention for below the knee angioplasty evaluation (DEBATE-BTK): a randomized trial in diabetic patients with critical limb ischemia. Circulation. 2013;128(6):615–21.
65. Zeller T, Micari A, Scheinert D, et al. The IN.PACT DEEP clinical drug-coated balloon trial: 5-year outcomes. JACC Cardiovasc Interv. 2020;13(4):431–43.
66. Katsanos K, Spiliopoulos S, Kitrou P, et al. Risk of death and amputation with use of paclitaxel-coated balloons in the infrapopliteal arteries for treatment of critical limb ischemia: a systematic review and meta-analysis of randomized controlled trials. J Vasc Interv Radiol. 2020;31(2):202–12.
67. Tosaka A, Soga Y, Iida O, et al. Classification and clinical impact of restenosis after femoropopliteal stenting. J Am Coll Cardiol. 2012;59(1):16–23.
68. Armstrong EJ, Singh S, Singh GD, et al. Angiographic characteristics of femoropopliteal in-stent restenosis: association with long-term outcomes after endovascular intervention. Catheter Cardiovasc Interv. 2013;82(7):1168–74.
69. Stabile E, Virga V, Salemme L, et al. Drug-eluting balloon for treatment of superficial femoral artery in-stent restenosis. J Am Coll Cardiol. 2012;60(18):1739–42.
70. Bague N, Julia P, Sauguet A, et al. Femoropopliteal in-stent restenosis repair: midterm outcomes after paclitaxel eluting balloon use (PLAISIR trial). Eur J Vasc Endovasc Surg. 2017;53(1):106–13.
71. Grotti S, Liistro F, Angioli P, et al. Paclitaxel-eluting balloon vs standard angioplasty to reduce restenosis in diabetic patients with in-stent restenosis of the superficial femoral and proximal popliteal arteries: three-year results of the DEBATE-ISR study. J Endovasc Ther. 2016;23(1):52–7.
72. Krankenberg H, Tübler T, Ingwersen M, et al. Drug-coated balloon versus standard balloon for superficial femoral artery in-stent restenosis: the randomized femoral artery in-stent restenosis (FAIR) trial. Circulation. 2015;132(23):2230–6.
73. Kinstner CM, Lammer J, Willfort-Ehringer A, et al. Paclitaxel-eluting balloon versus standard balloon angioplasty in in-stent restenosis of the superficial femoral and proximal popliteal artery: 1-year results of the PACUBA trial. JACC Cardiovasc Interv. 2016;9(13):1386–92.
74. Ott I, Cassese S, Groha P, et al. ISAR-PEBIS (paclitaxel-eluting balloon versus conventional balloon angioplasty for in-stent restenosis of superficial femoral artery): a randomized trial. J Am Heart Assoc. 2017;6(7):e006321.
75. Cassese S, Ndrepepa G, Kufner S, et al. Drug-coated balloon angioplasty for in-stent restenosis of femoropopliteal arteries: a meta-analysis. EuroIntervention. 2017;13(4):483–9.
76. Katsanos K, Spiliopoulos S, Karunanithy N, et al. Bayesian network meta-analysis of nitinol stents, covered stents, drug-eluting stents, and drug-coated balloons in the femoropopliteal artery. J Vasc Surg. 2014;59(4):1123–1133.e8.
77. Armstrong EJ, Saeed H, Alvandi B, et al. Nitinol self-expanding stents vs. balloon angioplasty for very long femoropopliteal lesions. J Endovasc Ther. 2014;21(1):34–43.
78. Micari A, Vadalà G, Castriota F, et al. 1-year results of paclitaxel-coated balloons for long femoropopliteal artery disease: evidence from the SFA-long study. JACC Cardiovasc Interv. 2016;9(9):950–6.
79. Brodmann M, Keirse K, Scheinert D, et al. Drug-coated balloon treatment for femoropopliteal artery disease: the IN.PACT global study De novo in-stent restenosis imaging cohort. JACC Cardiovasc Interv. 2017;10(20):2113–23.
80. Shammas NW, Coiner D, Shammas GA, et al. Percutaneous lower-extremity arterial interventions with primary balloon angioplasty versus Silverhawk atherectomy and adjunctive balloon angioplasty: randomized trial. J Vasc Interv Radiol. 2011;22:1223–8.
81. Shammas NW, Lam R, Mustapha J, et al. Comparison of orbital atherectomy plus balloon angioplasty vs. balloon angioplasty alone in patients with critical limb ischemia: results of the CALCIUM 360 randomized pilot trial. J Endovasc Ther. 2012;19:480–8.

82. Zeller T, Langhoff R, Rocha-Singh KJ, et al. Directional atherectomy followed by a paclitaxel-coated balloon to inhibit restenosis and maintain vessel patency: twelve-month results of the DEFINITIVE AR study. Circ Cardiovasc Interv. 2017;10(9):e004848.
83. Stavroulakis K, Schwindt A, Torsello G, et al. Directional atherectomy with antirestenotic therapy vs drug-coated balloon angioplasty alone for isolated popliteal artery lesions. J Endovasc Ther. 2017;24(2):181–8.
84. Dippel EJ, Makam P, Kovach R, et al. Randomized controlled study of excimer laser atherectomy for treatment of femoropopliteal in-stent restenosis: initial results from the EXCITE ISR trial (EXCImer Laser Randomized Controlled Study for Treatment of Femoropopliteal In-Stent Restenosis). JACC Cardiovasc Interv. 2015;8(1 Pt A):92–101.
85. Kokkinidis DG, Hossain P, Jawaid O, et al. Laser atherectomy combined with drug-coated balloon angioplasty is associated with improved 1-year outcomes for treatment of femoropopliteal in-stent restenosis. J Endovasc Ther. 2018;25(1):81–8.
86. Tzafriri AR, Garcia-Polite F, Zani B, et al. Calcified plaque modification alters local drug delivery in the treatment of peripheral atherosclerosis. J Control Release. 2017;264:203–10.
87. Kokkinidis DG, Jawaid O, Cantu D, et al. Two-year outcomes of orbital atherectomy combined with drug-coated balloon angioplasty for treatment of heavily calcified femoropopliteal lesions. J Endovasc Ther. 2020;27(3):492–501.
88. Shammas NW, Shammas GA, Jones-Miller S, et al. Long-term outcomes with Jetstream atherectomy with or without drug coated balloons in treating femoropopliteal arteries: a single center experience (JET-SCE). Cardiovasc Revasc Med. 2018;19(7 Pt A):771–7.
89. Gray WA, Granada JF. Drug-coated balloons for the prevention of vascular restenosis. Circulation. 2010;121(24):2672–80.
90. Duda SH, Bosiers M, Lammer J, et al. Drug-eluting and bare nitinol stents for the treatment of atherosclerotic lesions in the superficial femoral artery: long-term results from the SIROCCO trial. J Endovasc Ther. 2006;13(6):701–10.
91. Lammer J, Bosiers M, Zeller T, et al. First clinical trial of nitinol self-expanding everolimus-eluting stent implantation for peripheral arterial occlusive disease. J Vasc Surg. 2011;54(2):394–401.
92. Birkmeier KA, Kastrati A, Byrne RA, et al. Five-year clinical outcomes of sirolimus-eluting versus paclitaxel-eluting stents in high-risk patients. Catheter Cardiovasc Interv. 2011;77(4):494–501.
93. Marx SO, Marks AR. Bench to bedside: the development of rapamycin and its application to stent restenosis. Circulation. 2001;104(8):852–5.
94. Carter AJ, Aggarwal M, Kopia GA, et al. Long-term effects of polymer-based, slow-release, sirolimus-eluting stents in a porcine coronary model. Cardiovasc Res. 2004;63(4):617–24.
95. Zeller T, Brechtel K, Meyer DR, et al. Six-month outcomes from the first-in-human, single-arm SELUTION sustained-limus-release drug-eluting balloon trial in femoropopliteal lesions. J Endovasc Ther. 2020;27(5):683–90.
96. Katsanos K, Spiliopoulos S, Kitrou P, et al. Risk of death following application of paclitaxel-coated balloons and stents in the femoropopliteal artery of the leg: a systematic review and meta-analysis of randomized controlled trials. J Am Heart Assoc. 2018;7(24):e011245.
97. US Food & Drug Administration. Treatment of peripheral arterial disease with paclitaxel-coated balloons and paclitaxel-eluting stents potentially associated with increased mortality letter to health care providers; 2019.
98. Gray WA, Jaff MR, Parikh SA, et al. Mortality assessment of paclitaxel-coated balloons: patient-level meta-analysis of the ILLUMENATE clinical program at 3 years. Circulation. 2019;140(14):1145–55.
99. Schneider PA, Laird JR, Doros G, et al. Mortality not correlated with paclitaxel exposure: an independent patient-level meta-analysis of a drug-coated balloon. J Am Coll Cardiol. 2019;73(20):2550–63.
100. Whatley E. FDA presentation, circulatory system devices panel meeting, Gaithersburg, MD June 19, 2019; post vital status.

101. Rocha-Singh KJ, Duval S, Jaff MR, et al. Mortality and paclitaxel-coated devices: an individual patient data meta-analysis. Circulation. 2020;141(23):1859–69.
102. Bertges DJ, Sedrakyan A, Sun T, et al. Mortality after paclitaxel coated balloon angioplasty and stenting of superficial femoral and popliteal artery in the vascular quality initiative. Circ Cardiovasc Interv. 2020;13(2):e008528.
103. Secemsky EA, Kundi H, Weinberg I, et al. Association of survival with femoropopliteal artery revascularization with drug-coated devices. JAMA Cardiol. 2019;4(4):332–40.
104. Secemsky EA, Kundi H, Weinberg I, et al. Drug-eluting stent implantation and long-term survival following peripheral artery revascularization. J Am Coll Cardiol. 2019;73(20):2636–8.
105. Heidemann F, Peters F, Kuchenbecker J, et al. Long term outcomes after revascularisations below the knee with paclitaxel coated devices: a propensity score matched cohort analysis. Eur J Vasc Endovasc Surg. 2020;60(4):549–58.
106. Freisinger E, Koeppe J, Gerss J, et al. Mortality after use of paclitaxel-based devices in peripheral arteries: a real-world safety analysis. Eur Heart J. 2020;41(38):3732–9.
107. Behrendt CA, Sedrakyan A, Peters F, et al. Long term survival after femoropopliteal artery revascularisation with paclitaxel coated devices: a propensity score matched cohort analysis. Eur J Vasc Endovasc Surg. 2020;59(4):587–96.
108. Nordanstig J, James S, Andersson M, et al. Mortality with paclitaxel-coated devices in peripheral artery disease. N Engl J Med. 2020;383(26):2538–46.
109. Pietzsch JB, Geisler BP, Garner AM, et al. Economic analysis of endovascular interventions for femoropopliteal arterial disease: a systematic review and budget impact model for the United States and Germany. Catheter Cardiovasc Interv. 2014;84(4):546–54.
110. Salisbury AC, Li H, Vilain KR, et al. Cost-effectiveness of endovascular femoropopliteal intervention using drug-coated balloons versus standard percutaneous transluminal angioplasty: results from the IN.PACT SFA II trial. JACC Cardiovasc Interv. 2016;9(22):2343–52.
111. Kearns BC, Michaels JA, Stevenson MD, et al. Cost-effectiveness analysis of enhancements to angioplasty for infrainguinal arterial disease. Br J Surg. 2013;100(9):1180–8.

Chapter 13
Stenting in Infrainguinal Interventions

Steve Henao

A Brief History of Femoropopliteal Stenting

On January 16, 1964, Charles Dotter, an American vascular radiologist working at the Oregon Health & Science University, performed the first-in-man percutaneous transluminal angioplasty (PTA) procedure in a stenotic superficial femoral artery. Dr. Dotter's successful procedure was an important medical milestone that forever changed the way physicians treat vascular disease. Since that time, multiple technologies have been developed to treat atherosclerotic disease of the superficial femoral artery (SFA), including plain balloon angioplasty, atherectomy, drug-coated balloons, bare metal self-expanding stents, and drug-eluting self-expanding stents. Over the last two decades, stent technologies have evolved to address the specific anatomical and pathophysiological challenges unique to the femoropopliteal segment.

Challenge of the SFA

The femoropopliteal segment poses several mechanical challenges in the treatment of atherosclerotic disease in the SFA. The SFA is one of the longest arteries in the body and extends between the hip and the knee, two regions of the body that are subjected to a high amount of mechanical force. Because the SFA extends through a highly muscular segment of the leg and is unsupported by the surrounding tissue,

S. Henao (✉)
Presbyterian Hospital, Albuquerque, NM, USA

N. W. Shammas (ed.), *Peripheral Arterial Interventions*, Contemporary Cardiology, https://doi.org/10.1007/978-3-031-09741-6_13

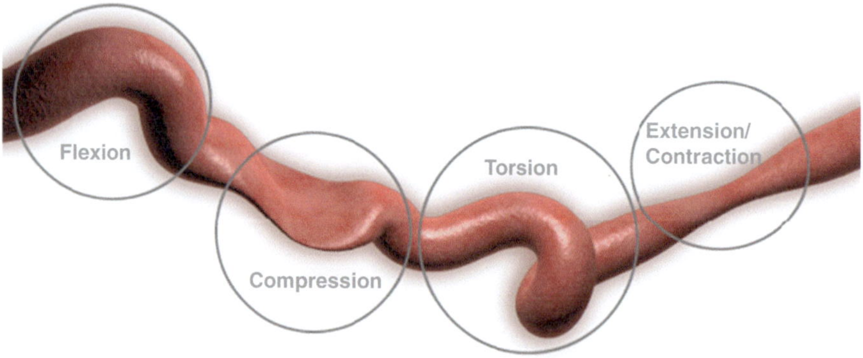

Fig. 13.1 Forces exerted on the SFA – flexion, compression, torsion, extension, and extension/contraction. (Abbott data on file)

it experiences a variety of intermittent mechanical stresses and deformations when performing activities such as walking, sitting, or climbing stairs. Forces exerted on the SFA include flexion, compression, torsion, extension, and contraction (Fig. 13.1) [1]. These forces, especially in the presence of a stent, are believed to cause constant injury to the vessel after an intervention, prolonging the duration of biological response to treatment and making the SFA more susceptible to restenosis.

The vascular wall of the femoropopliteal segment contains a higher density of vascular smooth muscle cells. Muscular arteries are more prone to develop extensive scar formation as a response to injury which can lead to restenosis [2]. Additionally, because the SFA is highly elastic, it undergoes longitudinal extension and axial distention which make it prone to deformation. From a pathophysiological perspective, the SFA is usually characterized by long, complex, heavily calcified lesions. This pattern of disease makes it more prone to acute PTA failure due to elastic recoil, vessel dissection, and residual restenosis.

Initial Treatment Approaches

Despite advances in balloon design and technique, the treatment of peripheral arterial disease (PAD) in the SFA with stand-alone PTA continues to demonstrate disappointing results with an estimated primary patency of less than 40% at 12 months [3]. Suboptimal clinical results and the risk of recoil and dissection have led to the adoption of stents for the treatment of SFA disease, both as a primary treatment therapy and as a bailout option in the case of acute PTA failure or complications. Balloon-expandable stents, like those used to treat coronary artery disease, were the first stents introduced to treat lesions in the SFA. However, these stents were short in length which limited their use to short femoral lesions, and because they were made of malleable metals, such as stainless steel or cobalt-based alloys, they were susceptible to stent crush by external forces. Additionally, multiple randomized trials failed to show a benefit with balloon-expandable stents compared to PTA [4–8].

The limitations of balloon-expandable stents in the treatment of femoropopliteal disease led to the development of self-expanding stents. Wallstent (Boston Scientific), one of the first self-expanding stents, was made of Elgiloy, a "superalloy" with high strength and ductility. Wallstent delivered good acute clinical results in the femoropopliteal artery but failed to sustain those results in the long term, and it was susceptible to stent fractures in the SFA [9, 10]. While Wallstent continues to be used in the venous anatomy today, it was eventually abandoned for the treatment of SFA lesions.

Nitinol-Based Self-expanding Stents

The development of self-expanding nitinol stents brought about an important advancement in the treatment of femoropopliteal disease providing strong radial force and resistance to crush. Nitinol, a super-elastic metal alloy of nickel and titanium, was invented in the early 1960s by William J. Buehler, a scientist at the US Naval Ordnance Laboratory who was experimenting with alloys for the development of aircraft nosecones. The unique mechanical properties of nitinol were immediately recognized, but it wasn't until the mid-1990s that nitinol self-expanding stents made their first appearance for the treatment of femoropopliteal disease. Multiple design factors, such as material selection, stent pattern, strut thickness, surface finish, connector geometry, and manufacturing process, are considered in the development of a nitinol stent, and each factor can have a profound impact on the acute performance of the stent as well as the longer-term clinical outcomes (Fig. 13.2) [11]. During the past two decades, manufacturers have made continuous advancements to nitinol stent design to improve stent performance and achieve better and more durable patient results.

Initially, nitinol was only available in a wire form, so the first nitinol stents consisted of coiled, knitted, or braided designs. These early designs tended to be thicker because of the crossing over of the wire, and they were more susceptible to

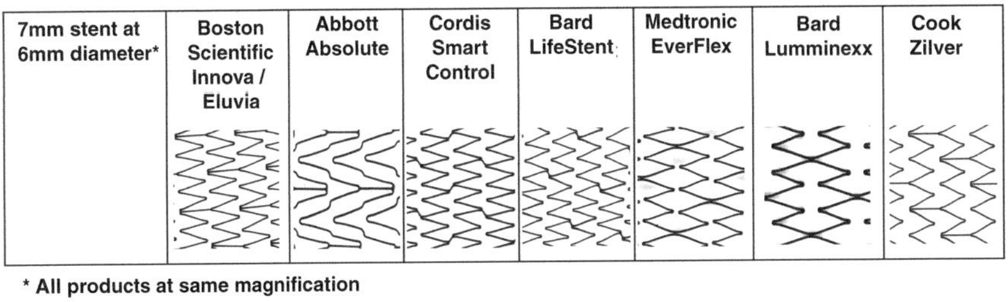
7mm stent at 6mm diameter*
Boston Scientific Innova / Eluvia
Abbott Absolute
Cordis Smart Control
Bard LifeStent
Medtronic EverFlex
Bard Lumminexx
Cook Zilver
* All products at same magnification

Fig. 13.2 Self-expanding stents produced by laser cutting of nitinol tubing (Boston Scientific data on file)

corrosion or wear at the crossover points. The first laser-cut nitinol stents were developed once nitinol sheets and tubing became available several years later. Most self-expanding stents today are produced by laser cutting of nitinol tubing.

First-Generation Stents

The first generation of nitinol stents was designed to provide good radial strength and crush resistance and to avoid permanent deformation, but they tended to be more rigid and were highly susceptible to stent fracture. Additionally, the early stents showed disappointing mid- and long-term clinical outcomes. In the Femoral Artery Stenting Trial (FAST), the Luminexx stent (Bard), a stent originally designed for treatment of the iliac arteries, was evaluated in the SFA. Despite the relatively short average lesion length in the study (45 mm), Luminexx failed to show an improvement in binary restenosis rates compared to stand-alone PTA, and stent fracture was reported in 12% of the patients [12]. The high fracture rate may be attributed to the rigidity of the stent and the suboptimal surface finish. The Vienna Absolute study (Abbott Dynalink/Absolute) was the first randomized trial to show superiority of nitinol self-expanding stents compared to PTA in the treatment of SFA lesions (63% vs 37% primary patency at 12 months, $p = 0.01$) [13]. These results represented a statistically significant improvement over stand-alone PTA, but they left room for improvement.

Issues with late mechanical fatigue and the resultant stent fractures were also observed in studies evaluating the performance of early-generation nitinol self-expanding stents. The SIROCCO I trial (drug-eluting versions of the Cordis SMART stent) reported fractures in 27% of the patients at 6 months. Despite reducing the allowed amounts of stents from three to two in the SIROCCO II trial, a study protocol that was intended to reduce the likelihood of fractures, investigators still observed a stent fracture rate of 11% [14].

Newer-Generation Stents

Manufactures sought to reduce fracture rates in newer-generation nitinol self-expanding stents by improving stent flexibility. This was achieved through several mechanisms: the quality of the nitinol was improved, open-cell designs were refined, and there were advancements in the stent surface finishing process, among other adaptations. Whereas many of the first-generation nitinol stents were designed to be implanted in less mechanically stressful anatomies (such as the biliary tract or iliac artery), newer, more flexible stents were designed to handle the unique biomechanical challenges experienced in the SFA. These stents demonstrated an improvement in patient outcomes and reduced fracture rates in the SFA. Randomized controlled trials evaluating these stents, including RESILIENT (Bard LifeStent), DURABILITY

II (Medtronic EverFlex), and SuperNOVA (Boston Scientific Innova), reported 12-month primary patency range from 74 to 81%, and fracture rates were below 5% [15–17]. The SUPERB trial, a single-arm study evaluating the Supera (Abbott) woven nitinol stent, reported an 86.3% primary patency at 12 months with no fractures. It is important to note that 50% of the stents in the SUPERB study were elongated and stent elongation was shown to reduce primary patency and freedom from target lesion revascularization [18].

Stent fractures have been found to occur more frequently in long stented segments with multiple overlapping stents [19]. In addition to improving stent design to minimize the likelihood of fracture, manufacturers also introduced longer stent lengths to the market to reduce the need to overlap stents when treating longer lesions. Other stent designs intended to increase conformability in the femoropopliteal artery are being investigated. The SMART Flex (Cordis/Cardinal) stent was designed with helical strut bands and "flex bridges" to reduce stent fractures. The BioMimics 3D stent (Veryan Medical) also has a three-dimensional helical shape which is intended to provide natural curvature in the SFA and to promote a laminar blood flow, which may have a protective effect on the endothelium.

Stent-Grafting in the SFA

Though initially reserved for treatment of traumatic lesions and exclusion of arterial aneurysms, adoption of covered stents as a treatment option for atherosclerotic disease of the SFA has increased with improvements in stent design. Early studies evaluating the performance of Dacron-covered stents in the SFA reported very low primary patency rates (23% at 12 months) [20]. The transition to stents covered with ePTFE improved primary patency rates and provided more favorable interaction with the vessel tissue. A physician-sponsored IDE trial evaluating the safety and efficacy of the Viabahn covered stent (Gore) reported a 73% primary patency at 12 months with an average lesion length of 26 cm [21].

Drug-Eluting SFA Stents

Initial efforts to bring drug-eluting stent technologies into the SFA were hindered by a lack of clinical improvement compared to bare metal stents. The SIROCCO II trial, which evaluated a sirolimus-eluting version of the SMART stent (Cordis), failed to show a statistically significant difference in efficacy between the sirolimus-eluting stent and the bare metal stent at 18 months [22]. The STRIDES trial, which evaluated an everolimus-eluting version of Abbott's Dynalink stent, demonstrated a concerning 32% restenosis rate at 12 months [23]. Efforts to commercialize these first DES stents were eventually abandoned. Results from the Zilver PTX randomized trial (Cook Medical) were more promising, showing an 83% primary patency rate at 12 months compared to 32% for the PTA arm. Zilver PTX is a self-expanding nitinol stent that releases paclitaxel without the use of a polymer or coating [24].

Results from the IMPERIAL study, a large randomized controlled trial comparing the Eluvia drug-eluting stent (Boston Scientific) to Zilver PTX, were recently reported. IMPERIAL demonstrated a 92% primary patency rate versus 82% for Zilver PTX at 1 year ($p = 0.0094$). Target lesion revascularization (TLR) rates were 13% for Eluvia and 20% for Zilver PTX at 2 years ($p = 0.0495$). The results for Eluvia represent some of the most impressive outcomes seen thus far in the treatment of SFA disease [25]. Eluvia is currently the only polymer-based drug delivery device for the treatment of femoropopliteal disease. Polymer-based drug delivery allows for a highly controlled and localized mechanism to deliver the lowest effective dose of drug to the site of treatment. It has been shown to significantly minimize downstream drug particulates, and it ensures that drug concentrations are sustained in the lesion long enough to match the restenotic physiologic process in the SFA [26].

Conclusion

Endovascular treatment of femoropopliteal lesions has seen dramatic advances since the advent of the first SFA stents. The transition from balloon-expandable stents to nitinol-based self-expanding stents, improvements in stent design, and the arrival of drug-eluting stents have led to better and more durable clinical outcomes with fewer adverse events.

References

1. Wood NB, Zhao SZ, Zambanini A, et al. Curvature and tortuosity of the superficial femoral artery: a possible risk factor for peripheral arterial disease. J Appl Physiol (1985). 2006;101(5):1412–8.
2. Schillinger M, Exner M, Mlekusch W, et al. Inflammatory response to stent implantation: differences in femoropopliteal, iliac, and carotid arteries. Radiology. 2002;224:529–35.
3. Rocha-Singh KJ, Jaff MR, Crabtree TR, et al. Performance goals and endpoint assessments for clinical trials of femoropopliteal bare nitinol stents in patients with symptomatic peripheral arterial disease. Catheter Cardiovasc Interv. 2007;69:910–9.
4. Zdanowski Z, Albrechtsson U, Lundin A, et al. Percutaneous transluminal angioplasty with or without stenting for femoropopliteal occlusions? A randomized controlled study. Int Angiol. 1999;18:251–5.
5. Vroegineweij D, Vos LD, Tielbeek AV, et al. Balloon angioplasty combined with primary stenting versus balloon angioplasty alone in femoropopliteal obstructions: a comparative randomized study. Cardiovasc Intervent Radiol. 1997;20:420–5.
6. Cejna M, Turnher S, Illiasch H, et al. PTA versus Palmaz stent in femoropopliteal artery obstructions: a multicenter prospective randomized study. J Vasc Interv Radiol. 2001;12:23–31.
7. Grimm J, Müller-Hülsbeck S, Jahnke T, et al. Randomized study to compare PTA with Palmaz stent placement for femoropopliteal lesions. J Vasc Interv Radiol. 2001;12:935–42.

8. Becquemin JP, Favre JP, Marzelle J, et al. Systematic vs. selective stent placement after superficial femoral artery balloon angioplasty: a multicenter prospective randomised study. J Vasc Surg. 2003;37:487–94.
9. Sabeti S, Schillinger M, Amighi J, et al. Patency of nitinol vs. wallstents in the superficial femoral artery—a propensity score adjusted analysis. Radiology. 2004;232:516–21.
10. Schlager O, Dick P, Sabeti S, et al. Stenting of the superficial femoral artery—the dark sides: restenosis, clinical deterioration and fractures. J Endovasc Ther. 2005;12:676–84.
11. Stoeckel D, Pelton A, Duerig T. Self-expanding nitinol stents: material and design considerations. Eur Radiol. 2004;14(2):292–301. Epub 2003 Sep 3.
12. Krankenberg H, Schluter M, Steinkamp HJ, et al. Nitinol stent implantation versus percutaneous transluminal angioplasty in superficial femoral artery lesions up to 10 cm in length: the femoral artery stenting trial (FAST). Circulation. 2007;116:285–92.
13. Schillinger M, Sabeti S, Loewe C, et al. Balloon angioplasty versus implantation of nitinol stents in the superficial femoral artery. N Engl J Med. 2006;354:1879–88.
14. Duda SH, et al. Drug-eluting and bare nitinol stents for the treatment of atherosclerotic lesions in the superficial femoral artery: long-term results from the SIROCCO trial. J Endovasc Ther. 2006;13(6):701–10. https://doi.org/10.1583/05-1704.1.
15. Laird JR, et al. Nitinol stent implantation vs. balloon angioplasty for lesions in the superficial femoral and proximal popliteal arteries of patients with claudication: three-year follow-up from the RESILIENT randomized trial. J Endovasc Ther. 2012;19(1):1–9. Absolute primary patency.
16. Matsumura JS, et al. The United States StuDy for EvalUating EndovasculaR TreAtments of lesions in the superficial femoral artery and proximal popliteal by usIng the Protégé EverfLex NitInol STent SYstem II (DURABILITY II). J Vasc Surg. 2013;58(1):73–83.e1.
17. Powell RJ, et al. Stent placement in the superficial femoral and proximal popliteal arteries with the innova self-expanding bare metal stent system. Catheter Cardiovasc Interv. 2017;89(6):1069–77. https://doi.org/10.1002/ccd.26976. Epub 2017 Mar 15.
18. Garcia L, Jaff MR, Metzger C, et al. Wire-interwoven nitinol stent outcome in the superficial femoral and proximal popliteal arteries: twelve-month results of the SUPERB trial. Circ Cardiovasc Interv. 2015;8(5):e000937. https://doi.org/10.1161/CIRCINTERVENTIONS.113.000937.
19. Scheinert D, et al. Prevalence and clinical impact of stent fractures after femoropopliteal stenting. J Am Coll Cardiol. 2005;45(2):312–5.
20. Ahmadi R, Schillinger M, Maca T, et al. Femoropopliteal arteries: immediate and long-term results with a Dacron-covered stent-graft. Radiology. 2002;223:345–50.
21. Viabahn instructions for use. https://www.accessdata.fda.gov/cdrh_docs/pdf4/P040037S060c.pdf. accessed 09/12/2022.
22. Duda SH, et al. Sirolimus-eluting versus bare nitinol stent for obstructive superficial femoral artery disease: the SIROCCO II trial. J Vasc Interv Radiol. 2005;16(3):331–8.
23. Lammer J, et al. First clinical trial of nitinol self-expanding everolimus-eluting stent implantation for peripheral arterial occlusive disease. J Vasc Surg. 2011;54(2):394–401. https://doi.org/10.1016/j.jvs.2011.01.047.
24. Dake MD, et al. Paclitaxel-eluting stents show superiority to balloon angioplasty and bare metal stents in femoropopliteal disease: twelve-month Zilver PTX randomized study results. Circ Cardiovasc Interv. 2011;4(5):495–504. https://doi.org/10.1161/CIRCINTERVENTIONS.111.962324. Epub 2011 Sep 27.
25. Gray W. Presented at LINC; 2020.
26. Data on file at Boston Scientific.

Chapter 14
Femoropopliteal Chronic Total Occlusions: Approach and Considerations for Crossing and Intervention

Michael H. Vu and Subhash Banerjee

Abbreviations

BTK	Below-the-knee
CA	Contrast angiography
CCD	CTO crossing device
CFA	Common femoral artery
CTA	Computed tomography angiography
CTO	Chronic total occlusion
DSA	Digital subtraction angiography
DUS	Duplex ultrasound
FP	Femoropopliteal
IVUS	Intravascular ultrasound
MRA	Magnetic resonance angiography
PCTO	Peripheral chronic total occlusion
RC	Rutherford classification
RCART	Reverse controlled antegrade-retrograde tracking
SFA	Superficial femoral artery
SI	Subintimal
STAR	Subintimal tracking and reentry
WC	Wire catheter

M. H. Vu
Methodist Health System of Dallas, Dallas, TX, USA
e-mail: MichaelVu@mhd.com

S. Banerjee (✉)
University of Texas Southwestern Medical Center, Dallas, TX, USA

Veterans Affairs North Texas Health Care System, Dallas, TX, USA
e-mail: Subhash.Banerjee@UTSouthwestern.edu

N. W. Shammas (ed.), *Peripheral Arterial Interventions*, Contemporary Cardiology, https://doi.org/10.1007/978-3-031-09741-6_14

Introduction

Femoropopliteal (FP) artery disease is responsible for a majority of lower extremity peripheral artery endovascular interventions. This accounts for approximately 55% of cases [1]. The FP artery crosses the hip and knee joints and courses through the adductor canal. This subjects the FP artery to increased mechanical stress resulting in a higher burden of atherosclerotic disease and restenosis [2]. Chronic total occlusions (CTOs) are a common finding in this vascular distribution and account for 40–50% of lesions treated [3, 4]. Therefore, it is necessary for an endovascular specialist to be adept at tackling FP-CTO lesions. Interventions on FP-CTOs are technically more challenging and are associated with higher complication rates, longer procedural time, and lower procedural success [5]. In this chapter, we will cover a framework for FP-CTO intervention with a systematic and step-by-step approach, which can lead to reproducible procedural success.

The following topics are covered in this section:

1. General principles
2. Procedure planning
3. Imaging
4. Vascular access
5. Treatment
    (a) Intraluminal and subintimal
    (b) Retrograde
    (c) Hybrid approaches
6. Below-the-knee chronic total occlusions

General Principles

A CTO is a completely occluded artery with thrombolysis in myocardial infarction (TIMI) 0 flow for a duration of at least 3 months. Without prior imaging, it can be clinically defined as an occluded artery without filling defects in the body to indicate an acute or subacute occlusion and no clinical history of acute lower extremity symptoms or acute limb ischemia [6, 7]. The CTO lesion length is defined as the angiographic distance between the proximal and distal caps and the CTO segment includes any additional lesions of ≥70% diameter stenosis compared to the reference vessel. Vascular calcifications associated with these lesions can be identified on angiography. They are classified as mild (isolated foci), moderate (contiguous segments on one or alternating sides), or severe (contiguous on both sides) [8]. Figure 14.1 displays an angiographic example of an SFA CTO with proximal and distal caps and collateral vasculature visualized.

Key decisions to make prior to FP-CTO intervention are vascular access, approach (antegrade, retrograde, or both), crossing strategy (guidewire or dedicated crossing

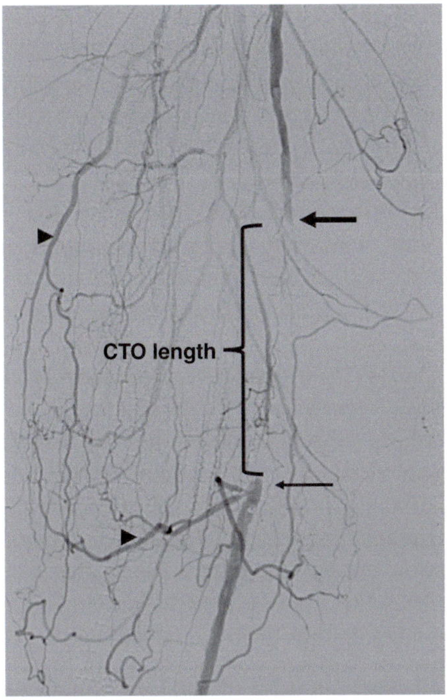

Fig. 14.1 Mid-superficial femoral artery chronic total occlusion (CTO). Thick arrow, proximal CTO cap; thin arrow, distal CTO cap; arrowhead, collateral vessels

device), and endovascular technique for intervention. Although a systematic and hierarchal approach is critical to successful crossing of FP-CTO lesions, it is important to maintain flexibility to account for intraprocedural findings and obstacles. This flexible strategy is termed the "hybrid approach." It refers to the utilization of all available techniques and approaches in order to achieve procedural success. This can be done by shifting the base of operations, the guidewire catheter complex, or the dedicated crossing device and attempting advanced crossing techniques. Advanced crossing techniques include but are not limited to reentry devices, reverse controlled antegrade-retrograde tracking (RCART), and subintimal tracking and reentry (STAR) [9, 10].

Procedure Planning

Preparation and planning for a FP-CTO procedure requires consideration of patient, angiographic, and technical factors. A patient's body habitus, renal function, current medications (antiplatelets or anticoagulants), surgical history, and comorbidities can influence body positioning during the said procedure and likelihood of procedural success or adverse events. Angiographically, lesion length, calcification, CTO cap characteristics (blunted or tapered), distal reconstitution, vessel course, and quality of target and vascular access vessel can be identified prior to the procedure. The chronic total occlusion crossing approach based on plaque cap morphology (CTOP) classification by Saab et al. is a useful guide (Fig. 14.2). It characterizes lesions based on proximal and distal cap morphology with type 1 being amendable to an anterograde approach and type IV lesions more suitable for a retrograde approach [11]. The scheme in the Percutaneous Crossing Algorithm for Femoropopliteal and Tibial Artery Chronic Total Occlusion (PCTO) algorithm described by Banerjee et al. incorporates lesion length, proximal cap features, and quality of target vessel and classifies them in three types with subgroups A, B, and C. An anterograde, antegrade or retrograde, or hybrid approach is recommended based on the classification (Fig. 14.3).

FP-CTO lesions tend to be heavily calcified, long (>150 mm), and multilevel [12]. Intervention on such lesions can be difficult as standard, luminal approaches are not sufficient. Failure to cross FP-CTOs is the primary reason for procedural failure. Failure rate can be as high as 30%. These lesions also carry a high risk of complications that include dissection, access site or retroperitoneal hematoma, embolization, perforation, bleeding diathesis, contrast-induced nephropathy, radiation injury, and others [5, 8]. As such, an ad hoc intervention on peripheral FP-CTOs is not advised. To maximize the likelihood of procedural success and to prepare for alternate techniques and approaches, thorough examination, lesion and vessel characterization through diagnostic testing, and planning cannot be overemphasized.

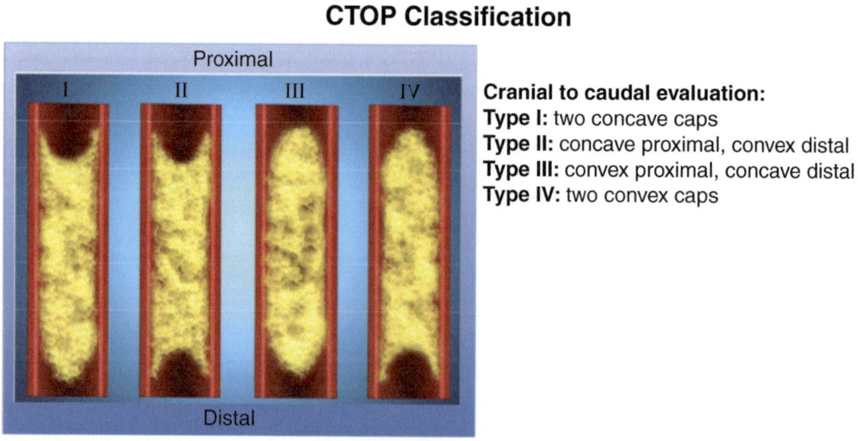

Fig. 14.2 The chronic total occlusion crossing approach based on plaque cap morphology (CTOP) classification

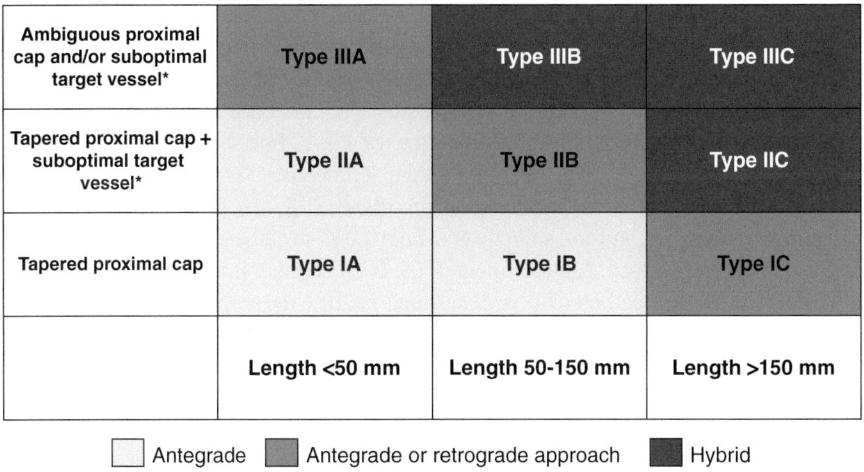
Ambiguous proximal cap and/or suboptimal target vessel*
Type IIIA
Type IIIB
Type IIIC
Tapered proximal cap + suboptimal target vessel*
Type IIA
Type IIB
Type IIC
Tapered proximal cap
Type IA
Type IB
Type IC
Length <50 mm
Length 50-150 mm
Length >150 mm
Antegrade
Antegrade or retrograde approach
Hybrid

Fig. 14.3 Schema in the Percutaneous Crossing Algorithm for Femoropopliteal and Tibial Artery Chronic Total Occlusion (PCTO) algorithm incorporating proximal cap features, quality of target vessel, and lesion length. (*Note*: From Banerjee S, Shishehbor MH, Mustapha JA, et al. A Percutaneous Crossing Algorithm for Femoropopliteal and Tibial Artery Chronic Total Occlusions (PCTO Algorithm). *The Journal of Invasive Cardiology*. 2019;31 [4]:18)

Imaging

Imaging modalities that are available for FP-CTO lesions include duplex ultrasound (DUS), computed tomography angiography (CTA), magnetic resonance angiography (MRA), digital subtraction angiography (DSA), and invasive contrast angiography (CA). CA remains the gold standard for diagnosis and endovascular treatment as it allows for optimal visualization of lesion length, lesion morphology, calcifications, patency of distal target, tibial vasculature, and contralateral iliac, profunda femoris, and pedal vessels [13]. DSA is preferred as it provides superior characterization of proximal and distal PCTO caps, side branches, collateral vessels, and distal vessel reconstitution [14]. CTA and MRA can provide valuable diagnostic information in regard to vascular anatomy and lesion morphology and are reliably accurate when compared to DSA [15, 16]. Proper selection of one or more of the aforementioned imaging techniques will provide the operator with an in-depth understanding of the target PCTO's anatomic features and help establish a safe, effective, and efficient strategy for crossing the occluded vascular segment.

For optimal CA, we advise beginning with an abdominal aortogram with the frame set to capture the infrarenal aorta, 10–20-mm superior to the aortic bifurcation. This can visualize multiple factors that can assist with case planning: aortoiliac disease, steepness of aortoiliac artery bifurcation, accessory renal artery takeoffs from common iliac arteries, external iliac tortuosity, presence of prior stents, and profunda femoris origin. A marker pigtail or RIM catheter (AngioDynamics, Latham, NY) can be used for this purpose.

The RIM catheter can be dropped to engage the contralateral common iliac artery origin. Imaging can be achieved by either (1) contrast injection into the contralateral common iliac artery to image the CFA bifurcation and capture the mid and distal superficial femoral artery segments or (2) using the CFA bifurcation image from the aortography and plan for selective injection of CFA. For the latter, a supportive hydrophilic 0.035-in guidewire (Advantage Glidewire, Somerset, NJ) can be advanced through the RIM catheter into the distal SFA, the RIM catheter is withdrawn and exchanged, and a straight tip end-hole 0.035-in catheter (CXI, Bloomington, IN) can then be advanced. Advancement of the RIM catheter into the distal SFA is not advised. The curved catheter tip is positioned against the vessel wall, and contrast injection can cause dissection or contrast staining. Selective cannulation of the SFA allows for FP and below-the-knee (BTK) angiography. It is important to note that if the ostial or proximal SFA is occluded, selective angiography of the CFA with filling of the profunda femoris can opacify distal reconstitution to evaluate distal FP, BTK, and distal foot perfusion. In patients with critical limb ischemia, visualization of pedal vessels is especially necessary. In claudicants, imaging up to the ankle vessels is highly recommended. It is best practice to evaluate foot perfusion in all cases if feasible. Selective DSA of distal FP or BTK angiography is preferred over runoffs in the absence of proximal or ostial SFA occlusion.

For FP and BTK CTOs, it is necessary to visualize the contralateral CFA, ipsilateral CFA bifurcation, and bilateral iliac vessels. The CFA bifurcation anatomy is relatively symmetrical, and an SFA origin with flush ostial occlusion can be estimated based on either its contralateral takeoff or linear calcification tracks that typically follow an occluded SFA course. Contralateral oblique projections are best for the iliac artery, whereas ipsilateral oblique projections are often needed for the CFA bifurcation. Anteroposterior and lateral oblique projections should be obtained in all cases in order to visualize the vascular anatomy of the foot.

The inferior epigastric artery origin is important to identify during CFA angiography. It serves as a landmark for the intrapelvic boundary of the external iliac artery and can be used during antegrade access of the SFA. Repeat diagnostic imaging of the SFA and BTK arteries is recommended if staged SFA intervention is planned after initial diagnostic angiogram or if initial diagnostic images are suboptimal. Finally, it is important to mention that the profunda femoris artery supplies most of the collaterals to the lower extremity, distal FP, and BTK vessels. Injury, dissection, embolization, ostial plaque shift, or obstruction must be avoided as failure to do so could result in acute ischemia of the lower extremity.

Vascular Access

Planning and obtaining adequate vascular access are crucial to the success of CTO crossing. Access selection should be based on choosing sites that support the operator's technical skill and an approach most appropriate for the given lesion. As detailed above, one may need to consider multiple or alternative access points to enable sufficient visualization of the primary lesion, delineation of distal and BTK vessels, account for surrounding atherosclerosis, and facilitation of the hybrid approach. Beginning with a 6- or 7-Fr vascular access sheath placed in the contralateral common femoral artery is frequently used to treat FP-CTO lesions. Of note, the tip of the 45-cm crossover sheath should be placed near the SFA-popliteal artery bifurcation as this will provide adequate support for additional guidewires and catheters.

Treatment

In patients with Rutherford Classification (RC) two to three symptoms who have failed or cannot tolerate exercise and pharmacologic therapy, with RC four to six symptoms, or critical limb ischemia, percutaneous intervention of FP-CTO lesions is advisable [17, 18]. Primary technical success is achieved when the initial strategy, wire catheter or crossing device, is successful in PCTO crossing. Secondary technical success includes switching from initial strategy to the other alternative. Provisional technical success refers to the use of a reentry device. When the CTO is crossed, it is important to confirm entry into the distal true lumen with intravascular ultrasound (IVUS) or angiography [8]. If the initial guidewire approach is unsuccessful in traversing the CTO segment, guidewire escalation or use of a crossing device is advised [19]. An escalation strategy should be attempted for approximately 10 min. If still unsuccessful, the operator should consider a retrograde approach [20].

Intraluminal and Subintimal

Intraluminal (IL) FP-CTO crossing is commonly used as an initial approach. A 0.014-, 0.018-, or 0.035-in hydrophilic guidewire is used with a support catheter or a CTO crossing device (CCD). CCDs are often only compatible with a 0.014 or 0.018 guidewire. The most frequently used wire catheter (WC) combination is a 0.035-in guidewire and microcatheter with a straight or angled tip. The operator advances the WC based on tactile feedback provided by the WC and the perceived vessel course. To prevent looping and dissection into the subintimal spice, the catheter tip must be kept close to the wire tip to limit the width of the guidewire loop [21]. Once the CTO is successfully crossed, the use of balloon angioplasty, atherectomy devices, or scoring balloons may be needed to debulk plaque material and create adequate space for larger stents or devices.

A subintimal (SI) crossing technique is when the WC is intentionally used to create a lumen between the intima and the adventitia of the artery (Fig. 14.4). The WC is advanced through the subintimal space until access to the distal true lumen is achieved. Again, a 0.035-in WC is frequently utilized [22]. The microcatheter should be flushed against the vessel wall, and the hydrophilic guidewire is advanced to create a loop. In order to maintain a narrow loop size, the two are advanced simultaneously, and the

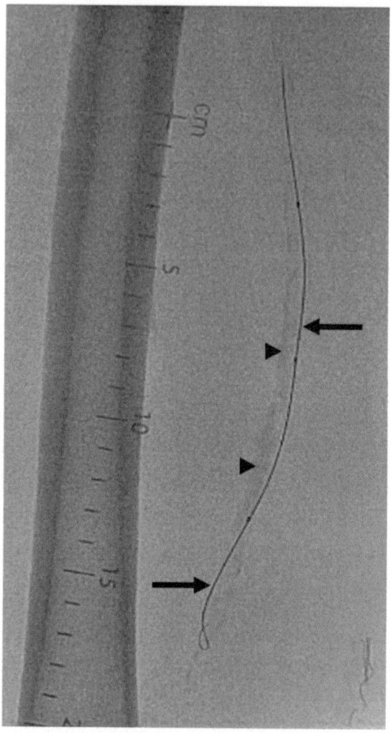

Fig. 14.4 Subintimal tracking of guidewire and catheter during crossing of a long and calcified superficial femoral artery chronic total occlusion (CTO). Thick arrows, subintimal tracking; arrowheads, extensive vascular calcification

catheter tip should be kept 10–20 mm away from the guidewire. If a specialized SI reentry device is needed, then it is delivered over the guidewire in the SI space, but a fresh guidewire should be passed into the true lumen through the reentry device. It is important to mention that SI passage limits the use of atherectomy catheters and is associated with a higher complication rate that includes perforation and loss of collateral vessels. Stenting is typically required to secure subintimal FP-CTO crossing.

Retrograde

Retrograde access to the SFA can be achieved through the popliteal or pedal arteries [23]. Traditionally, popliteal artery access requires the patient to be in the prone position, and this is not comfortable or ideal for the patient or operator. Pedal access is an option but is often limited by the length of available equipment for FP-CTOs. A retrograde approach via the supine position has been described by Shin et al. [24] A 15-mm, 21-gauge needle is used to penetrate the medial and ventral aspect of the patient's lower medial thigh which approximates the SFA, distal to the adductor canal. The puncture should be performed under fluoroscopy, and contrast injection through the sheath tip placed in the ipsilateral common femoral artery or proximal SFA may be necessary. The C-arm should be initially positioned in a contralateral oblique (30–45°) position. Once the puncture is made and the needle is advanced through the thigh muscles, the C-arm should be moved to a 90-degree orthogonal position to confirm if the needle is in line with the SFA. Once proper needle position is confirmed, the distal SFA can be punctured. A 0.018-in guidewire (V-18 Control, Boston Scientific, Natick, MA, USA) can be inserted through the needle followed by a 4- or 6-Fr, 10-cm sheath (Terumo) or support catheter. To deliver CCDs, a sheath may need to be inserted through the retrograde SFA puncture. Externalization and preferably antegrade delivery of balloons and stents complete FP-CTO recanalization. A retrograde guidewire can be advanced to engage the distal cap to serve as a distal cap marker when it is ambiguous or suboptimally visualized on angiographic imaging. This can assist with antegrade crossing. Pedal artery access is included in the section dedicated to below-the-knee CTO.

Hybrid Approaches

Antegrade reentry can be achieved with the knuckle wire technique. A looped polymer-jacketed guidewire is advanced toward the distal CTO cap through the SI space. This is done by avoiding excessive torqueing or rotation along with repeatedly retracting and advancing the guidewire in order to prevent a wide knuckled loop [25]. Subintimal tracking and reentry (STAR) technique is when a looped guidewire is advanced through the SI plan until it spontaneously enters the distal true lumen. The limited antegrade subintimal (LAST) technique utilizes an acute distal bend in the guidewire, approximately 45–60°.

Subintimal arterial flossing with antegrade-retrograde intervention (SAFARI) is a technique that can be utilized when antegrade SI approach is unsuccessful and retrograde access is in place. Retrograde SI dissection is performed until the SI space created by the antegrade attempt is reached. The retrograde guidewire is advanced through the antegrade sheath or catheter and externalized. Distal retrograde vascular access can be obtained via the popliteal, distal anterior tibial, distal posterior tibial, or dorsalis pedis arteries [26]. The rendezvous technique is a modified SI dissection technique where the antegrade SI space is kept very limited and is occupied by a support catheter. As seen in Fig. 14.5, a retrograde guidewire is advanced from the true or false lumen into the antegrade catheter, thereby creating a through-and-through guidewire connection [27]. Snares or balloon catheters can be used for distal or proximal vessel targeting.

With retrograde crossing, the knuckled loop guidewire technique is used to create and further dissect the SI space, similar to the antegrade approach. Reentry can be achieved through controlled antegrade-retrograde dissection or reentry (CART) or reverse CART (RCART). CART refers to when a balloon is inflated and then deflated over the retrograde guidewire when the antegrade guidewire is advanced into the distal true lumen. RCART is more frequently utilized and involves balloon inflation over the antegrade guidewire followed by advancement of the retrograde wire into the proximal true lumen. A detailed illustration is provided in Fig. 14.6. The most common reason for RCART failure is balloon undersizing. Therefore, performing this technique alongside IVUS is advised for correct balloon sizing [28].

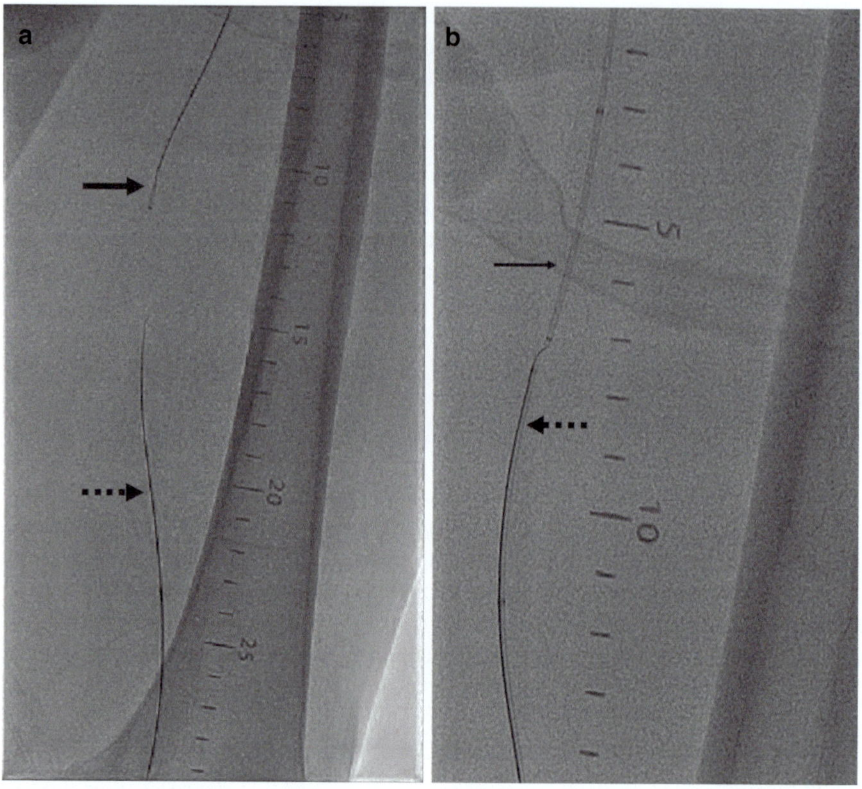

Fig. 14.5 Hybrid approach. (**a**) Antegrade guidewire and catheter enter the subintimal space (thick arrow). A 0.035-inch support catheter is placed in the narrow antegrade subintimal space (thin arrow). (**b**) Retrograde guidewire and catheter advanced via retrograde pedal access (dashed arrow). Retrograde guidewire penetrates the antegrade subintimal space into the receiving catheter present in the antegrade subintimal space and externalized to complete the procedure

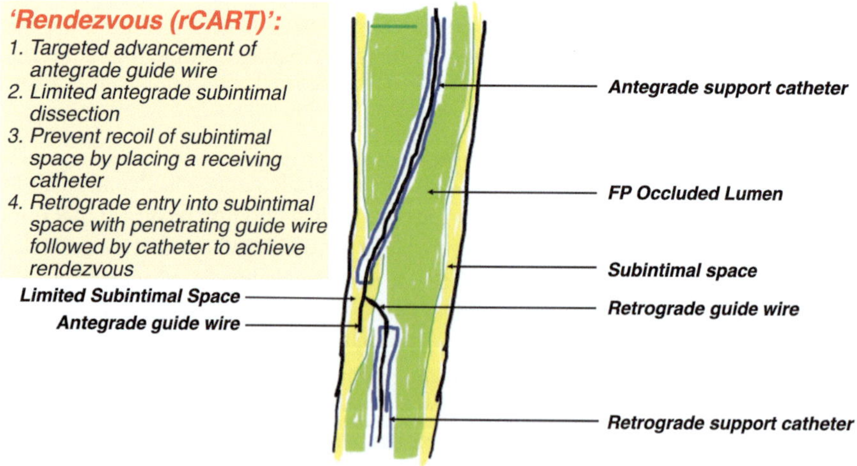

Fig. 14.6 Detailed illustration depicting concept of reverse controlled antegrade-retrograde dissection or reentry

"Tunneling" refers to passing a retrograde or antegrade guidewire from a respective retrograde or antegrade catheter into a receiving catheter on the contralateral side [29]. The re-back technique involves the use of a needle-based reentry device into a retrograde balloon [30]. Inflation of two balloon catheters over antegrade and retrograde guidewires in order to merge the subintimal places is referred to as the double-balloon technique. This can facilitate true lumen entry in either the antegrade or the retrograde direction [23]. Finally, controlled dissection reentry can be achieved through specialized reentry devices. Figure 14.7 highlights guidewire selection for FP-CTO crossing. Tables 14.1 and 14.2 depict preferred guidewires and crossing devices.

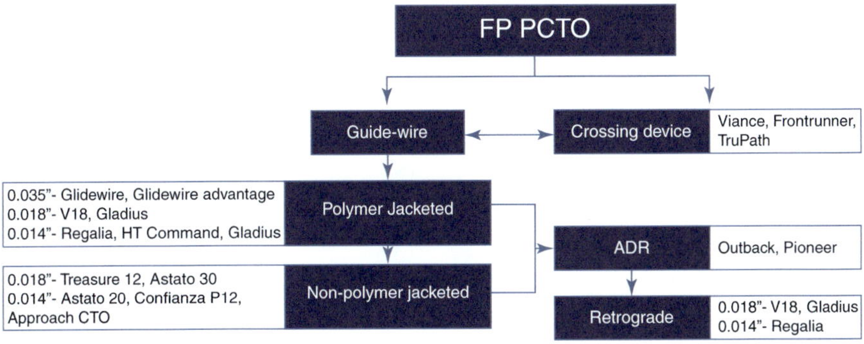

Fig. 14.7 Scheme for guidewire selection in femoropopliteal chronic total occlusion crossing. (*Note*: From Banerjee S, Shishehbor MH, Mustapha JA, et al. A Percutaneous Crossing Algorithm for Femoropopliteal and Tibial Artery Chronic Total Occlusions (PCTO Algorithm). *The Journal of Invasive Cardiology*. 2019;31 (4):18)

Table 14.1 Preferred guidewires with specifications for femoropopliteal chronic total occlusion crossing

Guidewire	Outer diameter [in]	Core material	Tip load	Description
0.035″ polymer jacket				
GlideWire 3 cm straight [Terumo]	0.035″	Nitinol	44.8 g	Supportive 0.035″ guidewire for delivering devices
GlideWire advantage 5 cm angled [Terumo]	0.035″	Nitinol	11.1 g	Nitinol guidewire with lower tip load for navigation
0.018″ polymer jacket				
V18—control wire/ short taper [Boston Scientific]	0.018″	Stainless	3 g	Supportive peripheral guidewire
Gladius [Asahi Intecc]	0.018″	Stainless	4 g	Composite core improves torque response with increased support for device delivery
Glide tip gold 3 cm straight/angled [Terumo]	0.018″	Stainless/ nitinol	4.1	Stainless-steel body with nitinol tip

(continued)

Table 14.1 (continued)

Guidewire	Outer diameter [in]	Core material	Tip load	Description
0.018″ non-polymer jacket				
Treasure 12 [Asahi Intecc]	0.018″	Stainless	12 g	Consistent response and tactile feedback for complex lesion navigation
Astato 30 [Asahi Intecc]	0.018″	Stainless	30 g	Tapered tip and high tip load for penetration
Platinum plus 0.018 [Boston Scientific]	0.018″	Stainless	NA	High support to deliver devices
SV5 [Cordis]	0.018″	Stainless	NA	High support to deliver devices
High-torque steel Core [Abbott Vascular]	0.018″	Stainless	NA	High support to deliver devices
0.014″ polymer jacket				
Regalia XS 1.0 [Asahi Intecc]	0.014″	Stainless	1 g	Balanced lubricity and trackability for below-the-knee procedures
Hi-torque command ES [Abbott vascular]	0.014″	Stainless/nitinol	3.5 g	Stainless-steel body with nitinol tip for durability
Gladius 0.014 [Asahi Intecc]	0.014″	Stainless	3 g	Composite core for improved torque and durability
GlideWire advantage 0.014 [Terumo]	0.014″	Nitinol	2.1 g	Stiff nitinol body with flexible nitinol tip
Victory 14 [Boston Scientific]	0.014″	Stainless	12/18/25/30 g	Non-tapered tip with varying tip loads for different penetration
0.014″ non-polymer jacket - specialty				
Halberd 0.014 [Asahi Intecc]	0.014″	Stainless	12 g	Non-tapered spring coil/tapered micro cone tip to improve penetration
Approach CTO [cook medical]	0.014″	Stainless	6/12/18/25 g	Non-tapered tip for complex lesion navigation
Astato 20 [Asahi Intecc]	0.014″	Stainless	20 g	Tapered spring coil for penetration
Confianza pro 12 [Asahi Intecc]	0.014″	Stainless	12 g	Tapered spring coil for penetration
0.014″ non-polymer jacket - support				
Hi-torque Spartacore [Abbott vascular]	0.014″	Stainless	NA	High support to deliver devices
Platinum plus [Boston Scientific]	0.014″	Stainless	7 g	High support to deliver devices

This list is not all-inclusive. Guidewire specifications sourced from published literature or manufacturer websites

Note: From Banerjee S, Shishehbor MH, Mustapha JA, et al. A Percutaneous Crossing Algorithm for Femoropopliteal and Tibial Artery Chronic Total Occlusions (PCTO Algorithm). *The Journal of Invasive Cardiology*. 2019;31 (4):18

Table 14.2 Preferred crossing devices with specifications for femoropopliteal chronic total occlusion crossing

Crossing device	Description
TruePath [Boston Scientific]	Creates microdissection in PCTOs to facilitate access into hard and calcified caps; 0.018 guidewire compatible with diamond-coated tip that rotates at 13,000 rpm. It has audible and visual alerts that are activated when excessive resistance is encountered. The tip may be bent up to 15° to help steer in different directions. Tabletop device without external console
Viance [Medtronic]	2.3 Fr coiled multiwire shaft and 3 Fr rounded atraumatic tip. Over-the-wire, 0.014″ guidewire compatible. Tip is advanced to the proximal PCTO cap and manually spun using a torque handle
Frontrunner [Cordis]	No guidewire lumen, advanced within a microguide. Consists of a proximal braided shaft for pushability and torque and a flexible distal shaft that can be shaped. Radiopaque distal actuating jaws for blunt microdissection through a PCTO
Crosser [C.R. Bard]	Comprised of an electronic generator, foot switch, high-frequency transducer, FlowMate injector, and crosser catheter; 0.014″ and 0.018″ guidewire compatible. Tip is either stainless-steel or titanium, uses high-energy vibration to penetrate hard caps. Catheter is advanced over the guidewire to the occlusion. Following guidewire removal, the device is activated and slowly advanced into the lesion
Wildcat [Avinger]	Rotatable tip with passive [wedges in] and active [wedges out] configurations. Passive mode is initial mode and active is for fibrocalcific lesions. Offers 0.014″ versions [Kittycat and Kittycat 2] for below-the-knee PCTOs
Ocelot [Avinger]	Over-the-wire device with optical coherence tomography [OCT] imaging; catheter shaft with crossing distal tip and a proximal handle. OCT identifies plaque morphology and provides continuous scans for navigating the tip within the PCTO. Intravascular tip position altered using directional markers that remain stationary in the display unless the outer shaft is rotated

This list is not all-inclusive. Guidewire specifications sourced from published literature or manufacturer websites

Peripheral chronic total occlusion [PCTO) re-entry devices

Crossing device	Description
Pioneer [Philips)	0.014″ guidewire compatible catheter with solid-state intravascular ultrasound [IVUS] and intraluminal hypotube with a curved retractable nitinol needle. After subintimal entry and reaching the desired true lumen entry point, the catheter is rotated so the true lumen is at 12 o'clock on the IVUS image. The curved needle tip is then plunged into the true lumen and the guidewire is advanced
Outback [Cordis]	Advanced over 0.014″ guidewire to desired re-entry site. Retractable curved nitinol needle positioned under fluoroscopy in two different orthogonal views: the Lradiopaque marker is oriented toward the lumen and after rotating the image intensifier 90° orthogonally, the T radiopaque marker is oriented over the lumen. Needle is then plunged into the true lumen and the guidewire is advanced

(continued)

Table 14.2 (continued)

Peripheral chronic total occlusion [PCTO) re-entry devices	
Crossing device	Description
Enteer [Medtronic)	0.018″guidewire compatible, flat, self-orienting balloon with two 180° offset exit ports. Barbed angle tip re-entry wire with different stiffness to enter true lumen through exit port located in the subintimal space
Offroad (Boston Scientific)	70 cm, over-the-wire, 0.035″ catheter with 5.4 mm conical balloon and a flexible neck that allows directing the balloon toward the true lumen, and 0.014″ compatible lancet for re-entry into the true lumen

Note: From Banerjee S, Shishehbor MH, Mustapha JA, et al. A Percutaneous Crossing Algorithm for Femoropopliteal and Tibial Artery Chronic Total Occlusions (PCTO Algorithm). *The Journal of Invasive Cardiology*. 2019;31 (4):18

Below-the-Knee Chronic Total Occlusions

Though a full, thorough discussion of below-the-knee (BTK) CTOs is beyond the scope of this chapter, they are important to briefly mention given their complexity, high prevalence, and role in critical limb ischemia (CLI). BTK atherosclerosis plays a large role in CLI and nonhealing diabetic foot ulcers. Supportive care, medical therapy, and adequate revascularization are all needed to achieve the maximum potential for limb salvage and healing. Multilevel CTOs are extremely prevalent in the BTK vasculature. They comprise 60–70% of lesions encountered with 50–60% coupled with multivessel disease [31]. The most commonly affected vessels are the anterior and posterior tibial arteries. The peroneal artery is typically spared [32].

Treatment of BTK disease can be based on an angiosome concept which refers to the phenomenon that areas of the foot supplied blood by an underlying source artery. These angiosomes are perfused by branches of the anterior tibial, posterior tibial, and peroneal arteries. Collaterals perfuse the tissue if the direct flow in the angiosome is compromised. Choke vessels allow perfusion of angiosomes by the adjacent one. Intervention should aim for direct revascularization, or at least indirect via collaterals, in order to achieve maximum clinical success [33]. As with FP-CTO lesions, obtaining high-quality angiographic imaging of the vasculature via digital subtraction is imperative in order to plan an approach suitable for the target lesion. This may require antegrade, retrograde, or simultaneous antegrade-retrograde contrast injection to adequately visualize the CTO caps, lesion length, distal vasculature, and dorsal and pedal arches.

Vascular access can be achieved through contralateral, antegrade, or retrograde approaches. The contralateral femoral artery is commonly used for above-the-knee lesions but is not favored for BTK disease. It does not provide as much sheath support as other approaches, is limited by device length, and produces suboptimal angiographic images. However, it can be suitable if a longer sheath (55, 65, or >70 cm) device is used along with adequate anticoagulation and intact inflow. Antegrade CFA, CFA-SFA junction, or proximal SFA access supplies substantial device support, can

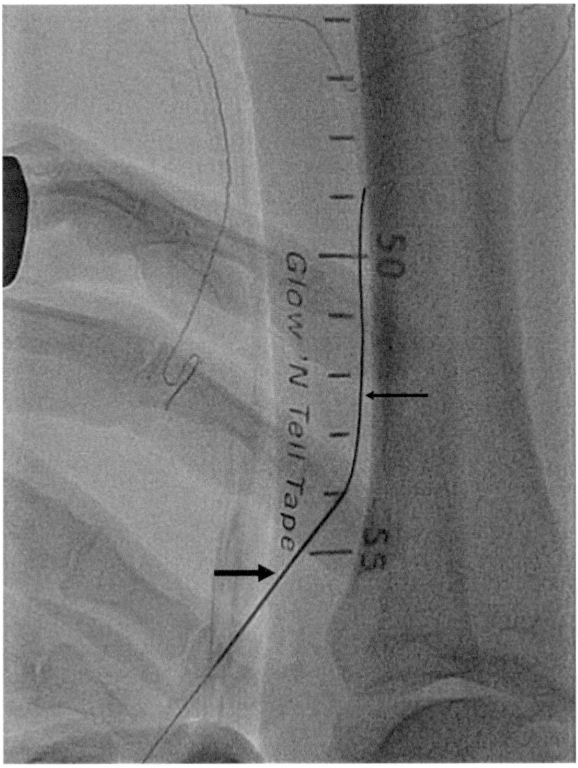

Fig. 14.8 Retrograde pedal access obtained under angiographic guidance by positioning the access needle first in an anteroposterior view and then in a lateral orthogonal view. Thick arrow indicates the needle inserted into the posterior tibial artery of the foot with guidewire advancement (thick arrow)

access distal vessels, and produces high-quality images. Retrograde pedal or tibial access can be achieved through the dorsalis pedis, posterior tibial (just above medial malleolus, Fig. 14.8), or distal anterior tibial arteries. Operators should consider this approach when intervention on a BTK-CTO lesion is planned as the proximal caps may not be well visualized and the presence of collaterals can complicate the procedure. Therefore, a retrograde pedal or tibial approach may improve BTK-CTO crossing success [34]. Direct ultrasound-guided micropuncture is advised rather than fluoroscopic or angiographic guidance. It is important to note that the peroneal artery can be accessed but, typically, is not given its deep course and potential for bleeding.

The tibio-pedal arterial minimally invasive retrograde revascularization (TAMI) approach utilizes retrograde tibial or pedal access for BTK lesions. It is centered on avoiding any femoral access. With a pure retrograde approach, this avoids any groin complications, improves crossing device support, and allows for improved visualization of distal vasculature. Of note, the TAMI approach depends on delivery of devices that are compatible with a pedal sheath as well as pedal access patency. The latter can be achieved with infusion of de-aired heparinized vasodilator solution (TAMI solution) through the sheath's side arm [35]. It is important to consider pedal loop revascularization and access as intact pedal vasculature plays a vital role in wound healing. Retrograde access can be obtained alongside ipsilateral antegrade access [36].

BTK-CTO lesions tend to be long and heavily calcified [37]. This proves to be a technical challenge, similar to FP-CTOs. As such, we advise that all aspects of the procedure including alternate techniques and vascular access points be planned prior to performing the intervention. However, the crossing approach to BTK-CTOs differs. Crossing the lesion through the true lumen is preferred compared to subintimal reentry or the hybrid approach. There is often a large plaque burden, and crossing through the true lumen allows debulking to be performed with atherectomy devices. Additionally, no stent placement is required. With an SI approach, stents are often needed to secure crossing, but due to the small diameter and length of BTK vessels, this limits the available choices for appropriate stents. We advise the use of IVUS to determine the degree of SI passage, confirm distal true lumen entry, and visualize segments that are amendable to atherectomy. However, SI and hybrid techniques such as CART and RCART as mentioned above can still be employed to achieve technical success. For both FP and BTK CTOs, the crossing technique greatly impacts the selection of final revascularization strategy (stent vs non-stent).

Acknowledgments We would like to thank the patients and members of the healthcare team who have allowed us to deliver care and to continue learning. Our deepest gratitude to prior innovators in the field so that we can continue to build upon their work and progress.

Disclosures Michael Vu—None; Subhash Banerjee: Consultant for Medtronic, Cordis, Kaneka and Institutional research grants from Boston Scientific Corporation and Chiesi.

Funding None.

References

1. Goodney PP, Beck AW, Nagle J, Welch HG, Zwolak RM. National trends in lower extremity bypass surgery, endovascular interventions, and major amputations. J Vasc Surg. 2009;50(1):54–60. https://doi.org/10.1016/j.jvs.2009.01.035.
2. Ho KJ, Owens CD. Diagnosis, classification, and treatment of femoropopliteal artery in-stent restenosis. J Vasc Surg. 2017;65(2):545–57. https://doi.org/10.1016/j.jvs.2016.09.031.
3. Hamur H, Onk OA, Vuruskan E, et al. Determinants of chronic total occlusion in patients with peripheral arterial occlusive disease. Angiology. 2017;68(2):151–8. https://doi.org/10.1177/0003319716641827.
4. Techniques in vascular and interventional radiology—Journal—Elsevier. https://www.journals.elsevier.com/journals.elsevier.com/techniques-in-vascular-and-interventional-radiology. Accessed 30 Aug 2021.
5. Kondapalli A, Jeon-Slaughter H, Lu H, et al. Comparative assessment of patient outcomes with intraluminal or subintimal crossing of infrainguinal peripheral artery chronic total occlusions. Vasc Med. 2018;23(1):39–45. https://doi.org/10.1177/1358863X17735192.
6. Guiding principles for chronic total occlusion percutaneous coronary intervention. Circulation. https://www.ahajournals.org/doi/10.1161/CIRCULATIONAHA.119.039797. Accessed 30 Aug 2021.
7. Banerjee S, Sarode K, Mohammad A, et al. Femoropopliteal artery stent thrombosis. Circ Cardiovasc Interv. 2016;9(2):e002730. https://doi.org/10.1161/CIRCINTERVENTIONS.115.002730.

8. Banerjee S, Sarode K, Patel A, et al. Comparative assessment of guidewire and microcatheter vs a crossing device-based strategy to traverse infrainguinal peripheral artery chronic total occlusions. J Endovasc Ther. 2015;22(4):525–34. https://doi.org/10.1177/1526602815587707.
9. Chou H-H, Huang H-L, Hsieh C-A, et al. Outcomes of endovascular therapy with the controlled antegrade retrograde subintimal tracking (CART) or reverse CART technique for long infrainguinal occlusions. J Endovasc Ther. 2016;23(2):330–8. https://doi.org/10.1177/1526602816630533.
10. Brilakis ES, Grantham JA, Rinfret S, et al. A percutaneous treatment algorithm for crossing coronary chronic total occlusions. JACC Cardiovasc Interv. 2012;5(4):367–79. https://doi.org/10.1016/j.jcin.2012.02.006.
11. Saab F, Jaff MR, Diaz-Sandoval LJ, et al. Chronic total occlusion crossing approach based on plaque cap morphology: the CTOP classification. J Endovasc Ther. 2018;25(3):284–91. https://doi.org/10.1177/1526602818759333.
12. Banerjee S, Shishehbor MH, Mustapha JA, et al. A percutaneous crossing algorithm for femoropopliteal and tibial artery chronic total occlusions (PCTO algorithm). J Invasive Cardiol. 2019;31(4):18.
13. Sheeran D, Wilkins LR. Long chronic total occlusions: revascularization strategies. Semin Interv Radiol. 2018;35(5):469–76. https://doi.org/10.1055/s-0038-1676343.
14. Manzi M, Cester G, Palena LM, Alek J, Candeo A, Ferraresi R. Vascular imaging of the foot: the first step toward endovascular recanalization. Radiographics. 2011;31(6):1623–36. https://doi.org/10.1148/rg.316115511.
15. Li X-M, Li Y-H, Tian J-M, et al. Evaluation of peripheral artery stent with 64-slice multidetector row CT angiography: prospective comparison with digital subtraction angiography. Eur J Radiol. 2010;75(1):98–103. https://doi.org/10.1016/j.ejrad.2009.03.032.
16. Liu J, Zhang N, Fan Z, et al. Image quality and stenosis assessment of non-contrast-enhanced 3-T magnetic resonance angiography in patients with peripheral artery disease compared with contrast-enhanced magnetic resonance angiography and digital subtraction angiography. PLoS One. 2016;11(11):e0166467. https://doi.org/10.1371/journal.pone.0166467.
17. Klein AJ, Pinto DS, Gray BH, et al. SCAI expert consensus statement for femoral-popliteal arterial intervention appropriate use. Catheter Cardiovasc Interv. 2014;84(4):529–38. https://doi.org/10.1002/ccd.25504.
18. Klein AJ, Jaff MR, Gray BH, et al. SCAI appropriate use criteria for peripheral arterial interventions: an update. Catheter Cardiovasc Interv. 2017;90(4):E90–E110. https://doi.org/10.1002/ccd.27141.
19. Niazi K, Farooqui F, Devireddy C, Robertson G, Shaw RE. Comparison of hydrophilic guidewires used in endovascular procedures. J Invasive Cardiol. 2009;21(8):397–400.
20. Venkatachalam S, Bunte M, Monteleone P, Lincoff A, Maier M, Shishehbor MH. Combined antegrade-retrograde intervention to improve chronic total occlusion recanalization in high-risk critical limb ischemia. Ann Vasc Surg. 2014;28(6):1439–48. https://doi.org/10.1016/j.avsg.2014.01.011.
21. Yilmaz S, Sindel T, Yegin A, Lüleci E. Subintimal angioplasty of long superficial femoral artery occlusions. J Vasc Interv Radiol. 2003;14(8):997–1010. https://doi.org/10.1097/01.rvi.000008261.05622.b8.
22. Fanelli F, Cannavale A. Retrograde recanalization of complex SFA lesions indications and techniques. J Cardiovasc Surg. 2014;55(4):465–71.
23. Schmidt A, Bausback Y, Piorkowski M, et al. Retrograde recanalization technique for use after failed antegrade angioplasty in chronic femoral artery occlusions. J Endovasc Ther. 2012;19(1):23–9. https://doi.org/10.1583/11-3645.1.
24. Shin S, Kim S, Ko Y-G, Hong M-K, Jang Y, Choi D. Retrograde distal superficial femoral artery approach in the supine position for chronic superficial femoral artery occlusion. Korean Circ J. 2014;44(3):184–8. https://doi.org/10.4070/kcj.2014.44.3.184.
25. Tasic M, Sreckovic MJ, Jagic N, Miloradovic V, Nikolic D. Knuckle technique guided by intravascular ultrasound for in-stent restenosis occlusion treatment. Postępy Kardiol Interwencyjnej. 2015;11(1):58. https://doi.org/10.5114/pwki.2015.49188.

26. Spinosa DJ, Leung DA, Harthun NL, et al. Simultaneous antegrade and retrograde access for subintimal recanalization of peripheral arterial occlusion. J Vasc Interv Radiol. 2003;14(11):1449–54. https://doi.org/10.1097/01.rvi.0000096764.74047.21.
27. Cao J, Lu H-T, Wei L-M, Zhao J-G, Zhu Y-Q. Rendezvous technique for recanalization of long-segmental chronic total occlusion above the knee following unsuccessful standard angioplasty. Vascular. 2016;24(2):157–65. https://doi.org/10.1177/1708538115589049.
28. Michael TT, Papayannis AC, Banerjee S, Brilakis ES. Subintimal dissection/reentry strategies in coronary chronic total occlusion interventions. Circ Cardiovasc Interv. 2012;5(5):729–38. https://doi.org/10.1161/CIRCINTERVENTIONS.112.969808.
29. Nihei T, Yamamoto Y, Kudo S, et al. Impact of the intracoronary rendezvous technique on coronary angioplasty for chronic total occlusion. Cardiovasc Interv Ther. 2017;32(4):365–73. https://doi.org/10.1007/s12928-016-0421-1.
30. Goltz JP, Anton S, Wiedner M, Barkhausen J, Stahlberg E. Simultaneous antegrade-retrograde subintimal revascularization of a femoropopliteal chronic total occlusion by a reentry device-facilitated puncture of a retrogradely inserted balloon. J Endovasc Ther. 2017;24(4):521–4. https://doi.org/10.1177/1526602817707742.
31. McCoach CE, Armstrong EJ, Singh S, et al. Gender-related variation in the clinical presentation and outcomes of critical limb ischemia. Vasc Med. 2013;18(1):19–26. https://doi.org/10.1177/1358863X13475836.
32. Iida O, Soga Y, Yamauchi Y, et al. Anatomical predictors of major adverse limb events after infrapopliteal angioplasty for patients with critical limb ischaemia due to pure isolated infrapopliteal lesions. Eur J Vasc Endovasc Surg. 2012;44(3):318–24. https://doi.org/10.1016/j.ejvs.2012.05.011.
33. Fujii M, Terashi H. Angiosome and tissue healing. Ann Vasc Dis. 2019;12(2):147–50. https://doi.org/10.3400/avd.ra.19-00036.
34. Ruzsa Z, Nemes B, Bánsághi Z, et al. Transpedal access after failed anterograde recanalization of complex below-the-knee and femoropoliteal occlusions in critical limb ischemia. Catheter Cardiovasc Interv. 2014;83(6):997–1007. https://doi.org/10.1002/ccd.25262.
35. Mustapha JA, Saab F, McGoff T, et al. Tibio-pedal arterial minimally invasive retrograde revascularization in patients with advanced peripheral vascular disease: the TAMI technique, original case series. Catheter Cardiovasc Interv. 2014;83(6):987–94. https://doi.org/10.1002/ccd.25227.
36. Palena LM, Manzi M. Extreme below-the-knee interventions: retrograde transmetatarsal or transplantar arch access for foot salvage in challenging cases of critical limb ischemia. J Endovasc Ther. 2012;19(6):805–11. https://doi.org/10.1583/JEVT-12-3998R.1.
37. Mustapha JA, Saab F, McGoff TN, Finton S, Adams G, Mullins JR. Chronic total occlusions: association between characteristics and mid-term outcomes in critical limb ischemia. J Crit Limb Ischem. 2021;1:7.

Chapter 15
Approach to Treatment of Iliac Artery Disease

Razan Elsayed and Beau M. Hawkins

Introduction

Peripheral artery disease (PAD) is a prevalent condition affecting roughly eight million individuals in the United States [1]. In addition to being associated with excess cardiovascular risk [2], many patients with PAD suffer from claudication or have critical limb ischemia (CLI) manifesting as ischemic rest or tissue loss. Epidemiologic studies report that over half of the patients with symptomatic PAD have iliac involvement [3]. This chapter summarizes the presentation and management of iliac artery disease, the cornerstone of which includes medical therapy and revascularization for select populations.

Clinical Presentation and Evaluation

While claudication most often originates in the calf segment, individuals with iliac disease may have symptoms involving the thigh or more proximal leg musculature. Moreover, the internal iliac artery supplies the pelvis, and disease in this segment or that involving the ipsilateral common iliac artery can result in symptoms localizing to the hip. Leriche syndrome is a unique manifestation of aortoiliac disease and is characterized by an abnormal femoral artery pulse exam, impotence, and claudication.

R. Elsayed · B. M. Hawkins (✉)
Section of Cardiovascular Disease, Department of Internal Medicine, University of Oklahoma Health Sciences Center, Oklahoma City, OK, USA
e-mail: razan-elsayed@ouhsc.edu; beau-hawkins@ouhsc.edu

N. W. Shammas (ed.), *Peripheral Arterial Interventions*, Contemporary Cardiology, https://doi.org/10.1007/978-3-031-09741-6_15

As with other forms of PAD, the evaluation of patients with iliac disease starts with obtaining a full clinical history with special attention paid to symptom description and presence of predisposing risk factors. Physical exam is of paramount importance and includes pulse examination and assessment for the presence of tissue changes including wounds, ulcers, and discoloration. A femoral bruit is often present but does not exclude the presence of significant ipsilateral iliac disease. Likewise, a relatively normal peripheral exam does not definitely exclude the presence of significant aortoiliac obstruction.

Multiple noninvasive testing modalities are available to evaluate for iliac artery disease. Arterial physiologic testing most often includes hemodynamic assessment with ankle pressures, pulse volume recordings, and segmental limb pressures and provides important information relating to diagnosis and severity of any existing PAD. It should be noted that the resting ankle-brachial index may be normal at baseline in individuals with isolated aortoiliac disease. In this situation, supplementing the baseline physiologic study with an exercise treadmill protocol may unmask hemodynamically significant inflow disease. In individuals with isolated internal iliac artery disease, physiologic testing will be normal necessitating alternative diagnostic modalities. Duplex ultrasonography (DUS) may not fully evaluate the proximal iliac arteries, particularly in individuals that are larger. Computed tomography angiography (CTA) and magnetic resonance angiography (MRA) do provide good anatomic assessment of the distal aorta and iliac arteries.

Treatment

Guideline-directed medical therapy (GDMT) is the first-line treatment for all individuals with iliac artery disease [4]. This includes antiplatelet agents, statins, smoking cessation, and glycemic and hypertension control. In addition, a walking program is an essential component of care for patients with PAD. Revascularization is indicated for patients with lifestyle-limiting claudication despite GDMT and in patients with chronic limb-threatening ischemia. The goal of revascularization in claudicants is to improve functionality and quality of life.

Several studies evaluated the effect of revascularization versus conservative management. The CLEVER study randomized 111 patients with intermittent claudication secondary to aortoiliac disease to one of the three arms: medical management alone, medical management plus supervised exercise program, and medical management plus stent revascularization [5]. The primary outcome was peak walking time (PWT). At 6 months of follow-up, both exercise and revascularization groups showed improvement in PWT and quality of life. The exercise group had more improvement in PWT, and the revascularization group had the greatest improvement in quality of life at 6 months [5]. The subsequent 18-month clinical and treadmill follow-up assessments, which included 79 patients, showed similar improvement in PWT in both exercise and revascularization groups as compared to medical management alone [6].

The IRONIC trial randomized 158 patients to receive either noninvasive medical management or revascularization (endovascular or open surgical) [7]. Thirty-one patients (20%) had aortoiliac disease, and another 31 patients (20%) had combined aortoiliac and femoropopliteal disease. Thirty-two percent had aortoiliac endovascular revascularization. There was a marked improvement in health-related quality of life and intermittent claudication distance in the invasive group compared to the noninvasive group after 1 year of follow-up.

Options for Revascularization

Revascularization options for aortoiliac disease include endovascular and open surgical approaches. The Trans-Atlantic Inter-Society Consensus (TASC) II classification scheme divides aortoiliac lesions into one of four types in increasing order of complexity (Table 15.1) [8]. Traditionally, the recommended approach was endovascular therapy for TASC A and B lesions, with surgery reserved for TASC C and D groups. However, endovascular techniques have substantially evolved, and

Table 15.1 TASC classification of aortoiliac lesions

Type A
• Unilateral or bilateral stenoses of the common iliac artery (CIA)
• Unilateral or bilateral single short (≤3 cm) stenosis of the external iliac artery (EIA)
Type B
• Short (≤3 cm) stenosis of the infrarenal aorta
• Unilateral CIA occlusion
• Single or multiple stenoses totaling 3–10 cm involving EIA not extending into the common femoral artery (CFA)
• Unilateral EIA occlusion not involving origins of the internal iliac artery or CFA
Type C
• Bilateral CIA occlusions
• Bilateral EIA stenoses 3–10 cm long not extending into the CFA
• Unilateral EIA stenosis extending into the CFA
• Unilateral EIA occlusion that involves origins of the internal iliac and/or CFA
• Heavy calcified unilateral EIA occlusion with or without involving origins of the internal iliac and/or CFA
Type D
• Infrarenal aortoiliac occlusion
• Diffuse disease involving the aorta and both iliac arteries
• Diffuse multiple stenoses involving the unilateral CIA, EIA, and CFA
• Unilateral occlusions of both CIA and EIA
• Bilateral occlusions of EIA
• Iliac stenoses in patients with AAA requiring treatment and not amenable to endograft placement or other lesions requiring open aortic or iliac surgery

Adapted from [8]

several studies have now shown equivalent rates of success, limb salvage, and improvement in symptoms in TASC C and D lesions. Additionally, an endovascular approach is associated with lower procedural risk, fewer complications, and quicker recovery time when compared to surgery, which allows for inclusion of high-risk patients who would not be ideal surgical candidates [9–12].

Ichihashi et al. retrospectively compared outcomes of endovascular stenting in TASC A/B versus TASC C/D iliac disease in 413 patients [12]. Median follow-up was 72 months. Technical success rates were 99% for both groups, and both groups had comparable long-term patency rates (88% for A/B and 83% for C/D at 5 years, p 0.17). The C/D group had higher complication rates (9% vs 3%; p 0.014) and longer procedural times. Another analysis of over 2000 patients compared outcomes in TASC C/D lesions to A/B subgroups and demonstrated slightly lower procedural success rates, similar 5-year primary patency rates, and nominally higher rates of procedure complications [12].

To summarize, an endovascular approach has become the first line revascularization option for most patients with iliac artery disease. Surgical revascularization remains an effective therapy in patients with suitable operative risk with lesion subsets of increased complexity.

Considerations for Endovascular Therapy

Access determination depends predominantly on lesion location. Commonly used sites include the common femoral, radial, and brachial arteries. An ipsilateral retrograde CFA approach is ideal for common iliac lesions, but may not be feasible if there is concurrent severe distal iliac disease. In these scenarios, a radial or brachial approach may be used, understanding that these sites require appropriate length equipment. An anterograde "up-and-over" approach via contralateral CFA access is suitable for external iliac or distal common iliac disease. When bilateral common iliac disease is present, dual access is used to allow for kissing angioplasty and stenting.

Iliac revascularization techniques include angioplasty with or without selective stenting, and primary stenting. Several studies have evaluated success and long-term patency between these two techniques. In the Dutch iliac stent trial, 279 patients were randomized to either primary stenting or angioplasty with bailout stenting when the residual mean pressure gradient was >10 mmHg across the treated site. No differences in ankle-brachial index, patency, or quality of life were identified between groups. It is worth mentioning that 43% of patients in the angioplasty arm actually had provisional stent placement [13].

In contrast, the randomized STAG trial results favored primary stenting over angioplasty. While there was no significant difference in patency at 2 years, technical success was higher, and complications were lower in the stent arm (98% vs 84%, $p = 0.007$, 5% vs 11% $p = 0.01$, respectively) [14]. Owing to better procedural success and lower complications, primary stenting has become the strategy of choice for most iliac lesions.

Commonly used stents for iliac endovascular therapy include balloon-expandable and self-expanding bare-metal stents. Both types come in bare and covered platforms. Balloon-expandable stents are usually rigid, have high radial force, and allow for precise deployment. They are ideal for ostial common iliac and highly calcified lesions. In contrast, self-expanding stents are flexible and are better suited for tortuous vessels like the external iliac artery.

Several studies evaluated different types of stents for iliac artery disease. The COBEST trial randomized 125 patients with aortoiliac occlusive disease (168 lesions) to either covered balloon-expandable or bare-metal stenting. Patients were followed up to 18 months. Covered stents had better long-term patency for TASC C and D lesions, but there was no difference between the two for TASC B lesions [15]. A subsequent 5-year post hoc analysis of the COBEST trial showed higher patency in the covered stent group (74.7 vs 62.5%; p 0.01), but this difference was again most pronounced in TASC C and D groups. There was also less target lesion revascularization (TLR) in the covered stent group [16]. These data suggest that covered stents are more beneficial in complex aortoiliac lesions.

The ICE trial sought to determine if balloon-expandable or self-expanding stents were more efficacious for iliac artery disease [17]. In total, 660 patients were randomized to either balloon-expandable or self-expanding stents. Sixteen percent of lesions were chronic total occlusions (CTOs), and 25% were heavily calcified. At 12 months, the primary outcome of binary restenosis was significantly lower in the self-expanding stent group (6.1% vs 14.9%; $p < 0.006$); the self-expanding group also had lower rates of TLR. There was no difference between the two groups in terms of walking impairment, amputations rate, all-cause death, or procedural complications.

Intravascular ultrasound (IVUS) is a helpful tool in the diagnosis and management of iliac disease. In addition to characterizing lesions, IVUS can also help with determining angioplasty diameter, and with assessing adequacy of stent deployment. One such study evaluated stent deployment in 71 limbs (52 patients) using IVUS compared to arteriography alone [18]. Primary patency estimates at 3 and 6 years were significantly higher in the IVUS-guided group. There was also a significantly higher secondary intervention rate in the non-IVUS group. Another more recent study of 154 patients identified IVUS-detected small minimum stent area and stent-edge dissection as predictors of TLR and long-term patency [19]. In this sense, IVUS may be helpful in optimizing technical results during iliac interventions.

Iliac chronic total occlusions (CTO) are more complex and challenging with a higher incidence of complications at the time of revascularization. An endovascular approach has been shown to be an effective and safe approach to CTO revascularization. One retrospective analysis of 48 patients demonstrated good long-term primary and secondary patency along with high rates of limb salvage at 36 months of follow-up [20]. Another analysis of 120 patients with iliac CTOs reported a success rate of 84% with 14% of lesions requiring reentry devices. A significant proportion of the lesions were TASC C and D. Good patency and limb salvage rates were demonstrated [21]. These studies, along with others, further emphasize the important role of endovascular therapies in the treatment of complex iliac disease.

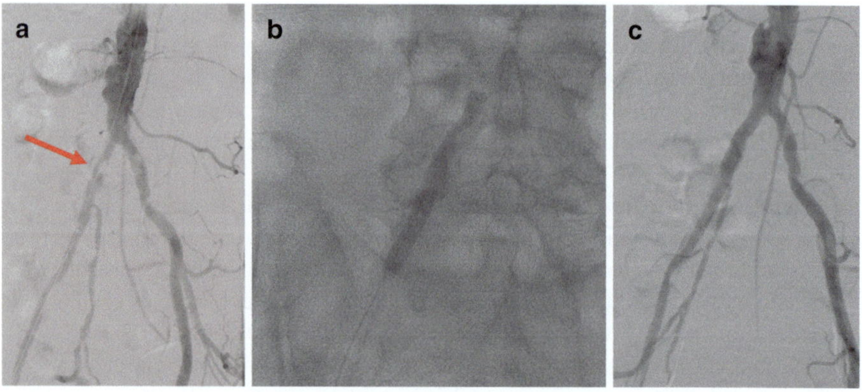

Fig. 15.1 (**a**) A 64-year-old male presents with lifestyle-limiting right lower extremity claudication. Angiography reveals a severely calcified right common iliac stenosis (arrow). (**b**) Lithotripsy is performed followed by angioplasty. (**c**) A balloon-expandable stent is deployed with excellent results

Intravascular lithotripsy is a new therapeutic modality to treat heavily calcified, stenotic iliac artery lesions (Fig. 15.1). This technology utilizes ultrasonic energy to fracture calcium within atherosclerotic plaque, thereby facilitating successful dilation with angioplasty balloons. The safety and efficacy of this technique have been shown in the Disrupt PAD III study which reported outcomes in 118 patients with 200 iliac lesions [22]. Technical success was 100%, and complication rates were remarkably low. On the basis of these and other data, increased utilization of this technology can be anticipated in the near future.

Complications of Endovascular Revascularization

Although the overall rates of complications, morbidity, and mortality are low with endovascular therapy, serious and sometimes fatal complications can occur. In general, complication risk is highest in more complex lesion subsets and, in particular, those lesions that are heavily calcified. In addition to commonly encountered complications with arteriograms, such as those related to contrast media, access site, and intra-procedural sedation, there are a specific subset of complications unique to iliac and other peripheral interventions. These include arterial dissection, arterial rupture (Fig. 15.2), thrombosis, and distal embolization (Fig. 15.3). When recognized quickly, the majority of these vascular complications can be treated endovascularly at the time of index procedure. Such treatments include balloon dilation and covered stenting of hemodynamically significant iliac dissections and arterial ruptures, thrombectomy or catheter-directed thrombolysis for vessel thrombosis, and additional stenting with kissing techniques for contralateral iliac artery occlusion following index lesion stenting [23].

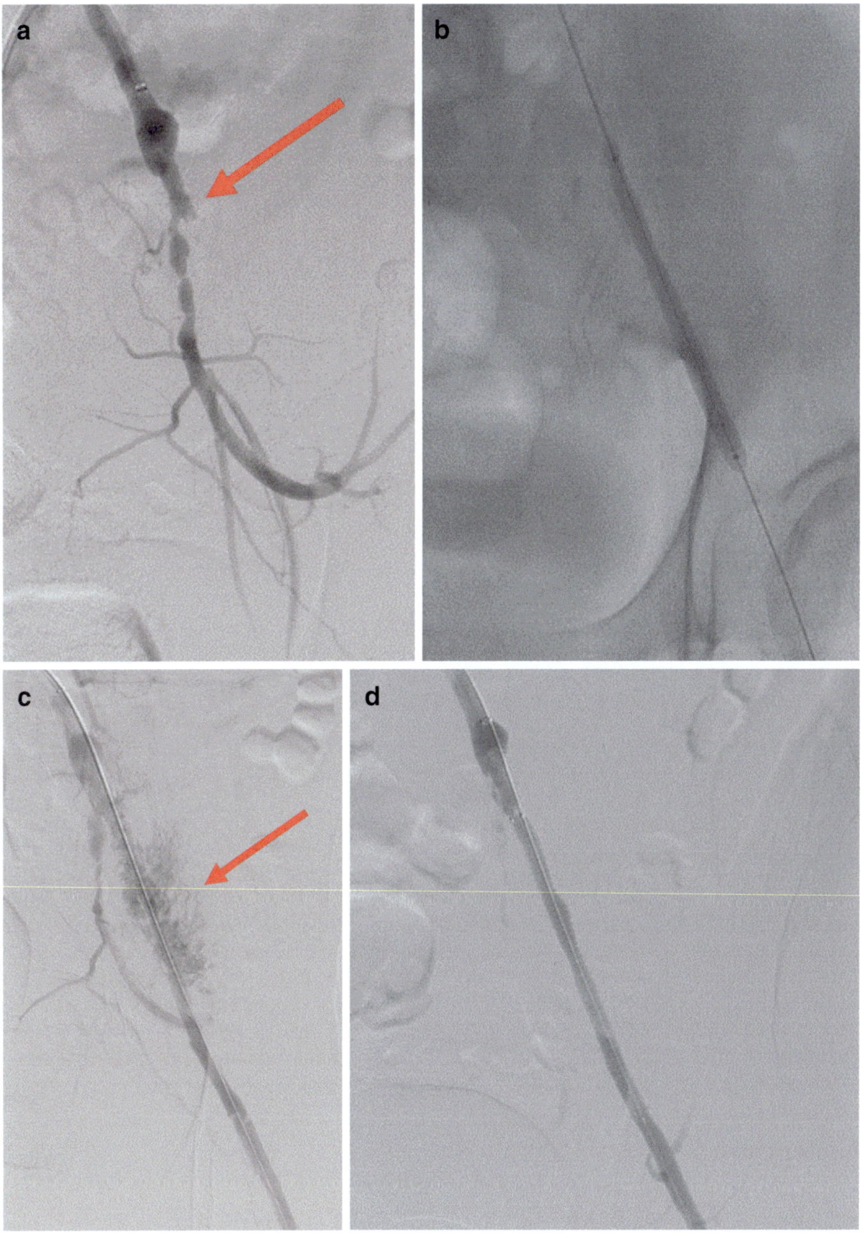

Fig. 15.2 (**a**) A 60-year-old male present with a left plantar foot wound. Angiography demonstrates a left external iliac occlusion (arrow) with reconstitution in the common femoral artery. (**b**) The lesion is crossed and angioplasty is performed. (**c**) A perforation is present (arrow). (**d**) A covered stent is deployed with successful resolution of the perforation

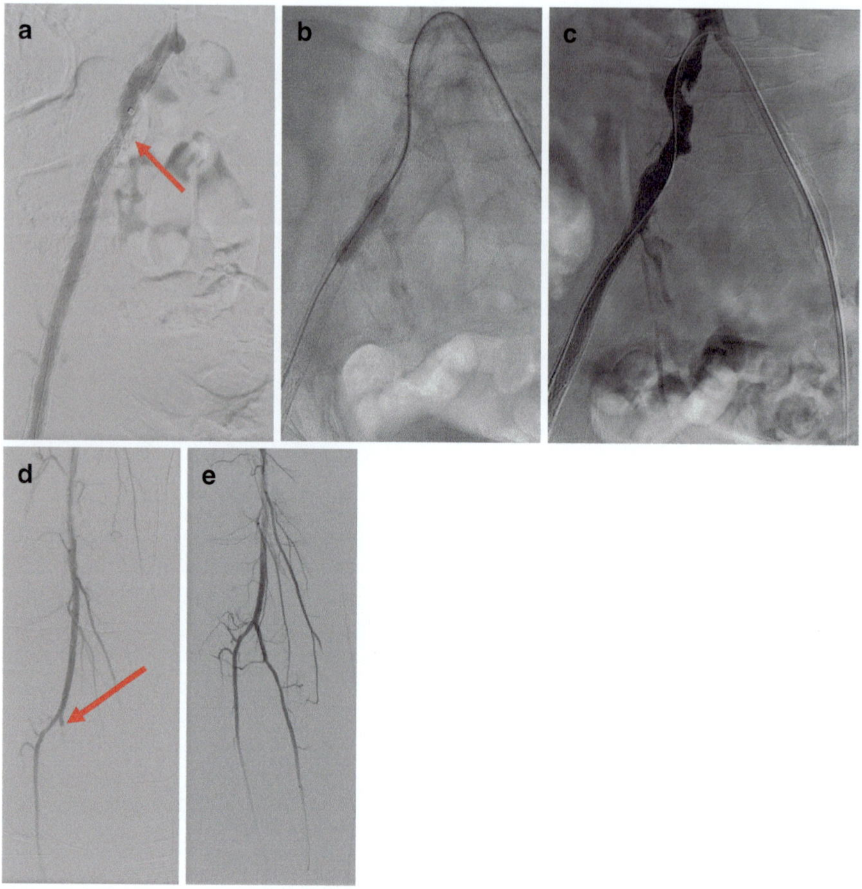

Fig. 15.3 (**a**) A 72-year-old male with prior iliac stenting presents with recurrent right leg claudication. Angiography demonstrates stent underexpansion in the right external iliac artery (arrow). There is a 60-mmHg pressure gradient across this lesion. (**b**) Laser atherectomy and angioplasty are performed. (**c**) The stenosis is reduced to 30%, and there is abolishment of the preexisting hemodynamic gradient. (**d**) Completion angiography reveals acute occlusion of the right anterior tibioperoneal trunk from embolization (arrow). (**e**) Aspiration thrombectomy and angioplasty result in restoration of flow through the tibioperoneal trunk into the posterior tibial artery

Conclusion

Iliac arterial disease is one of the common subtypes of PAD. Management of iliac arterial disease includes optimal medical therapy and an exercise program in all patients. Patients with life-limiting claudication despite these interventions along with patients who have limb-threatening ischemia may require revascularization. An endovascular first approach is now the technique of choice in most iliac lesions and can be effectively performed in most complex lesions with excellent success rates and a low risk of periprocedural complications.

References

1. Benjamin EJ, Virani SS, Callaway CW, Chamberlain AM, Chang AR, Cheng S, et al. Heart disease and stroke statistics-2018 update: a report from the American Heart Association. Circulation. 2018;137(12):e67–e492.
2. Grenon SM, Vittinghoff E, Owens CD, Conte MS, Whooley M, Cohen BE. Peripheral artery disease and risk of cardiovascular events in patients with coronary artery disease: insights from the heart and soul study. Vasc Med. 2013;18(4):176–84.
3. Aboyans V, Desormais I, Lacroix P, Salazar J, Criqui MH, Laskar M. The general prognosis of patients with peripheral arterial disease differs according to the disease localization. J Am Coll Cardiol. 2010;55(9):898–903.
4. Gerhard-Herman MD, Gornik HL, Barrett C, Barshes NR, Corriere MA, Drachman DE, et al. 2016 AHA/ACC guideline on the management of patients with lower extremity peripheral artery disease: a report of the American College of Cardiology/American Heart Association task force on clinical practice guidelines. Circulation. 2017;135(12):e726–79.
5. Murphy TP, Cutlip DE, Regensteiner JG, Mohler ER, Cohen DJ, Reynolds MR, et al. Supervised exercise versus primary stenting for claudication resulting from aortoiliac peripheral artery disease: six-month outcomes from the claudication: exercise versus endoluminal revascularization (CLEVER) study. Circulation. 2012;125(1):130–9.
6. Murphy TP, Cutlip DE, Regensteiner JG, Mohler ER 3rd, Cohen DJ, Reynolds MR, et al. Supervised exercise, stent revascularization, or medical therapy for claudication due to aortoiliac peripheral artery disease: the CLEVER study. J Am Coll Cardiol. 2015;65(10):999–1009.
7. Fakhry F, Spronk S, van der Laan L, Wever JJ, Teijink JA, Hoffmann WH, et al. Endovascular revascularization and supervised exercise for peripheral artery disease and intermittent claudication: a randomized clinical trial. JAMA. 2015;314(18):1936–44.
8. Norgren L, Hiatt WR, Dormandy JA, Nehler MR, Harris KA, Fowkes FG, et al. Inter-society consensus for the management of peripheral arterial disease (TASC II). J Vasc Surg. 2007;45(Suppl S):S5–S67.
9. de Donato G, Bosiers M, Setacci F, Deloose K, Galzerano G, Verbist J, et al. 24-month data from the BRAVISSIMO: a large-scale prospective registry on iliac stenting for TASC a & B and TASC C & D lesions. Ann Vasc Surg. 2015;29(4):738–50.
10. Gabel JA, Kiang SC, Abou-Zamzam AM Jr, Oyoyo UE, Teruya TH, Tomihama RT. Trans-atlantic inter-society consensus class D aortoiliac lesions: a comparison of endovascular and open surgical outcomes. AJR Am J Roentgenol. 2019;213(3):696–701.
11. Suzuki K, Mizutani Y, Soga Y, Iida O, Kawasaki D, Yamauchi Y, et al. Efficacy and safety of endovascular therapy for aortoiliac TASC D lesions. Angiology. 2017;68(1):67–73.
12. Ichihashi S, Higashiura W, Itoh H, Sakaguchi S, Nishimine K, Kichikawa K. Long-term outcomes for systematic primary stent placement in complex iliac artery occlusive disease classified according to trans-atlantic inter-society consensus (TASC)-II. J Vasc Surg. 2011;53(4):992–9.
13. Klein WM, van der Graaf Y, Seegers J, Spithoven JH, Buskens E, van Baal JG, et al. Dutch iliac stent trial: long-term results in patients randomized for primary or selective stent placement. Radiology. 2006;238(2):734–44.
14. Goode SD, Cleveland TJ, Gaines PA, STAG Trial Collaborators. Randomized clinical trial of stents versus angioplasty for the treatment of iliac artery occlusions (STAG trial). Br J Surg. 2013;100(9):1148–53.
15. Mwipatayi BP, Thomas S, Wong J, Temple SE, Vijayan V, Jackson M, et al. A comparison of covered vs bare expandable stents for the treatment of aortoiliac occlusive disease. J Vasc Surg. 2011;54(6):1561–70.
16. Mwipatayi BP, Sharma S, Daneshmand A, Thomas SD, Vijayan V, Altaf N, et al. Durability of the balloon-expandable covered versus bare-metal stents in the covered versus balloon expandable stent trial (COBEST) for the treatment of aortoiliac occlusive disease. J Vasc Surg. 2016;64(1):83–94 e1.

17. Krankenberg H, Zeller T, Ingwersen M, Schmalstieg J, Gissler HM, Nikol S, et al. Self-expanding versus balloon-expandable stents for iliac artery occlusive disease: the randomized ICE trial. JACC Cardiovasc Interv. 2017;10(16):1694–704.
18. Buckley CJ, Arko FR, Lee S, Mettauer M, Little D, Atkins M, et al. Intravascular ultrasound scanning improves long-term patency of iliac lesions treated with balloon angioplasty and primary stenting. J Vasc Surg. 2002;35(2):316–23.
19. Miki K, Fujii K, Fukunaga M, Nishimura M, Horimatsu T, Saita T, et al. Impact of intravascular ultrasound findings on long-term patency after self-expanding nitinol stent implantation in the iliac artery lesion. Heart Vessel. 2016;31(4):519–27.
20. Papakostas JC, Chatzigakis PK, Peroulis M, Avgos S, Kouvelos G, Lazaris A, et al. Endovascular treatment of chronic total occlusions of the iliac arteries: early and midterm results. Ann Vasc Surg. 2015;29(8):1508–15.
21. Chen BL, Holt HR, Day JD, Stout CL, Stokes GK, Panneton JM. Subintimal angioplasty of chronic total occlusion in iliac arteries: a safe and durable option. J Vasc Surg. 2011;53(2):367–73.
22. Armstrong EJ, Soukas PA, Shammas N, Chamberlain J, Pop A, Adams G, et al. Intravascular lithotripsy for treatment of calcified, stenotic iliac arteries: a cohort analysis from the disrupt PAD III study. Cardiovasc Revasc Med. 2020;21(10):1262–8.
23. Ozkan U, Oguzkurt L, Tercan F. Technique, complication, and long-term outcome for endovascular treatment of iliac artery occlusion. Cardiovasc Intervent Radiol. 2010;33(1):18–24.

Chapter 16
Chronic Limb-Threatening Ischemia: Evaluation and Management

Timir K. Paul and Subhash Banerjee

Introduction

Critical limb-threatening ischemia (CLTI) is an advanced stage of peripheral artery disease (PAD) that leads to limb loss/amputation. In the USA, the prevalence of CLTI is estimated to be between 2 and 3.4 million, and these numbers are projected to increase to 4.7 million by 2030 [1]. Approximately 29% of CLTI patients suffer a major amputation or die within the first year, and the risk of mortality is about 54% over 4 years [2]. In 2011, data from CLTI Medicare beneficiaries revealed that per CLTI patient, there was an average total cost of $93,800 over a 4-year follow-up period [2]. However, there is no consensus on the optimal management strategies of CLTI. The terms CLTI and critical limb ischemia (CLI) are often used interchangeably. In general, CLTI management aims pain reduction, wound healing, prevention of major amputation, and reduction of mortality [3]. Although revascularization whether endovascular or surgical bypass is regarded as an essential part of CLTI management [4], there is inconsistency in treatment approaches among providers as to the optimal initial and ongoing management of this complex subset of PAD.

T. K. Paul (✉)
University of Tennessee at Nashville, Nashville, TN, United States

S. Banerjee
Department of Medicine, University of Texas Southwestern Medical Center at Dallas, VA North Texas Health Care System, Dallas, TX, USA
e-mail: Subhash.Banerjee@utsouthwestern.edu

N. W. Shammas (ed.), *Peripheral Arterial Interventions*, Contemporary Cardiology, https://doi.org/10.1007/978-3-031-09741-6_16

Definition and Diagnosis

Chronic limb-threatening ischemia (CLTI) is the updated terminology of CLI, the advanced form of PAD characterized by rest pain, nonhealing ulcer/wound, or gangrene and categorized as Rutherford classes 4–6 [5]. The first test to diagnose CLTI is the ankle-brachial index (ABI) which is recommended as class I [6]. If ABI is between ≤0.9 and >0.70, additional perfusion assessment such as toe-brachial index (TBI) with waveform, transcutaneous oxygen pressure (TcPO2), and skin perfusion pressure (SPP) is reasonable to perform (IIa) [6]. TBI is indicated for non-compressible arteries (ABI >1.40). The likelihood of wound healing decreases with toe pressure <30 mmHg, and SPP ≥30–50 mmHg is associated with increased odds of wound healing [6]. Other noninvasive imaging such as duplex ultrasound, computed tomography angiography (CTA), or magnetic resonance angiography (MRA) are recommended as class I for the diagnosis of CLTI [6].

Invasive angiography including selective digital subtraction angiography (DSA) is the gold standard for detecting CLTI. However, only approximately 25% of patients undergo invasive angiography at time of diagnosis and less than one-third receive optimal medical therapy (OMT) [7, 8]. Studies have shown that the majority of the CLTI patients who underwent primary amputation had no diagnostic angiography or revascularization procedure prior to the amputation [8, 9]. Although considered gold standard, the invasive angiography predominantly allows for evaluation of the lumen, without the ability to fully examine the vessel wall. Lately, intravascular ultrasound (IVUS) has been used for the diagnosis of CLTI that provides information on the vessel wall, plaque morphology, plaque burden, and the extent of disease. The CLI Global Society has recently published an interdisciplinary expert recommendation for superselective DSA of the ankle and foot with an algorithm in appropriately indicated CLTI patients to optimize limb salvage and reduce the incidence of primary amputation [10]. A superselective digital subtraction angiography (DSA) should be utilized to determine a salvageable limb prior to amputation, and primary amputation should not be the first line of treatment for CLTI unless the limb is deemed nonviable [10]. This Society also recommends for the evaluation of CLTI patients by an interdisciplinary specialty care team and determination of whether a CLTI limb is salvageable or not.

Treatment Modalities

Medical Management

Although maintaining direct arterial blood flow with revascularization remains the key for the treatment of CLTI, concomitant guideline-directed medical therapy is equally important to prevent future major adverse limb events (MALE) and cardiovascular events. Ongoing aggressive cardiovascular risk factors modification, and regular exercise are essential parts of CLTI management similar to the management of any other forms of PAD. The 2016 American Heart Association/American College of Cardiology (AHA/ACC) guidelines on PAD stated that there are critical evidence gaps to support the determination of optimal antiplatelet and statin therapy [6]. There is limited evidence on statin therapy for CLTI patients. A meta-analysis including 19 studies with 26,985 CLTI patients demonstrated that patients treated with statin were 25% less likely to have amputation and 38% less chance of having a fatal event [11]. With current evidence, all patients with CLTI should be treated with statin and one antiplatelet therapy along with other guideline-directed therapies for hypertension and diabetes. Unfortunately, regardless of guideline recommendations for OMT with antiplatelet, antidiabetic, antihypertensive, and lipid-lowering medical therapy, less than one-third receive OMT [7, 8].

Revascularization

Although revascularization is the key for managing CLTI patient [12], whether surgical bypass or endovascular therapy as a first approach is still a matter of debate. However, endovascular approach is gaining popularity and has been proven to be an effective and safe approach and probably the better approach as compared to surgical revascularization for CLTI patients. Patients with CLTI often present with multilevel disease, and >70% have some degree of infrapopliteal disease for which [13] treatment of both inflow and outflow diseases is necessary for proper would healing. Progression of intermittent claudication to CLTI is rare; therefore, preemptive revascularization of claudicants to prevent progression to CLTI is not indicated [6].

Endovascular Approach

Technical Aspects of Endovascular Intervention

The complete discussion of the technical aspects of the endovascular therapy is beyond the scope of this chapter. Briefly, we discuss the key points of the endovascular approaches.

Access Site

Like any endovascular intervention, choosing an appropriate arterial access site is the key. Several factors that play roles in selecting access site are severity of disease including calcification in common femoral artery, tortuosity of the femoral and iliac arteries, bifurcating angle of the abdominal aorta, the lesion length and site, obesity, infection in the groin area, previous surgery, and available endovascular device compatibility. Antegrade access in the common femoral artery is one of the commonly used approaches to perform tibial and foot artery revascularization. This approach provides excellent wire pushability and other devices for crossing the lesions especially the chronic total occlusion (CTO) as this access site is closer to the lesions. Ultrasound-guided access may reduce radiation doses and vascular complications. However, if antegrade access fails to cross the lesion retrograde, pedal or tibial access is usually successful. The ultrasound-guided retrograde tibiopedal arterial access is becoming one of the popular and successful alternatives for endovascular interventions in CLTI patients. Saab et al. showed that pedal access was required in up to 67% of cases based on the findings of the CTOP (chronic total occlusion crossing approach based on plaque cap morphology) classification particularly if the disease involves the popliteal and tibial vessels [14]. Retrograde tibiopedal arterial minimally invasive (TAMI) technique was used to treat CLTI patients for whom common femoral artery access was not favorable [15]. This retrograde access was used to cross the lesion, and atherectomy, balloon angioplasty, and stenting were performed as well via this access [15].

Guidewire

The tip load, tip stiffness, hydrophilic coating of the tip and body (polymer-jacketed), guidewire flexibility, ability to shape, shaping memory, shaft support, torque transmission, trackability, and pushability are all critical components of a guidewire for a below-the-knee intervention [16]. Selection of the guidewire depends on the lesion location, lesion length, severity of stenosis, calcification, and CTO. Non-hydrophilic guidewires allow better tactile feedback and greater torque response and are less likely to cause dissection compared with hydrophilic wires. However, these guidewires have the lower chance of crossing a lesion particularly a CTO or severely calcified stenosis. Contrary, hydrophilic wire provides good maneuverability in tortuous and long vessels with minimal resistance but with higher chance of vessel dissection and reduced tactile feeling. Guidewires with higher tip stiffness increase penetration ability. Both 0.014-in and 0.018-in wires have been successfully used in below-the-knee interventions, but the selection of the wires is usually operator-dependent with some operators start with 0.018-in wires for CTOs.

Balloon/Support Catheter

There are many low-profile balloons of various sizes and lengths with either a 0.014-in or 0.018-in platform available for the below-the-knee (BTK) intervention. A 0.018-in over-the-wire (OTW) angioplasty balloon with increased shaft strength provides adequate pushability and wire support to cross a complex CTO. An OTW balloon catheter system with 0.018-in platform allows good control of the wire and allows a smooth exchange of the 0.018 in with a 0.014-in wire when needed. It also allows wire exchange without sacrificing the progress made through the lesion, and their lumen can be used to inject contrast as well for the verification of position and distal flow suggesting true lumen entry. There are various 0.018-in and 0.014-in compatible support catheters available and can be used for the similar purposes as OTW balloon.

The Concept of Angiosome in Treating CLTI

The foot and ankle area is composed of six demarcated angiosomes supplied by the anterior tibial artery, posterior tibial artery, and peroneal artery [17, 18]. The anterior tibial artery supplies the dorsal side of the foot and toes and the posterior tibial artery supplies the plantar side of the foot, toes, interdigital web spaces, and inner side of the heel, while the peroneal artery supplies the lateral ankle and lateral side of the heel. There are extensive connections between below-the-knee arteries supplying the foot with inter-angiosome supplying vessels. Whether angiosome-guided endovascular revascularization is necessary is not yet well validated as there is no objective method to evaluate foot perfusion after successful revascularization. The current AHA/ACC guidelines give class IIb recommendations for the use of angiosome-directed endovascular therapy for patients with CLTI and nonhealing wound or gangrene [6].

Different Endovascular Modalities

During the past decade, the catheter-based revascularization technologies have been profoundly advanced, replacing surgical bypass as the initial therapy in most cases especially with Rutherford class 5 and 6 diseases. This paradigm shift toward endovascular revascularization results in higher repeat interventions due to high restenosis rates and progression of disease. There are several endovascular access strategies for BTK/CLTI/CTO patients such as contralateral, antegrade, retrograde, and loop technique via the pedal arch, and choosing one of them as an initial approach depends on the operators' experience and preference. One of the important aspects of BTK CTO procedures is being flexible for switching from one approach to another and having a backup plan. Usually if one strategy is unsuccessful within 10 min, it is better to switch to alternate approach for successful recanalization and avoid the risks of injury to the BTK arteries for future attempts even it fails for the first time.

There is no consensus on evidence-based endovascular revascularization modalities for CLTI. Percutaneous transluminal angioplasty (PTA) with plain old balloon angioplasty (POBA)/conventional balloon angioplasty (BA), drug-coated balloon (DCB), scoring/cutting balloons, stents, and atherectomy devices either alone or in combination are used as the revascularization options for infrainguinal vessels. Patients with CLTI tend to have severely calcified arteries that pose significant challenges to endovascular techniques. Additionally, calcification decreases the effect of antiproliferative drugs delivered by current DCB and drug-eluting stent (DES) due to physical barrier to reach the endothelium proper. Although cheap, BA alone is not always sufficient/successful in these complex calcified lesions due to frequent vessel recoil, potential for spiral dissections, and perforations and tends to have the worst outcomes among all endovascular options [19].

Although stents provide better acute results, it is associated with in-stent restenosis, thrombosis, and stent fracture, poses a challenge to reintervention, and hinders for future surgical anastomotic sites [20]. A meta-analysis by Katsanos et al. demonstrated that infrapopliteal intervention with DES was associated with significantly reduced rates of restenosis, target lesion revascularization (TLR), and amputations and improved wound healing when compared with BA and bare-metal stent (BMS) [21]. In addition, DES was associated with significantly reduced amputations compared with paclitaxel-coated balloon [21].

Although associated with less TLR, DCBs are expensive, and like conventional BA, they also present with suboptimal results due to early recoil and flow-limiting dissections especially in calcified lesions if debulking/plaque modifications are not performed. Paclitaxel-based DCBs (IN.PACT Admiral, Lutonix, Stellarex, and Ranger balloons) are widely accepted interventional approaches after several randomized trials (RCT) showing benefit over conventional BA. Both IN.PACT SFA (Admiral™ DCB) [22] and LEVANT 2 trials (Lutonix DCB) [23, 24] revealed higher primary patency over conventional BA alone. IN.PACT SFA trial revealed superior primary patency and lower TLR with DCB compared with BA (69.5% vs 45.1% and 15.2% vs 31.1%, respectively) [25]. At 12 months, the rate of primary patency with DCB was higher as compared with conventional BA (65.2% vs 52.6%, $p = 0.02$) [24]. However, controversies arise after the publication of the meta-analysis by Katsanos et al. in 2018 showing increased risk of mortality in patients treated with paclitaxel-coated balloons [26]. A meta-analysis of individual level data (2185 subjects) from 8 RCTs that used paclitaxel containing devices with 4-year median follow-up demonstrated an absolute 4.6% increased mortality risk associated with the use of these devices [27]. However, several studies/analyses have showed no evidence of increased mortality with the use of paclitaxel-coated devices including in the treatment of CLTI patients [28–32]. Discussing the results of all these studies in detail is beyond the scope of our discussion. Results from a recent meta-analysis showed that there was no significant difference in short-term to midterm mortality in a predominately CLTI patients treated with paclitaxel-coated balloons or stents compared with uncoated balloons [29]. An unplanned analysis from the multicenter, randomized, open-label, registry-based SWEDEPAD (Swedish Drug-Elution Trial in Peripheral Arterial Disease) clinical trial demonstrated no significant difference in all-cause mortality between treatment with paclitaxel-coated or paclitaxel-uncoated devices between 1 and 4 years of follow-up [33]. This study randomized 2289 patients to drug-coated devices (1149 patients) or drug-uncoated devices (1140 patients). During a mean follow-up of 2.49 years, there was no significant difference in the incidence of death between the treatment groups among patients with CLTI. Results from the ILLUMENATE EU RCT and ILLUMENATE pivotal RCT were presented by Marianne Brodmann (University of Graz, Graz, Austria) at LINC 2021 (Leipzig Interventional Course; 25–29 January, virtual). These two RCTs which comprised of 600 patients showed that at 5 years, there was no difference in all-cause mortality (19.3% with the Stellarex DCB vs 19.4% with BA).

Atherectomy devices have been used for challenging calcified lesions for preparing vessels by debulking or modifying plaque for conventional BA or DCB angioplasty, but it is associated with higher cost. The available atherectomy devices for infrainguinal vessels are rotational, orbital, and directional atherectomy (DA) (Jetstream, Rotablator, Phoenix, ROTAREX®S, Diamondback 360, SilverHawk™, TurboHawk, and HawkOne™) and laser atherectomy (excimer and B-laser). However, for BTK vessels SilverHawk/TurboHawk, laser and Diamondback 360 orbital atherectomy are indicated. Each device has its unique properties with advantages, disadvantages, and contraindications and usually selected as per operators' experience, cost, and availability at individual institution. There are no head-to-head comparisons of these devices, and some atherectomy devices need concomitant distal embolic protection to capture atheroembolic debris. The individual description with specific advantages and disadvantages of each atherectomy device is beyond the scope of this section. The DEFINITIVE LE study, a large prospective study of 800 patients (1022 target lesions) with PAD including CLTI patients with infrapopliteal lesions, has demonstrated the safety and effectiveness of directional atherectomy [34]. In CLTI patients, the patency at 12 months was 68% for the superficial femoral artery, 67% for the popliteal artery, and 78% for the infrapopliteal artery [34]. Bailout stenting rate in DEFINITIVE LE trial was 3.2% and in DEFINITIVE Ca++ study was 4.1% in short, calcified femoropopliteal disease [34, 35]. A study by Rastan et al. revealed that the freedom from major amputation rate at 1 year was 97.1% in the infrapopliteal CLTI cohort [36]. A recent analysis of 36,860 Medicare patients with CLTI who had revascularization demonstrated that the rate of mortality and major amputation over 4 years were lower in atherectomy group compared with other modalities, including surgical bypass [19]. Intravascular shockwave lithotripsy is an alternate strategy without the need for distal protection and was used to treat moderate or severe calcification in DISRUPT PAD II trial with a technical success rate of 100% and residual stenosis of 24.2% [37].

The combination of atherectomy with balloon angioplasty alone or DCB or DES has showed improved clinical outcomes as compared to BA alone. In the randomized DEFINITIVE AR trial, the SilverHawk and TurboHawk atherectomy devices were used comparing DA plus DCB versus DCB alone [38]. Grade C/D dissections were seen less frequently in the DA group (2.1% vs 18.5%; $p = 0.01$) with a need for bailout stenting in 3.7% versus none in patients who received a DCB alone vs DA, respectively, and the rate of flow-limiting dissections was 19% for DCB alone and 2% for DA plus DCB ($p = 0.01$) [38]. Another study revealed primary patency rate at 1 year was significantly higher in the DA + DCB group compared to DCB alone (65% vs 82%; $p = 0.021$) in isolated popliteal lesions [39]. The REALITY (DiRectional AthErectomy + Drug CoAted BaLloon to Treat Long, CalcifIed FemoropopliTeal ArterY Lesions) study prospectively enrolled 102 patients with 8- to 36-cm femoropopliteal stenoses or occlusions with bilateral vessel wall calcification treated with DA prior to DCB angioplasty. The results were presented at

VIVA (Vascular InterVentional Advances) annual meeting, November 6–8, 2020. This study revealed that provisional stents were implanted in 9% of patients, the 12-month primary patency rate was 77%, and the freedom from clinically driven TLR rate was 93%.

Despite adequate vessel preparation, some patients still may have flow-limiting dissections or recoil, resulting in severe residual stenosis that need stenting. A "spot-stenting" approach with short stents using Tack Endovascular System (Intact Vascular, Inc.) rather than using full metal jacket will allow the future interventional technique simpler than those required to intervene typical long in-stent restenosis [40].

Surgical Approach

Several factors may be considered as favorable for surgical revascularization: (1) patients with a life expectancy of >2 years and potential to have good functional capacity after revascularization; (2) long segment tibial occlusion (TASC D), femoral bifurcation disease, and popliteal (P2, P3) occlusive disease; (3) failed endovascular treatment; (4) lack of healing or symptom relief despite endovascular therapy; and (5) significant tissue loss >2 cm. Although conducted in remote past, the results of the BASIL trial indicated that patients with relatively good functional capacity and expected to live >2 years should be considered for surgical bypass given the apparent improved durability and reduced reintervention rate of surgery, whereas those with significant comorbidities or a life expectancy <2 years should be offered endovascular therapy when possible [41]. Larger areas of tissue loss (>2-cm transverse diameter) may heal more often and more rapidly with bypass [42]. Bypass may be better for patients with chronic total occlusions (TASC D lesions), with involvement of the common femoral bifurcation especially if the profunda femoris artery is diseased, and with long, complex tibial artery occlusion, particularly if an autogenous conduit is available [43]. Of course, surgical bypass is warranted after failed endovascular therapy [44]. Availability of appropriate bypass graft conduit particularly the autologous conduit is the key for long-term patency. The great saphenous vein remains the ideal choice, either ipsilateral or contralateral, with 80% good patency and limb preservation at 5 years [45]. On the other hand, the prosthetic bypass conduit showed a 52% and 35% limb preservation rates at 2 and 5 years, respectively, for femoropopliteal revascularization, and the rate for tibial arteries is much lower [46].

Endovascular Versus Surgical First

There is no consensus on the evidence-based endovascular-first versus surgical-first modality for treating patients with CLTI. The "endovascular first" is considered as the preferred revascularization approach for symptomatic infrainguinal atherosclerotic disease [47]. Currently, endovascular intervention for BTK vessel is a preferable first-line treatment for patients with CLTI due to high technical success and better clinical outcomes with a low complication rate. The main purpose for tibial and pedal artery intervention in CLTI patients is limb salvage and prevention of amputations. As many CLTI patients have severe comorbidities, the endovascular-first approach generally preferred in view of the reduction of surgical site infection, recovery time, and other potential systemic complications.

Evidence by randomized data is lacking to guide us in choosing optimal mode of revascularization for patients with CLTI and the waited BEST-CLI [48] and BASIL-2 [49]. RCTs would provide further evidence for clarity in managing these subsets of patients. Two recent retrospective studies revealed equivocal results between surgical and endovascular means of revascularization. A retrospective analysis of 108 patients with infrageniculate disease comparing surgical and endovascular modalities demonstrated no significant difference in MALE, overall survival, or amputation-free survival (AFS) at 3 years [50]. However, an endovascular strategy was associated with increased revascularization rate during the follow-up period [50]. Another retrospective study including 264 CLTI patients who underwent bypass or percutaneous transluminal angioplasty in femoropopliteal vessels showed similar technical success and limb preservation rates between the two approaches [51]. However, angioplasty was associated with a shorter hospital stay and fewer reinterventions for procedural complications [51]. The National Surgical Quality Improvement Program (NSQIP) database included patients with CLTI and isolated infrageniculate disease who underwent bypass-first or endovascular-first revascularization [52]. The results demonstrated that patients who had bypass first as compared with endovascular first had lower amputation rate (4.3% vs 7.4%; 95% CI, 0.36–0.98). There were no differences in MALE, 30-day loss of patency, reintervention, readmissions, or reoperations between two groups [52]. However, there was increased wound complication rates (9.7% vs 3.7%; 95% CI, 1.71–4.42), major adverse cardiovascular events (6.9% vs 2.6%; 95% CI, 2.18–6.88), and higher 30-day mortality rates (3.23% vs 1.8%; 95% CI, 1.26–6.11) in surgical bypass patients [52]. The limitation of this database analysis is that no follow-up beyond perioperative period. An observational study using Medicare claims data ($N = 36{,}860$) with propensity-match analysis on CLTI patients revealed all-cause mortality rate was 54.7% for angioplasty, 53.7% for stent deployment, and 51.4% for surgical bypass ($p < 0.05$ for all pairwise comparisons) [19]. The higher amputation was observed in surgical bypass patients (10.8%) versus angioplasty (8.1%) and stent deployment (7.8%) ($p < 0.05$ for all pairwise comparisons except angioplasty vs stent) [19].

Novel Treatment Modalities

Deep Venous Arterialization (DVA)

End-stage CLTI or "dessert foot" was observed in up to 20% of CLTI patients who have no bypass or endovascular revascularization options aka "no options" due to the uncrossable severely calcified lesions, extensive comorbidities, and especially absence of or very poor distal target vessels [53, 54]. Major amputation remains as the only viable option in these patients unless percutaneous deep vein arterialization (pDVA) can be performed as a last resort if not a surgical DVA candidate [53, 54]. The LimFlow pDVA System (LimFlow, Inc.) is a promising revascularization option for this end-stage CLTI population. The PROMISE I (the United States) early feasibility study included 32 "no-option" CLTI patients who were indicated for major amputation presented by Clair D at VIVA (November 5–6, 2019, Las Vegas). The study demonstrated that 67% of patients wound had healed or healing with 74% major amputation-free survival at 6 months. A study published recently demonstrated that pDVA with the LimFlow device is associated with 97% technical success rate and 83.9%, 71.0%, and 67.2% amputation-free survival at 6, 12, and 24 months, respectively [55]. In addition, limb salvage was 86.8%, 79.8%, and 79.8% at 6, 12, and 24 months, respectively, and complete wound healing was achieved with 36.6%, 68.2%, and 72.7% of patients at 6, 12, and 24 months, respectively [55].

Endovascular Bypass Technology

Approximately two-thirds of CLTI patients present with a combination of femoropopliteal and infrapopliteal disease [56], making endovascular treatment outcomes for these long lesions suboptimal with prohibitively high surgical risk in these critically ill high comorbid patients [6]. The PQ Bypass System (PQ Bypass, Inc.) is an endovascular approach to femoropopliteal bypass that aims to provide long-term durability and minimize surgical risks. The safety and effectiveness of this device will be investigated in the prospective, international DETOUR II study (NCT03119233).

Postrevascularization CLTI Management

Wound Care

After reestablishment of arterial blood flow, a comprehensive wound care management is a part and parcel for limb preservation and wound healing. Innovative wound care treatment methods are being developed and utilized (e.g., amniotic membrane grafts), and ongoing investigation is essential to advance the wound healing process.

Future Perspectives

Future studies are needed investigating systematically on medication, dietary, and exercise therapy to optimize and sustain successful revascularization outcomes with the aim of reducing mortality, improving quality of life, and preventing amputation.

More trials are needed to compare different endovascular treatment modalities among devices and combination of devices such as atherectomy plus BA, DCB, and DES versus these devices alone or combinations for choosing appropriate devices and defining optimal outcomes.

Conclusion

Screening PAD and early diagnosis of CLTI are essential to prevent amputation, improve quality of life, and reduce mortality. Multidisciplinary team approach with a joint decision-making including patients, caregivers, and physicians is crucial, and close communication between interventionalists and vascular surgeons is paramount to providing the optimal care for patients with CLTI. Aggressive management of cardiovascular risk factors, standardized and advanced wound care, and close surveillance of perfusion status are essential as well. There is a gap in evidence, and current guidelines are lacking in providing clear recommendations for the management of CLTI. pDVA is emerging as promising treatment modality in "no-option" CLTI patients. Prospective BEST-CLI and BASIL-2 RCTs will provide further evidence in managing CLTI patients.

References

1. Yost M. Epidemiology of critical limb ischemia (CLI): prevalence and comorbidities. CLI Global. 2019;1:6.
2. Mustapha JA, Katzen BT, Neville RF, Lookstein RA, Zeller T, Miller LE, et al. Determinants of long-term outcomes and costs in the management of critical limb ischemia: a population-based cohort study. J Am Heart Assoc. 2018;7(16):e009724.
3. Gray BH, Diaz-Sandoval LJ, Dieter RS, Jaff MR, White CJ. SCAI expert consensus statement for infrapopliteal arterial intervention appropriate use. Catheter Cardiovasc Interv. 2014;84(4):539–45.
4. Bailey SR, Beckman JA, Dao TD, Misra S, Sobieszczyk PS, White CJ, et al. ACC/AHA/SCAI/SIR/SVM 2018 appropriate use criteria for peripheral artery intervention: a report of the American College of Cardiology Appropriate use criteria task force, American Heart Association, Society for Cardiovascular Angiography and Interventions, Society of Interventional Radiology, and Society for Vascular Medicine. J Am Coll Cardiol. 2019;73(2):214–37.
5. Duff S, Mafilios MS, Bhounsule P, Hasegawa JT. The burden of critical limb ischemia: a review of recent literature. Vasc Health Risk Manag. 2019;15:187–208.
6. Gerhard-Herman MD, Gornik HL, Barrett C, Barshes NR, Corriere MA, Drachman DE, et al. 2016 AHA/ACC guideline on the management of patients with lower extremity peripheral artery disease: a report of the American College of Cardiology/American Heart Association task force on clinical practice guidelines. J Am Coll Cardiol. 2017;69(11):e71–e126.
7. Chung J, Timaran DA, Modrall JG, Ahn C, Timaran CH, Kirkwood ML, et al. Optimal medical therapy predicts amputation-free survival in chronic critical limb ischemia. J Vasc Surg. 2013;58(4):972–80.
8. Henry AJ, Hevelone ND, Belkin M, Nguyen LL. Socioeconomic and hospital-related predictors of amputation for critical limb ischemia. J Vasc Surg. 2011;53(2):330–9.e1.

9. Goodney PP, Travis LL, Nallamothu BK, Holman K, Suckow B, Henke PK, et al. Variation in the use of lower extremity vascular procedures for critical limb ischemia. Circ Cardiovasc Qual Outcomes. 2012;5(1):94–102.
10. Mustapha JA, Saab FA, Martinsen BJ, Pena CS, Zeller T, Driver VR, et al. Digital subtraction angiography prior to an amputation for critical limb ischemia (CLI): an expert recommendation statement from the CLI global society to optimize limb salvage. J Endovasc Ther. 2020;27(4):540–6.
11. Kokkinidis DG, Arfaras-Melainis A, Giannopoulos S, Katsaros I, Jawaid O, Jonnalagadda AK, et al. Statin therapy for reduction of cardiovascular and limb-related events in critical limb ischemia: a systematic review and meta-analysis. Vasc Med. 2020;25(2):106–17.
12. Uccioli L, Meloni M, Izzo V, Giurato L, Merolla S, Gandini R. Critical limb ischemia: current challenges and future prospects. Vasc Health Risk Manag. 2018;14:63–74.
13. Graziani L, Silvestro A, Bertone V, Manara E, Andreini R, Sigala A, et al. Vascular involvement in diabetic subjects with ischemic foot ulcer: a new morphologic categorization of disease severity. Eur J Vasc Endovasc Surg. 2007;33(4):453–60.
14. Saab F, Jaff MR, Diaz-Sandoval LJ, Engen GD, McGoff TN, Adams G, et al. Chronic total occlusion crossing approach based on plaque cap morphology: the CTOP classification. J Endovasc Ther. 2018;25(3):284–91.
15. Mustapha JA, Saab F, McGoff TN, Adams G, Mullins JR, Al-Dadah A, et al. Tibiopedal arterial minimally invasive retrograde revascularization (TAMI) in patients with peripheral arterial disease and critical limb ischemia. On behalf of the peripheral registry of endovascular clinical outcomes (PRIME). Catheter Cardiovasc Interv. 2020;95(3):447–54.
16. Godino C, Sharp AS, Carlino M, Colombo A. Crossing CTOs-the tips, tricks, and specialist kit that can mean the difference between success and failure. Catheter Cardiovasc Interv. 2009;74(7):1019–46.
17. Taylor GI, Palmer JH. The vascular territories (angiosomes) of the body: experimental study and clinical applications. Br J Plast Surg. 1987;40(2):113–41.
18. Taylor GI, Palmer JH. Angiosome theory. Br J Plast Surg. 1992;45(4):327–8.
19. Mustapha JA, Katzen BT, Neville RF, Lookstein RA, Zeller T, Miller LE, et al. Propensity score-adjusted comparison of long-term outcomes among revascularization strategies for critical limb ischemia. Circ Cardiovasc Interv. 2019;12(9):e008097.
20. Yu JS, Park KM, Jeon YS, Cho SG, Hong KC, Shin WY, et al. Midterm outcome of femoral artery stenting and factors affecting patency. Vasc Specialist Int. 2015;31(4):115–9.
21. Katsanos K, Kitrou P, Spiliopoulos S, Diamantopoulos A, Karnabatidis D. Comparative effectiveness of plain balloon angioplasty, bare metal stents, drug-coated balloons, and drug-eluting stents for the treatment of infrapopliteal artery disease: systematic review and Bayesian network meta-analysis of randomized controlled trials. J Endovasc Ther. 2016;23(6):851–63.
22. Tepe G, Laird J, Schneider P, Brodmann M, Krishnan P, Micari A, et al. Drug-coated balloon versus standard percutaneous transluminal angioplasty for the treatment of superficial femoral and popliteal peripheral artery disease: 12-month results from the IN.PACT SFA randomized trial. Circulation. 2015;131(5):495–502.
23. Ouriel K, Adelman MA, Rosenfield K, Scheinert D, Brodmann M, Peña C, et al. Safety of paclitaxel-coated balloon angioplasty for femoropopliteal peripheral artery disease. JACC Cardiovasc Interv. 2019;12(24):2515–24.
24. Rosenfield K, Jaff MR, White CJ, Rocha-Singh K, Mena-Hurtado C, Metzger DC, et al. Trial of a paclitaxel-coated balloon for femoropopliteal artery disease. N Engl J Med. 2015;373(2):145–53.
25. Schneider PA, Laird JR, Tepe G, Brodmann M, Zeller T, Scheinert D, et al. Treatment effect of drug-coated balloons is durable to 3 years in the femoropopliteal arteries: long-term results of the IN.PACT SFA randomized trial. Circ Cardiovasc Interv. 2018;11(1):e005891.
26. Katsanos K, Spiliopoulos S, Kitrou P, Krokidis M, Karnabatidis D. Risk of death following application of paclitaxel-coated balloons and stents in the femoropopliteal artery of the leg:

a systematic review and meta-analysis of randomized controlled trials. J Am Heart Assoc. 2018;7(24):e011245.
27. Rocha-Singh KJ, Duval S, Jaff MR, Schneider PA, Ansel GM, Lyden SP, et al. Mortality and paclitaxel-coated devices: an individual patient data meta-analysis. Circulation. 2020;141(23):1859–69.
28. Behrendt CA, Sedrakyan A, Peters F, Kreutzburg T, Schermerhorn M, Bertges DJ, et al. Editor's choice—long term survival after femoropopliteal artery revascularisation with paclitaxel coated devices: a propensity score matched cohort analysis. Eur J Vasc Endovasc Surg. 2020;59(4):587–96.
29. Dinh K, Gomes ML, Thomas SD, Paravastu SCV, Holden A, Schneider PA, et al. Mortality after paclitaxel-coated device use in patients with chronic limb-threatening ischemia: a systematic review and meta-analysis of randomized controlled trials. J Endovasc Ther. 2020;27(2):175–85.
30. Freisinger E, Koeppe J, Gerss J, Goerlich D, Malyar NM, Marschall U, et al. Mortality after use of paclitaxel-based devices in peripheral arteries: a real-world safety analysis. Eur Heart J. 2020;41(38):3732–9.
31. Secemsky EA, Kundi H, Weinberg I, Jaff MR, Krawisz A, Parikh SA, et al. Association of survival with femoropopliteal artery revascularization with drug-coated devices. JAMA Cardiol. 2019;4(4):332–40.
32. Shishehbor MH, Secemsky EA, Varcoe RL. Is there a real association between paclitaxel devices and mortality? Time to pause and re-evaluate what we know about this statistical finding. J Am Heart Assoc. 2019;8(10):e012524.
33. Nordanstig J, James S, Andersson M, Andersson M, Danielsson P, Gillgren P, et al. Mortality with paclitaxel-coated devices in peripheral artery disease. N Engl J Med. 2020;383(26):2538–46.
34. McKinsey JF, Zeller T, Rocha-Singh KJ, Jaff MR, Garcia LA. Lower extremity revascularization using directional atherectomy: 12-month prospective results of the DEFINITIVE LE study. JACC Cardiovasc Interv. 2014;7(8):923–33.
35. Roberts D, Niazi K, Miller W, Krishnan P, Gammon R, Schreiber T, et al. Effective endovascular treatment of calcified femoropopliteal disease with directional atherectomy and distal embolic protection: final results of the DEFINITIVE Ca^{++} trial. Catheter Cardiovasc Interv. 2014;84(2):236–44.
36. Rastan A, McKinsey JF, Garcia LA, Rocha-Singh KJ, Jaff MR, Noory E, et al. One-year outcomes following directional atherectomy of infrapopliteal artery lesions: subgroup results of the prospective, multicenter DEFINITIVE LE trial. J Endovasc Ther. 2015;22(6):839–46.
37. Brodmann M, Werner M, Holden A, Tepe G, Scheinert D, Schwindt A, et al. Primary outcomes and mechanism of action of intravascular lithotripsy in calcified, femoropopliteal lesions: results of disrupt PAD II. Catheter Cardiovasc Interv. 2019;93(2):335–42.
38. Zeller T, Langhoff R, Rocha-Singh KJ, Jaff MR, Blessing E, Amann-Vesti B, et al. Directional atherectomy followed by a paclitaxel-coated balloon to inhibit restenosis and maintain vessel patency: twelve-month results of the DEFINITIVE AR study. Circ Cardiovasc Interv. 2017;10(9):e004848.
39. Stavroulakis K, Schwindt A, Torsello G, Stachmann A, Hericks C, Bosiers MJ, et al. Directional atherectomy with antirestenotic therapy vs drug-coated balloon angioplasty alone for isolated popliteal artery lesions. J Endovasc Ther. 2017;24(2):181–8.
40. Gray WA, Cardenas JA, Brodmann M, Werner M, Bernardo NI, George JC, et al. Treating post-angioplasty dissection in the femoropopliteal arteries using the tack endovascular system: 12-month results from the TOBA II study. JACC Cardiovasc Interv. 2019;12(23):2375–84.
41. Adam DJ, Beard JD, Cleveland T, Bell J, Bradbury AW, Forbes JF, et al. Bypass versus angioplasty in severe ischaemia of the leg (BASIL): multicentre, randomised controlled trial. Lancet. 2005;366(9501):1925–34.
42. Neville RF, Capone A, Amdur R. A single center experience comparing tibial bypass with heparin-bonded ePTFE vs saphenous vein. J Vasc Surg. 2010;52:1746–7.

43. Giles KA, Pomposelli FB, Spence TL, Hamdan AD, Blattman SB, Panossian H, et al. Infrapopliteal angioplasty for critical limb ischemia: relation of TransAtlantic InterSociety consensus class to outcome in 176 limbs. J Vasc Surg. 2008;48(1):128–36.
44. Joels CS, York JW, Kalbaugh CA, Cull DL, Langan EM 3rd, Taylor SM. Surgical implications of early failed endovascular intervention of the superficial femoral artery. J Vasc Surg. 2008;47(3):562–5.
45. Neville RF, Capone A, Amdur R, Lidsky M, Babrowicz J, Sidawy AN. A comparison of tibial artery bypass performed with heparin-bonded expanded polytetrafluoroethylene and great saphenous vein to treat critical limb ischemia. J Vasc Surg. 2012;56(4):1008–14.
46. Hobson RW 2nd, Lynch TG, Jamil Z, Karanfilian RG, Lee BC, Padberg FT Jr, et al. Results of revascularization and amputation in severe lower extremity ischemia: a five-year clinical experience. J Vasc Surg. 1985;2(1):174–85.
47. Garg K, Kaszubski PA, Moridzadeh R, Rockman CB, Adelman MA, Maldonado TS, et al. Endovascular-first approach is not associated with worse amputation-free survival in appropriately selected patients with critical limb ischemia. J Vasc Surg. 2014;59(2):392–9.
48. Menard MT, Farber A, Assmann SF, Choudhry NK, Conte MS, Creager MA, et al. Design and rationale of the best endovascular versus best surgical therapy for patients with critical limb ischemia (BEST-CLI) trial. J Am Heart Assoc. 2016;5(7):e003219.
49. Popplewell MA, Davies H, Jarrett H, Bate G, Grant M, Patel S, et al. Bypass versus angioplasty in severe ischaemia of the leg - 2 (BASIL-2) trial: study protocol for a randomised controlled trial. Trials. 2016;17:11.
50. Biagioni RB, Nasser F, Matielo MF, Burihan MC, Brochado Neto FC, Ingrund JC, et al. Comparison of bypass and endovascular intervention for popliteal occlusion with the involvement of trifurcation for critical limb ischemia. Ann Vasc Surg. 2020;63:218–26.
51. Altreuther M, Mattsson E. Long-term limb salvage and amputation-free survival after femoropopliteal bypass and femoropopliteal PTA for critical ischemia in a clinical cohort. Vasc Endovasc Surg. 2019;53(2):112–7.
52. Dayama A, Tsilimparis N, Kolakowski S, Matolo NM, Humphries MD. Clinical outcomes of bypass-first versus endovascular-first strategy in patients with chronic limb-threatening ischemia due to infrageniculate arterial disease. J Vasc Surg. 2019;69(1):156–63.e1.
53. Faglia E, Clerici G, Clerissi J, Gabrielli L, Losa S, Mantero M, et al. Long-term prognosis of diabetic patients with critical limb ischemia: a population-based cohort study. Diabetes Care. 2009;32(5):822–7.
54. Mustapha JA, Saab FA, Clair D, Schneider P. Interim results of the PROMISE I trial to investigate the LimFlow system of percutaneous deep vein arterialization for the treatment of critical limb ischemia. J Invasive Cardiol. 2019;31(3):57–63.
55. Schmidt A, Schreve MA, Huizing E, Del Giudice C, Branzan D, Ünlü Ç, et al. Midterm outcomes of percutaneous deep venous arterialization with a dedicated system for patients with no-option chronic limb-threatening ischemia: the ALPS multicenter study. J Endovasc Ther. 2020;27(4):658–65.
56. Mustapha JA, Diaz-Sandoval LJ, Saab F. Infrapopliteal calcification patterns in critical limb ischemia: diagnostic, pathologic and therapeutic implications in the search for the endovascular holy grail. J Cardiovasc Surg. 2017;58(3):383–401.

Chapter 17
Distal Embolization in the Treatment of Peripheral Arterial Disease

Michael H. Wholey

Historical Background

In early interventional radiology literature, writers reported a rate of distal embolization rates between 3.8 and 37% related to angioplasty of arteries in the iliac and femoropopliteal system [1–3]. In 2005, we submitted the first publications on the use of distal embolic protection with atherectomy devices used in the femoropopliteal artery and recorded a high incidence (10/10) of embolic plaque ranging in size from 0.5 to 10 mm [4, 5]. We did not expect the ensuing controversy about the creation and the treatment options for distal emboli during peripheral arterial interventions of the lower extremities [5, 6]. For nearly 16 years, this debate has continued with several studies and reviews despite the highly charged economic forces involved. There are multiple variables in addressing the problem, the most important being how relevant are the distal emboli.

The Problem: Distal Embolization from Endovascular Procedures

All arterial interventions be it crossing an atherosclerotic lesion with a wire, ballooning, stenting, or debulking all can result in distal embolic material [7]. (Refer to Fig. 17.1a–c). This distal embolization includes material ejected off the atherosclerotic plaque as well as thromboemboli. Distal embolization occurs in all arterial beds including the coronary, carotid, and intracerebral, renal, aortic, and pelvic and lower extremities. The clinical significance and the ability to diagnose the

M. H. Wholey (✉)
Audie L. Murphy Memorial Veterans Hospital, San Antonio, TX, USA

N. W. Shammas (ed.), *Peripheral Arterial Interventions*, Contemporary Cardiology, https://doi.org/10.1007/978-3-031-09741-6_17

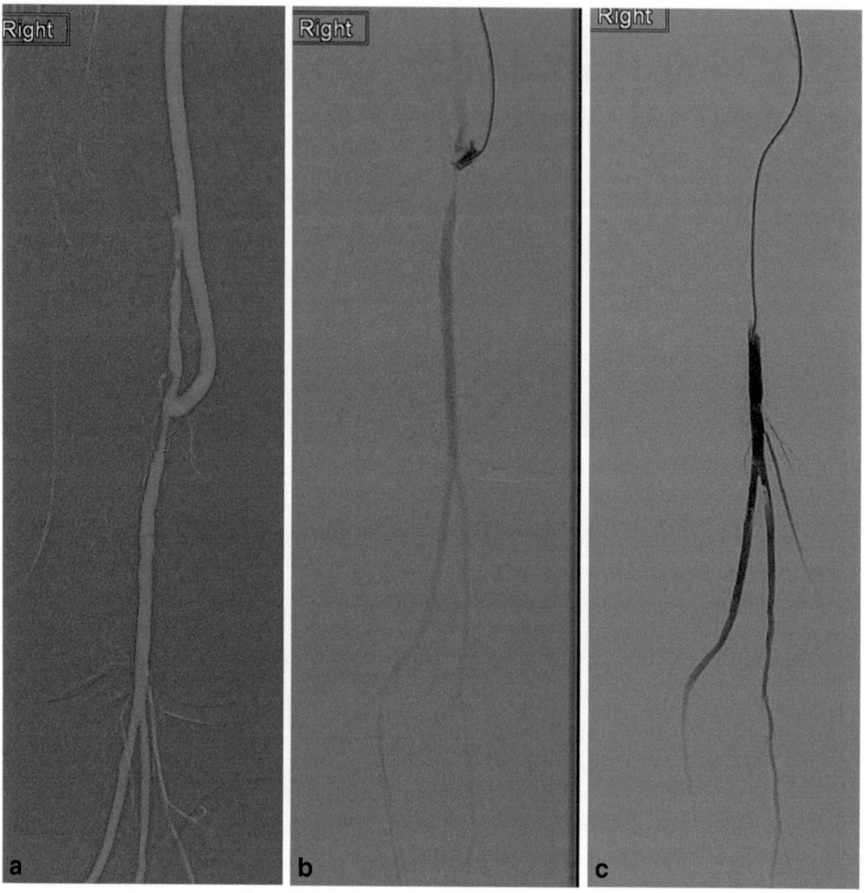

Fig. 17.1 (**a**) Initial carbon dioxide angiogram revealing moderate disease at the distal end of the fem-pop bypass graft. (**b**) Contrast injection with a 4-Fr Glide catheter near the distal anastomosis revealing greater stenosis along native popliteal artery and patent three vessels distally (not shown). (**c**) With the Glidecath across the stenosis, contrast injection reveals the new filling defect in the tibial peroneal artery (arrow)

occurrence of the distal emboli depend upon the region treated and the imaging available. For example, with carotid artery angioplasty and stent placement, the diagnosis of distal emboli depended much upon the use of diffusion-weighted MR images documenting the multiple ischemic insults. Neurological correlation would then be provided to determine the resultant clinical significance.

So how is distal embolization determined in PAD cases? This ranges from the following:

- Increased Doppler signals that occur distal to the treated area during a case.
- Whether there is material retained within the embolic protection device (EPD) basket if used. The material has been delineated to visible and macroscopic

material or as microscopic; the determining diameter of microscopic versus macroscopic material varies to under 2 mm in some studies and under diameter <100 μm in other studies [8, 9].
- Angiographic findings of distal embolization pre- and post-intervention which usually pertains to those large vessels of the trifurcation; there has been little written about the loss of the small arteries in the foot. Likewise, most studies did not employ an independent core lab. The quality of conventional digital subtraction angiography can vary resulting in different resolution and detection of small emboli [10].
- Whether further intervention is needed. Some studies have used "distal emboli" to denote the need for TLR or other interventions.

What are the Rates of Distal Embolization?

As the table below reveals, there is a wide range of reported distal emboli that occurs with PAD inventions depending upon a multitude of factors including:

1. Target location: Aortoiliac which has had larger vessel diameter with more chronic disease, femoropopliteal which has the largest series of data with extensive use of distal protection (DP), and below the knee (BTK) with generally less plaque volume and vessels too small for DP.
2. Acuteness of symptoms: Acute ischemia traditionally had higher fresh clot and clot burden with larger and more disastrous distal embolization downstream. Most studies deal with chronic ischemic disease with older plaque and established thromboemboli.
3. Whether EDP is used and how is the debris counted: Microemboli or macroemboli in the basket.
4. Who measures the severity of the distal emboli? (Table 17.1).

Incidence of Distal Emboli

The incidence of distal embolization during lower extremity arterial intervention is easily determined by visible or macroscopic debris particles, usually greater than 2 mm, retained in the EDP basket. In Krishnam's study of 508 patients, he had 62% of cases with macroscopic debris [14]. Yet in Shammas' study of 557 patients, there were only 2.4% [13]. This variation in incidence from two respective centers with similar procedures and patient types may reflect the random nature of the embolic debris created. Microscopic debris found in the filter baskets was highly prevalent in some studies such as Spiliopoulos and Lewis' studies showing 100% and 87%, respectively [9, 10]. Müller et al. evaluated the safety and effectiveness of EPD in reducing distal embolization during percutaneous lower extremity interventions

Table 17.1 Review of distal embolization incidence in major PAD studies

Author	Targ sites	Years	Pt no.	Lesion no.	Device	EDP filter?	% Distal emboli	% Clinical significance
Cassius [11]	Iliac/ SFA-POP	2017		10,875	All	Angio	1.7%	66%req'd treatment
Shirankde [12]	SFA-POP	2011	1029 18 18 55 570 740 736	2137	Jetstream CSI Laser PTA PTA/Stent SilverHawk	Angio	1.6% 22% 22% 3.6% 0.9% 0.7% 0.1%	
Shammas [13]	SFA-POP	2009	557	1183	All types	Yes	2.4%	2.4%
Krishnan [14]	SFA-POP	2017	508		All		62% macro	15% filter overflow
Balzer [15]	Iliac	2010	195	285	PTA/Stent	Yes	4.2%	
Definitive CA study [16]	SFA-POP	2014	133	168	SilverHawk	Yes	97.5%	3 cases
Milnerowicz [17]	Iliac/ SFA	2019	74		Rotarex	Angio.	8.1%	
PROTECT registry [18]	SFA-POP	2008	40	43 13	PTA/Stent SilverHawk	Yes Yes	28% 91%	>2 mm
DEEP Emboli [8]	SFA-POP	2009	20	44	Laser spectra	Yes	66%	Macrodebris in 12 cases
Spiliopoulos [9]	SFA-POP	2014	40		PTA/Stent	Yes	100%micro	No angio-occlusions
Lewis [10]	SFA-POP	2010	35	64	PTA/Stent	Yes	87% micro	3 DP baskets completely full
Hadidi [19]	SFA-POP	2012	30	36	All	Balloon	89%	Angiographic 5.5%

including angioplasty/stenting and directional atherectomy [20]. All patients undergoing directional atherectomy with the SilverHawk device demonstrated significant macroembolization, and 37.9% of patients undergoing angioplasty and/or stenting demonstrated significant macroembolization [20].

The incidence of distal embolization detected angiographically or clinically was reported between 1.6 and 8.1%; however, contemporary studies have demonstrated a much higher incidence of 3.8–67% [1, 10, 18, 21–24]. As for other modalities, Lam et al. used a transcranial Doppler to detect signals related to DE during superficial femoral artery (SFA) interventions and found 100% occurrence [25]. So why would the angiographic detection be so much lower for distal emboli detection compared to filter retention studies? It may be due to equipment used, limited views of the foot and distal circulation, and economic forces: Why look for trouble?

As the above chart shows, the incidence of distal emboli is difficult to determine from the various registries and single-center studies. In PTA/stent procedures involving the SFA-POP, distal emboli occurred from 0.7 to 100%. For atherectomy usage, the range for distal embolization was from 0.1 to 97.5%. Obviously, the rate of distal embolization is higher with atherectomy and other invasive means of treating atherosclerotic disease compared to angioplasty and stenting. In the PROTECT registry, basket captured distal embolization occurred in 28% of the PTA/stent cases versus 91% of the atherectomy (FoxHollow SilverHawk) [18]. In Shirankde's study, there was a 22% angiographic rate of embolization with the CSI and Jetstream versus 0.9% for PTA/stent [12].

A special risk is treating acute arterial occlusions: high rate of distal embolization often resulting in complete occlusions downstream. The rate of distal embolization during thrombolytic therapy in limb-threatening ischemia has been reported as 3.8–37% [22, 24].

The Clinical Relevance of Distal Emboli

All arterial interventions can cause distal embolic complications. For the PAD, positive embolic debris findings are reported either with distal protection devices with full or partially full baskets, with angiographic findings of distal vessels occluded, or by ultrasound. But for PAD cases, it is difficult to determine how significant the loss of a peroneal, anterior, or a posterior tibial artery following an embolic shower. These lost vessels raise questions: Does distal emboli result in discoloration? Does it result in the poor healing of a wound? Does it clear in time? Does the patient have worsening claudication, ABI, or other parameters? These are all questions with vague answers, which are easily overlooked, and which are why it is hard to justify and to subsequently provide adequate reimbursement for the use of distal protection and why after 16 years we ask the same question: Do we really need distal protection for PAD cases?

Muller et al. reported performing 30 lower extremity revascularizations for the femoropopliteal artery and used an embolic protection device (DP) in all of the cases. All of the filters were found to have debris under microscope examination, and 90% were deemed "clinically significant" because they were visible by the naked eye [20]. In our limited series in 2005, we were surprised by the large size of the fragments of plaque for the diameters of the tibial vessels are often under 2–3 mm [5]. As Shammas et al. said, large debris >2 mm do occur at a high frequency, ranging from 20 to >90% depending on lesions and devices used [18]. Thus, it would not take much to totally occlude the infrapopliteal vessels.

The pathological features of the captured distal emboli have been interesting to study. We found that when angioplasty and stent placement were performed in high-risk patients, the debris tended to be small fragments or microembolization. Treatment with atherectomy devices led to larger or more visible fragments. According to published data, embolic material during peripheral endovascular procedures consists of plaque and vessel lumen components, such as fibrin, calcified deposits, cholesterol clefts, and inflammatory and endothelial cells [26, 27]. In Karnabatidis et al.'s study, they found in their 50 cases the total area of occlusion was 2.76 ± 6.5 mm^2 with 12% of the particles greater than 3 mm [27]. Collected particles included platelets, fibrin conglomerates, trapped RBC, inflammatory cells, and extracellular matrix which compose atherosclerotic plaque and thrombosed elements [27]. Hence, with such material occluding infrapopliteal arteries, it will be hard to succeed with standard thrombolytic therapy with tPA that only works on a thrombus 2–3 weeks or less.

The peripheral microcirculation in ischemic patients has been compromised, and any further downstream embolization may result in worsening or persistent ischemia [12]. This is supported by the findings of Karnabatidis in which histologic analysis demonstrated a greater amount of collected particles in the filter baskets positively correlating with increased lesion length and reference vessel diameter, acute thrombosis, and total vessel occlusion [4, 10]. All of these factors could lead to disastrous consequences for our typical CLI patient.

A main issue in the endovascular community has been the lack of consensus for the definition of "clinically significant" distal emboli and when, how, and in whom this should be treated. Operators at present might differ in their approach in defining and treating distal emboli [13]. However, it appears that only a small fraction (2.4% in Shammas et al.'s study) of these debris requires further treatment [13]. Limb-threatening distal embolization occurred in approximately 2% of patients during routine intervention in other major studies [28, 29] Given the previous discussion on the unreported incidence of distal emboli and the size and pathological features of these emboli, it is hard to understand why there are not more limb-threatening events. The consequence of distal embolization resulting in occlusion of the vascular bed in patients with poor arterial inflow, poor collateralization, or poor runoff may be devastating.

Possible reasons include the durability of the distal circulation of "healthy" PAD patients such as claudicants, patients with three vessel runoff, and nondiabetics. Namely, if the patient has limited reserve in the distal circulation, then he or she can take less embolic insult. Also, despite increased debris from our procedures, many patients seem to clear these obstructions over a week or 2 weeks. Possibly, the patients develop collaterals, the spasm reduces, or the inflammation improves allowing the flow to return.

This complication may require the use of additional intervention including thrombectomy or thrombolysis, resulting in longer procedure time, greater volumes of contrast administered, and increased radiation exposure [10, 18]. The acute outcomes are less symptom relief, worsening of symptoms, and increased emergent surgical bypass. Long-term outcomes are also adversely affected with decreased symptom relief at 2 years and increased above-the-knee, below-the-knee, and below-the-ankle amputations [13, 25, 30].

Freeman et al. defines high-risk patients as those with limited distal runoff, vulnerable or unstable plaque, history of thromboembolic disease, or aneurysmal disease [31]. Features separating patients with stable claudication from those with ongoing ischemia include the length of the stenosis and the length of the lesion, presence of distal runoff, and chronicity of disease [30]. Embolism has also been reported in patients with concentric stenoses [26, 27]. However, Shammas et al. state that predicting which vessels will embolize based on lesion characteristics is not always possible [13].

Shirkande et al. showed some lesion types that are more prone to embolization [12]. TASC C and D lesions had higher rates of embolization than TASC A and B lesions (2.2% vs 0.9%, $p = 0.018$) [12]. In a study by Lam et al., there was no difference in sonographically detected embolic signals between TAIC classifications [25]. Shirkande et al. showed total occlusions (2.4%) or ISR (3.2%) had a higher rate of DE than native stenotic lesions (0.9%; $p<0.01$) [12]. The higher rate of distal emboli in ISR could reflect the nature of the material within the stent, which may be softer and more friable than standard atherosclerotic plaque [25]. Shammas provided a good review of patients with a high risk of distal emboli are those with a prior history of amputation, TASC D lesions, and the presence of angiographic thrombus. In his study, thrombotic lesions had 5.9 times greater odds of embolization than nonthrombotic ones [13]. Also, patients presenting with acute thrombotic occlusions (within 24 h of symptom onset) showed a trend toward more distal emboli than those presenting subacutely/chronically [13].

Indications for the Use of Distal Embolic Filters

Common sense indicates that EPD use may be of value in a lesion with vulnerable or unstable plaque, acute thrombosis, chronic total occlusions, or aneurysmal disease [10]. It is safe to generalize that all CTO, ISR, and thrombotic lesions treated with atherectomy merit the use of embolic protection devices because of high risk of embolization. Current recommendations support the use of these filters in cases of significant calcification, although operator discretion plays a pivotal role in their deployment. The decision for the use of EPD in calcific lesions and atherosclerotic lesions is dependent on lesion length. Lesions >140 mm when atherosclerotic and >40 mm when calcific warrant the use of an embolic protection device to prevent complications.

Although embolization is a potential complication of any atherectomy device, it remains unclear whether certain devices or techniques predispose patients to distal embolization. Further, certain devices may be preferred in a given lesion morphology, and additional research may be necessary to address this question. Third, the incremental cost of EPD is significant (often in the range of $1000), and additional cost-benefit analyses could help clarify the optimal clinical scenarios for both atherectomy and embolic protection device uses. Although the proposed algorithm is therefore a useful guide, it is not clear that this algorithm would apply to every clinical scenario in which atherectomy is being used [32].

Krishnan et al. prepared a good algorithm for the use of EPD with atherectomy devices depending upon lesion characteristics [30]. Once the diagnostic angiogram is performed, the operator assesses the following morphology and anatomic characteristics: thrombotic, calcific, restenotic, CTO, lesion length, and runoff [30].

EPD filters are recommended for the following:

- Calcium with length greater than 4 cm.
- In-stent restenosis, thrombus, and complete total occlusions.
- Atherosclerotic lesions in lesions longer than 14 cm and with distal runoffs of less than 2 vessels.

Current Status of Distal Protection

Currently, there is no consensus for the use of EPD during atherectomy, and the only Food and Drug Administration-approved device with an indication in the femoropopliteal segment is the SpiderFX for use in conjunction with directional atherectomy in heavily calcified lesions [16].

There are currently two available EPD filter protections in treating PAD. The SpiderFX Embolic Protection Device (Medtronic, Minneapolis, Minnesota) is indicated for use as a guidewire and embolic protection system to contain and remove embolic material in conjunction with the TurboHawk (Medtronic, Minneapolis, MN), either during standalone procedures or together with PTA and/or stenting, in the treatment of severely calcified lesions in arteries of the lower extremities. The SpiderFX device (Fig. 17.2) has a braided nitinol filter that conforms to the vessel wall and maintains apposition. The pore size is 167–209 μm. The capture wire rotates and moves longitudinally independent of the filter and is available in diameter sizes 3–7 mm.

Advantages for the SpiderFX device include:

- The ease of use with the ability to cross a lesion with a 0.014–0.018″ wire of choice followed by the delivery catheter or the ability to deliver it through a 4-Fr compatible catheter.
- The EPD filter allows flow through the vessel while deployed reducing the chance of fibrin buildup to occlude flow.
- Recovery catheter (opposite end of the delivery catheter) is very easy to use and captures efficiently.

Disadvantages for the SpiderFX device and for many EPD include:

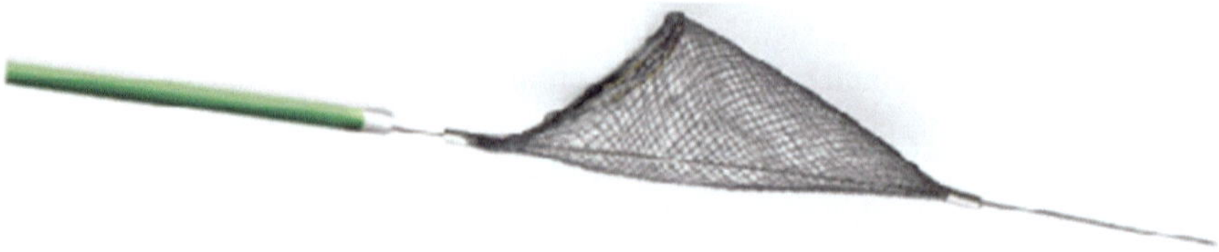

Fig. 17.2 SpiderFX embolic protection device

- The pore size is rather large and lets smaller debris (200 μm) flow through.
- The proximal busing holding the strut for the basket is susceptible to become stuck with coaxial balloon catheters, stents, and other devices.
- The filter basket with the nitinol basket design can easily become ensnared with self-expandable stents.
- When the filter becomes full of debris, it is very hard to get a catheter down to basket to aspirate the debris out, and if a solid plaque is captured, it may not be withdrawn into the overlying sheath.
- Then the length of the filter and diameter is limited, so it will not capture the large iliac vessels well.
- It is useful primarily with the FoxHollow (Medtronic line) atherectomy line.
- Once the system is retracted, a second wire must be passed to the treated lesion.

A second EPD filter is the Mednova later Abbott Emboshield Nav [6] (Plymouth, MN) (Fig. 17.3) which is indicated for use as a guidewire and embolic protection system to contain and remove embolic material (thrombus/debris) while performing angioplasty and stenting procedures while performing atherectomy, during stand-alone procedures or together with PTA and/or stenting, in lower extremity arteries. The diameter of the artery at the site of the filtration element placement should be between 2.5 and 7.0 mm. It has a centered wire design to prevent bias against the vessel wall; circumferential nitinol frame maintains optimal wall apposition.

Advantages for the Abbott Emboshield Nav [6] system include:

- The unique wire technology allows the wire to rotate and advance freely, independent of the filter. This allows the device to be used with most of the atherectomy devices.
- The filter is designed to stay in place during device delivery.
- Continued wire access, after the filter is fully retracted, allows for easy delivery of additional therapy.

Disadvantages of the Abbott Emboshield Nav [6] system include:

- The filter can be pulled back but cannot be easily pushed forward without recapturing it.

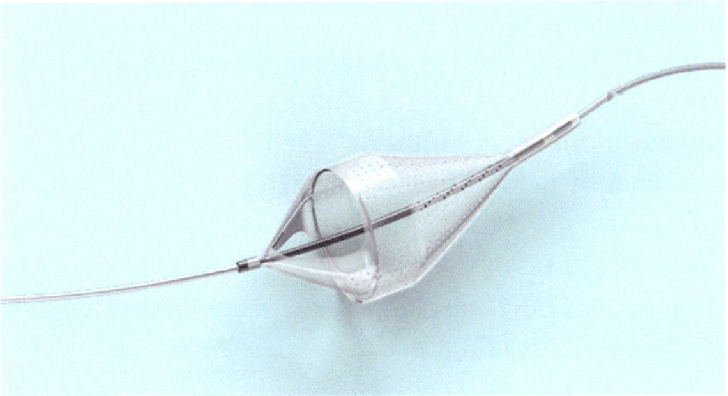

Fig. 17.3 Abbott Emboshield Nav [6]

- The two struts with plastic covering can deflect plaque to sides and can fail to capture them.
- The filter has 140 μm pore size which is very efficient in capturing small debris but can lead to a full basket.

Technique of Distal Protection

The standard technique for use of distal protection is simple. After an angiogram is performed involving the pelvis and/or lower extremity from either retrograde or antegrade approach, the site of EPD filter deployment is selected. Selection is based upon a region well enough distal to the targeted treatment zone. Other considerations include trying to preserve as many main vessels and collateral vessels as possible (Fig. 17.4a–g). Deployment is best if the vessel does not have extensive plaque and is fairly straight.

If the lesion is not terribly tight and we cross with our 4-Fr catheter or complete target occlusion (CTO) catheter which utilizes a 0.035″ wire, then we will simply remove the 0.035″ wire and advance our filter and deploy it. If we use a 0.014″ wire and are worried about the plaque/thrombus, we will use the special rapid exchange catheter to allow deployment of the filter. Once the filter is in place, we will move swiftly to perform the needed intervention. For atherectomy, we will be more vigilant for a full basket. After the procedure is done, we advance the filter recovery catheter quite slowly in the smaller vessel, capture the ringlike structure, and then remove the catheter and filter very carefully especially with a sent in the path of the filter and recovery system.

There are several inherent limitations with the use of EPD through selected lesions including chronic total occlusions which may pose a challenge. The EPD devices are routinely mounted on medium support wires, which are not intended to function as primary crossing wires.

EPD typically requires a rather long length of vessel for safe implantation, which may pose a challenge since many patients with CLI have extensive and diffuse atherosclerotic disease. Incomplete apposition of the device to the vessel wall may allow side escape of engendered debris. Furthermore, arterial spasm, arterial injury (including dissection), and de novo thrombus may occur as a result of the EPD device itself [27].

Revascularization procedures often result in the production of large amounts of macroscopic debris. The size of the filter basket may be inadequate for collection of debris. Extreme care must be taken since filter wire retrieval may also result in dislodgment of debris due to squeezing of the basket. Larger clots may also remain outside the struts of the EPD filter and are too large to be removed by filter closing and standard re-sheathing techniques. EPD provides no protection to the collateral circulation. Therefore, the collateral vessels are vulnerable to the sequelae of distal embolization should it occur.

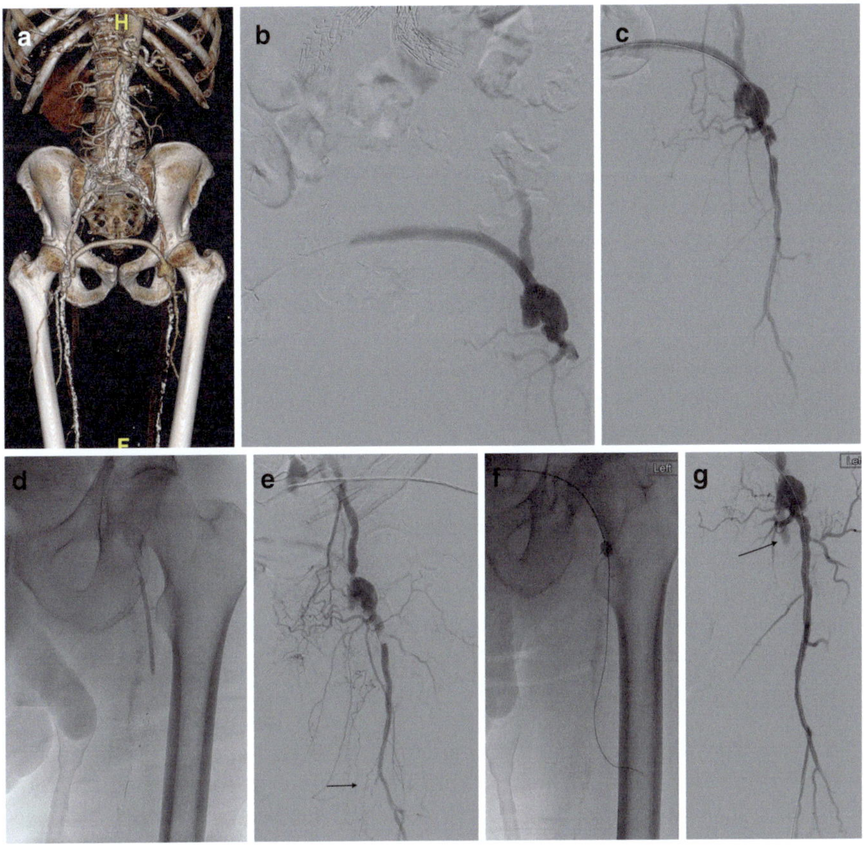

Fig. 17.4 (**a**) Complicated left leg rest pain in a patient with occluded native left iliac, SFA, and fem-pop bypass graft with a patent fem-fem bypass graft. CTA had been performed several months earlier. (**b**) Initial angiogram from the right end of bypass graft showing the occluded left main PFA. (**c**) Lesion was crossed and TPA administered overnight. High-grade stenosis seen at PFA origin. (**d**) The lesion is crossed with a 4-Fr Glidecath over the 0.035″ Wholey wire. Once across, a 6-mm-diameter SpiderFX is deployed in a distal portion. Penumbra aspiration and 4-mm PTA are then performed. (**e**) After the above intervention, increased collaterals are now seen, but PFA plaque or probable clot persists. The distal filter can be seen with wire extending into the medial side branch now with debris in the basket (arrow). Filter was removed with the recovery catheter. (**f**) With the native SFA open at the stump, decision was made to use a Fogarty balloon over the wire to pull the recalcitrant plaque/clot back into the CFA and have it float into the occluded SFA. (**g**) Final angiogram after additional angioplasty showing the improved flow to the PFA and its branches. The plaque/clot of the PFA can be seen in the SFA stump (arrow)

Conclusion and Future of Distal Protection

The role of distal protection in PAD cases has remained an enigma for most interventionalists. EPD is extremely useful in treating large caliber vessels such as the iliac, CFA, SFA, PFA, and popliteal arteries especially when atherectomy are being used. EPD are useful in treating high-risk lesions such as thrombotic segments, long segment occlusions, in-stent restenosis, and heavy calcified lesions all complicated by limited distal runoff.

If not useful, why are EPD not used more frequently in treating PAD? There appears to be three main factors. Firstly, as the various studies, corporate-sponsored registries, and few randomized trials have shown, it is difficult to obtain standard complication rates. The fact that distal embolization occurs cannot be denied, but the rate of significant events related to the distal emboli is hard to determine; there are many variables that involve assessing and treating PAD patients; it is hard to determine what is successful and what is not in treating the PAD population.

Secondly, EPD are not perfect and have faults. You lose wire access when you need to get distal to the filter, filter baskets can get full and hard to clean out, and, importantly, filters cannot prevent distal emboli from getting past or through the filter. There is much improvement that can be done with EPD technology. Possibly, as EPD are used more frequently in the cerebral, coronary, and other circulations, there will be improvements in its use and design in the PAD.

Finally, after 20 years since their invention, EPD for PAD are still not reimbursed in the US market. We looked into creating a randomized trial for one of the EPD in 2006, but it was not possible to establish reliable endpoints. Strangely, the reimbursement of PTA and atherectomy in outpatient facilities is $11,000 versus $3500 for PTA alone (CPT 37,225–37,224). So with EPD costing approximately $1600–$2000 per device, there is much hesitation for interventionists especially at outpatient facilities to employ EPD use, especially in cases without atherectomy use.

In summary, distal embolization can occur with any intervention in treating PAD. When it does occur, it results in longer case time, contrast, and fluoroscopy at the minimum. Worse cases will result in worsened claudication, rest pain, amputation, and even death. The best approach to avoid distal embolization is to prevent its occurrence: though EPD filters are not perfect, they do provide protection from harmful embolic debris.

References

1. McDermott JC, Crummy AB. Complications of angioplasty. Semin Interv Radiol. 1994;11:145–9.
2. Rickard MJ, Fisher CM, Soong CV, et al. Limitations of intra-arterial thrombolysis. Cardiovasc Surg. 2013;1997:634–40.
3. Chalmers RT, Hoballah JJ, Kresowik TF, et al. Late results of a prospective study of direct intraarterial urokinase infusion for peripheral arterial and bypass graft occlusions. Cardiovasc Surg. 1995;2013:293–7.
4. Suri R, Wholey MH, Postoak D, Hagino RT, Toursarkissian B. Distal embolic protection during femoropopliteal atherectomy. Catheter Cardiovasc Interv. 2006;67(3):417–22.
5. Wholey MH, Suri R, Postoak D, Hagino RT, Toursarkissian B. Plaque excision in 2005 and beyond: issues of the past have yet to be resolved. Endovasc Today; 2005.
6. Wholey M, Teitelbaum G. State of the art: distal protection filters. Scientific session and scientific poster abstracts. J Vasc Interv Radiol. 2002;13((2) Supplement):P158–9.

7. Allie DE. To PROTECT or not to PROTECT? In lower extremity angioplasty procedures, "why not?" is the question! J Endovasc Ther. 2008;15:277–82.
8. Shammas NW, Coiner D, Shammas GA, Christensen L, Dippel EJ, Jerin M. Distal embolic event protection using excimer laser ablation in peripheral vascular interventions: results of the DEEP EMBOLI registry. J Endovasc Ther. 2009;16(2):197–202.
9. Spiliopoulos S, Theodosiadou V, Koukounas V, et al. Distal macro- and microembolization during subintimal recanalization of femoropopliteal chronic total occlusions. J Endovasc Ther. 2014;21(4):474–81.
10. Lewis S, Lookstein R. Is there a role for embolic protection during treatment of critical limb ischemia? Review article. Interv Cardiol. 2010;2:1–3. https://www.openaccessjournals.com/journals/interventional-cardiology-citations-report.html
11. Ochoa Chaar CI, Shebl F, Sumpio B, Dardik A, Indes J, Sarac T. Distal embolization during lower extremity endovascular interventions. J Vasc Surg. 2017;66(1):143–50.
12. Shrikhande GV, Khan SZ, Hussain HG, Dayal R, McKinsey JF, Morrissey N. Lesion types and device characteristics that predict distal embolization during percutaneous lower extremity interventions. J Vasc Surg. 2011;53(2):347–52.
13. Shammas NW, Shammas GA, Dippel EJ, Jerin M, Shammas WJ. Predictors of distal embolization in peripheral percutaneous interventions: a report from a large peripheral vascular registry. J Invasive Cardiol. 2009;21(12):628–31.
14. Krishnan P, Tarricone A, Purushothaman K, Purushothaman M, Vasquez M, Kovacic M, et al. An algorithm for the use of embolic protection during atherectomy for femoral popliteal lesions. J Am Coll Cardiol Intv. 2017;10:403–10.
15. Balzer JO, Thalhammer A, Khan V, Zangos S, Vogl TJ, Lehnert T. Angioplasty of the pelvic and femoral arteries in PAOD: results and review of the literature. Eur J Radiol. 2010;75(1):48–56.
16. Roberts D, Niazi K, Miller W, Krishnan P, Gammon R, Schreiber T, Shammas NW, Clair D, DEFINITIVE Ca++ Investigators. Effective endovascular treatment of calcified femoropopliteal disease with directional atherectomy and distal embolic protection: final results of the DEFINITIVE Ca++ trial. Catheter Cardiovasc Interv. 2014;84(2):236–44.
17. Milnerowicz A, Milnerowicz A, Kuliczkowski W, Protasiewicz M. Rotational atherectomy plus drug-coated balloon angioplasty for the treatment of total in-stent occlusions in iliac and infrainguinal arteries. J Endovasc Ther. 2019;26(3):316–21.
18. Shammas NW, Dippel EJ, Coiner D, Shammas GA, Jerin M, Kumar A. Preventing lower extremity distal embolization using embolic filter protection: results of the PROTECT registry. J Endovasc Ther. 2008;15(3):270–6.
19. Hadidi OF, Mohammad A, Zankar A, Brilakis ES, Banerjee S. Embolic capture angioplasty in peripheral artery interventions. J Endovasc Ther. 2012;19(5):611–6.
20. Müller-Hülsbeck S, Schäfer PJ, Hümme TH, et al. Embolic protection devices for peripheral application: wasteful or useful? J Endovasc Ther. 2009;16(Suppl. 1):I163–9.
21. Becker GJ, Katzen BT, Dake MD. Noncoronary angioplasty. Radiology. 1989;170:921–40.
22. Rickard MJ, Fisher CM, Soong CV, et al. Limitations of intra-arterial thrombolysis. Cardiovasc Surg. 1997;5:634–40.
23. Chalmers RT, Hoballah JJ, Kresowik TF, et al. Late results of a prospective study of direct intra-arterial urokinase infusion for peripheral arterial and bypass graft occlusions. Cardiovasc Surg. 1995;3:293–7.
24. Wholey MH, Maynar MA, Wholey MH, et al. Comparison of thrombolytic therapy for lower extremity acute, subacute, and chronic arterial occlusions. Catheter Cardiovasc Diagn. 1998;44:159–69.
25. Lam RC, Shah S, Faries PL, McKinsey JF, Kent KC, Morrissey NJ. Incidence and clinical significance of distal embolization during percutaneous interventions involving the superficial femoral artery. J Vasc Surg. 2007;46:1155–9.
26. Wholey M. The role of embolic protection in peripheral arterial atherectomy. Tech Vasc Interv Radiol. 2011;14(2):65–74.

27. Karnabatidis D, Katsanos K, Kagadis GC, et al. Distal embolism during percutaneous revascularization of infra-aortic arterial occlusive disease: an underestimated phenomenon. J Endovasc Ther. 2006;13:269–80.
28. Belli AM, Cumberland DC, Knox AM, et al. The complication rate of percutaneous peripheral balloon angioplasty. Clin Radiol. 1990;41(6):380–3.
29. Matsi PJ, Manninen HI. Complications of lower limb percutaneous transluminal angioplasty: a prospective analysis of 410 procedures on 295 consecutive patients. Cardiovasc Intervent Radiol. 1998;21(5):361–6.
30. Krishnan P, Tarricone A, Purushothaman KR, Purushothaman M, Vasquez M, Kovacic J, Baber U, Kapur V, Gujja K, Kini A, Sharma S. An algorithm for the use of embolic protection during atherectomy for femoral popliteal lesions. JACC Cardiovasc Interv. 2017;10(4):403–10.
31. Freeman HJ, Rundback JH. Embolic protection in femoropopliteal artery intervention. Endovasc Today. 2006;5:65–9.
32. Armstrong EJ, Waldo SW. Prevention of distal embolization during peripheral vascular interventions: filtering the evidence. J Am Coll Cardiol Intv. 2017;10(4):411–2.

Chapter 18
Management of Aortic Aneurysms

Mel J. Sharafuddin and Jeanette H. Man

Introduction

Abdominal aortic aneurysms (AAA) are a common disorder with an estimated incidence of 4–7% in western countries [1–5]. It is the 13th leading cause of death in the United States, with 15,000 deaths yearly. Ruptured AAA carry an operative mortality of 40–70% and overall mortality of 80–90% [6–11]. Risk factors include smoking, hypertension, hyperlipidemia, and family history of aneurysms. Screening is recommended to adults >65 years who have smoked or have a family history of aneurysms.

AAA are defined as an enlargement of the aorta 1.5 times the normal diameter, which has led to conventional diameter requirement >3 cm. The risk of rupture increases dramatically with increasing aortic size. Therefore, elective repair is indicated when the aortic diameter is >5.5 cm in men and >5.0 cm in women or when the growth rate is faster than average, >0.3 cm/year.

Traditionally, open repair was the gold standard of repair. Endovascular repair of aortic aneurysm (EVAR) has since revolutionized the treatment of AAA and has become the new standard. EVAR is associated with decreased morbidity, operative times, hospital stay, and perioperative mortality [12]. The idea of using vascular endoprosthesis to exclude aneurysms originated in the late 1960s with animal experimentation. The first landmark deployment of an aortic stent to exclude a human AAA was reported by Parodi et al. in 1991 [13]. Straight grafts consisting of polyester tubes were used and reinforced with Palmaz stents. Today, this design has

M. J. Sharafuddin (✉) · J. H. Man
Division of Vascular Surgery, Department of General Surgery, University of Iowa Hospitals and Clinics, Iowa City, IA, USA
e-mail: mel-sharafuddin@uiowa.edu

N. W. Shammas (ed.), *Peripheral Arterial Interventions*, Contemporary Cardiology, https://doi.org/10.1007/978-3-031-09741-6_18

evolved into modular grafts. Furthermore, with the constant evolution of endovascular technology, variations of EVAR are also being used to treat increasingly complicated aneurysms. Patients who are poor candidates for open repair have the option of treatment with fenestrated EVAR (FEVAR), chimney EVAR (ch-EVAR), and physician-modified endografts (PMEG) [14–16].

There have been several randomized trials demonstrating the early advantage of EVAR compared to open repair. The EVAR 1 trial demonstrated that EVAR offered a 30-day mortality benefit over open repair [12]. The DREAM and OVER trials demonstrated that although this early benefit was not sustained long term, EVAR patients still had a similar survival rate compared to the open group at 6 and 9 years, respectively, despite having long-term problems related to graft durability such as endoleaks that may require reintervention [17, 18]. Meanwhile, the IMPROVE trial showed that patients with ruptured AAA were more likely to discharge to home when compared to those who underwent open repair [19].

Indications for EVAR

The ideal candidate for EVAR must have the anatomy amendable for stent grafts. This includes having adequately sized access vessels, good proximal and distal fixation zones (with special attention to the aortic neck and iliac arteries), good aortic wall quality without excessive calcification, and non-severe angulation. Different devices will have different anatomical criteria based on their instructions for use. However, in general, the ideal candidates for EVAR will have a neck length >15 mm, neck diameter <32 mm, neck angulation <60°, iliac artery diameter <22 mm, and iliac artery length >20 mm. Below are graphs comparing some of the criteria of different devices currently available (Table 18.1). With the constant technological developments, there are also several newer devices that continue to push boundaries. Gore Excluder Iliac Branch Endoprosthesis is the first off-the-shelf aortic branch solution approved in the United States that allows for preservation of blood flow to the external and internal iliac arteries. Furthermore, currently in trial is Gore Excluder Conformable AAA Endoprosthesis with Active Control System that can be used for AAA with a shorter neck length of 10 mm, high neck angulation up to 90°, and smaller diameter neck of 16 mm. Meanwhile, other indications for EVAR include ineligibility to open repair due to reduced cardiac reserve, reduced pulmonary capacity, hostile abdomen, or multiple comorbidities. EVAR may also be used a bridge to open repair in patient who are too sick to undergo emergent open repair, such as those with aorto-enteric fistulas.

Table 18.1 Comparison of currently available stent grafts for endovascular repair of AAA

Device	Profile OD (main body)	Profile OD (limb)	Distal iliac diameter range	Stent material	Graft material	Neck indication (angle and diameter)	Active fixation	Advantages
TriVascular ovation prime	14–15 Fr	13–15 Fr	8–20 mm	Nitinol	PTFE	≤60° if neck ≥10 mm, ≤45° if neck <10 mm. 16–30	Suprarenal stent with barbs	Small profile of delivery system
Medtronic endurant II	18–20 Fr	14–15 Fr	8–25 mm	Nitinol	Multi-filament polyester	Suprarenal neck <45°, infrarenal neck <60°. 19–32 mm	Suprarenal fixation with barbs	Overcame issues of earlier-generation stent grafts
Gore excluder C3	16–18 Fr	12–15 Fr	8–25 mm	Nitinol	ePTFE	≤60°. Infrarenal neck 19–32 mm	Infrarenal barbs	User friendly, less steps in deployment
Gore excluder conformable with active control	15–18 Fr	12–15 Fr	8–25 mm	Nitinol	ePTFE	≤90°. 16–32 mm	Nitinol anchors, ePTFE sealing cuff	Good for angulated short necks
cook zenith flex	18–22 Fr	14–16 Fr	7.5–20 mm	Stainless steel	Polyester	Suprarenal neck <45°, infrarenal neck <60°. 18–32 mm	Suprarenal fixation with barbs	Allows for small, large, or scalloped fenestrations
Endologix AFX	17–19 Fr	11 Fr	10–23 mm	Cobalt chromium	ePTFE	≤60°. 18–32 mm	Suprarenal fixation	Preservation of aortic bifurcation
Treo	18–19 Fr	13–14 Fr	8–20 mm	Nitinol	Polyester	Suprarenal neck <45°, infrarenal neck <75°. 16–30 mm	Suprarenal and infrarenal fixation barb	Dual proximal fixation and lock stent

OD outer diameter

Preoperative Assessment and Planning

Imaging plays in an important role in sizing aneurysms to allow for the appropriate choice of stent grafts. A CTA abdomen/pelvis should be obtained at 2.5-mm intervals. MRA abdomen/pelvis with time of flight can be obtained instead in patients with renal disease. After obtaining the proper imaging, one can use 3D reconstruction programs and centerline calculations to obtain accurate measurements. The key areas of focus include dimensional details of angles, areas of wall irregularity, existence of any thrombus, the shape and diameter of the flow lumen, the level of tortuosity, the severity of calcification, and the relationship with the lowest renal artery. Once these measurements are performed, most endovascular device companies recommend oversizing by 10–15% to allow for good seal. However, beware of excessive oversizing which can cause excessive radial expansile force and graft migration (Fig. 18.1).

Fig. 18.1 Clinical example. Here is an example of an EVAR we performed. It was complicated by a right iliac artery aneurysm and distal tortuosity that required us to perform a right internal iliac artery embolization to allow for extension of the stent graft limb into the right external iliac artery. (**a**) Preoperative scan. Preoperative measurements for the stent graft were performed using a CTA with fine cuts. Centerline measurements were then made through the aorta, right iliac artery, and left iliac artery. (**b**) Intraoperative. Access was gained with a 12-Fr sheath in the right common femoral artery and 18-Fr sheath in the left common femoral artery. An Active Control Conformable Excluder Device was chosen for the repair. A 28-mm × 14.5-mm × 16-cm device was deployed in the recommended manner. The contralateral gate was cannulated and then extended into the expected position of the right iliac bifurcation using a 16-mm × 12-mm × 7-cm iliac extension. Angiography revealed extreme deformity of the straightened tortuous iliac segment with the common iliac aneurysm as well as the hypogastric artery readily filling. It became obvious that achieving seal in the distal right common iliac artery right above the bifurcation would not be accomplishable with the excluder limb. We therefore proceeded with embolization of the internal iliac artery and extension of the right iliac limb into the distal external iliac artery. A 14-mm Amplatzer plug was used to occlude the ostium of the internal iliac artery and then extended using a 13-mm × 100-mm Viabahn stent graft. The interfaces were dilated with a 14-mm balloon angiography which revealed persistent endoleak which we felt might represent a junctional endoleak. Because of that and because of the now improved accessibility across that segment, we decided to reline the entire limb using a 14.5-mm × 16-cm excluder limb. The ipsilateral limb of the device was then deployed, and we extended further to the level of the bifurcation using a 16-mm × 13.5-cm excluder limb. The proximal seal zone and the overlap segments were all dilated with either a CODA balloon or 14- or 12-mm angioplasty balloons. Angiography revealed excellent position of the endograft with exclusion of the aneurysm and maintained patency of both renal arteries and the left hypogastric artery. Occlusion of the plugged right internal iliac artery was confirmed. There was no evidence of type I or III endoleak. (**c**) Postoperative scan (1 year after). On 1-year follow-up, the patient remained asymptomatic. CTA scan showed interval mild regression of his sac diameter. There was a small type II endoleak emanating from the inferior mesenteric artery that we will continue to monitor

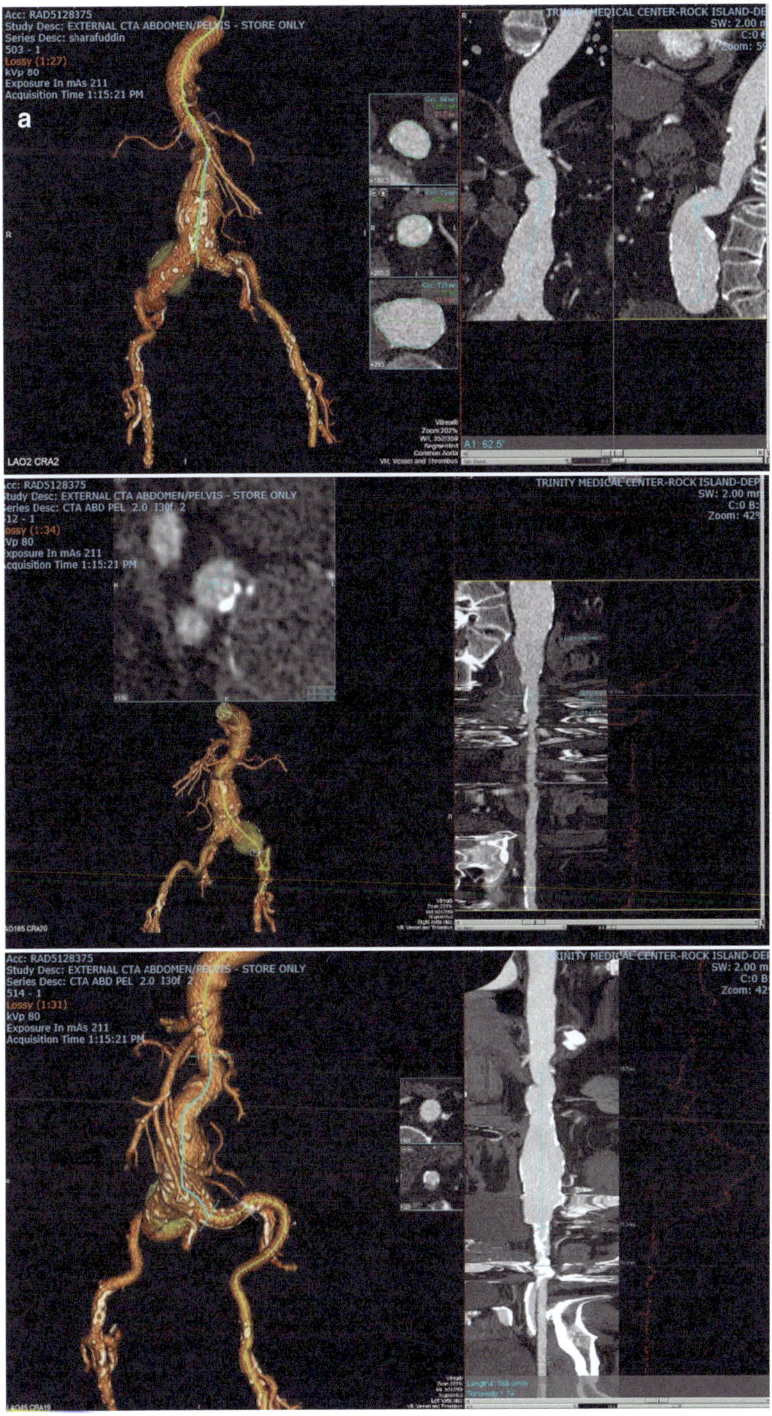

Acc: RAD5128375
Study Desc: EXTERNAL CTA ABDOMEN/PELVIS - STORE ONLY
Series Desc: sharafuddin
503 - 1
Lossy (1:27)
kVp 80
Exposure In mAs 211
Acquisition Time 1:15:21 PM
a
LAO2 CRA2
TRINITY MEDICAL CENTER-ROCK ISLAND-DE
SW: 2.00
A1 62.5°
Study Desc: EXTERNAL CTA ABDOMEN/PELVIS - STORE ONLY
Series Desc: CTA ABD PEL 2.0 130f 2
Exposure In mAs 211
Acquisition Time 1:15:21 PM
TRINITY MEDICAL CENTER-ROCK ISLAND-DEP
SW: 2.00
Acc: RAD5128375
Study Desc: EXTERNAL CTA ABDOMEN/PELVIS - STORE ONLY
Series Desc: CTA ABD PEL 2.0 130f 2
514 - 1
Lossy (1:31)
kVp 80
Exposure In mAs 211
Acquisition Time 1:15:21 PM
TRINITY MEDICAL CENTER-ROCK ISLAND-DE
SW: 2.00

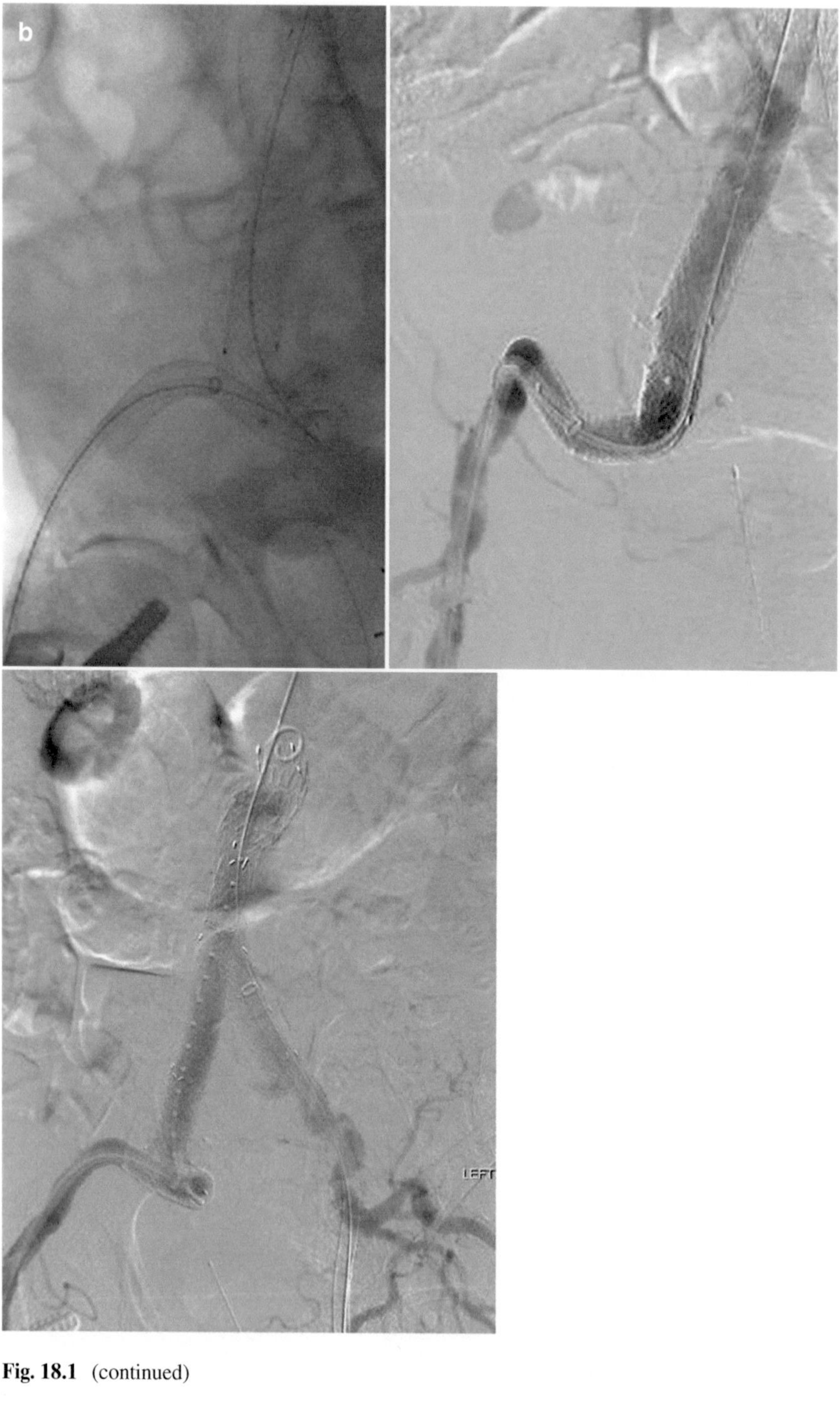

Fig. 18.1 (continued)

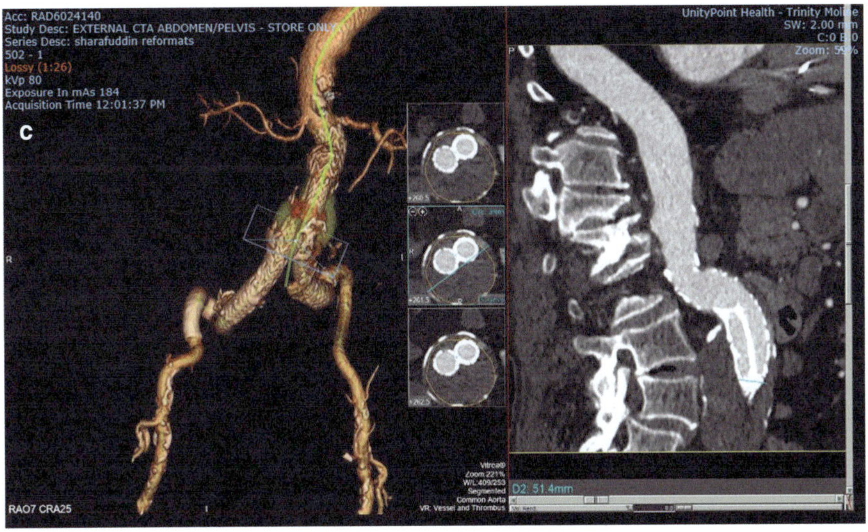

Fig. 18.1 (continued)

Operative Technique

Several different types of anesthesia can be used when performing EVAR. If the patient can tolerate lying flat, monitored anesthesia cares and local anesthetic are sufficient and quite common. However, if the patient has more worrisome risk factors, general anesthesia can also be used. An epidural is another option in frail and sick patient who cannot undergo general anesthesia.

The following steps for an EVAR are for modular devices. The patient is prepared from the xiphoid to the bilateral knees, in case there is a need for emergent conversion to open repair. First, obtain percutaneous access in the bilateral common femoral arteries with ultrasound guidance, and use preclose technique. Next, introduce the wire into the descending abdominal aorta. Upsize the sheaths based on the stent graft being used and if a sheath is required for the device. Heparinize the patient to keep ACT >200–250. Perform an aortogram using a flush catheter. Angulate the C-arm and mark where the lowest renal artery is. Introduce the main body, position just the lowest renal artery, and deploy. An additional piece may or may not be needed depending on the length to the ipsilateral common iliac artery. Afterward, cannulate the contralateral gate. Introduce the contralateral iliac delivery system, and deploy with care to not cover the internal iliac artery. Once the stent grafts are in place, use a molding balloon to ensure good expansion of the stent grafts. Lastly, perform a completion angiogram to assess for stent graft apposition, exclusion of the aneurysm, and the presence of any endoleaks.

Postoperative Surveillance and Complications

Postoperative surveillance is performed at 30 days, 6 months, 1 year, and then annually afterward. EVAR complications can be grouped into access complications, graft-related complications, and organ system failure [20–22]. Access-related complications can include hematoma, pseudoaneurysm, infection, lymphocele, dissection, and distal limb emboli. Graft-related complication includes endoleaks, limb kinking or thrombosis, graft migration, and graft infection. Endoleaks are a common complication and can be further subdivided into five types. A type I endoleak occurs when there is an inadequate seal at either the proximal or the distal seal zone. A type II endoleak occurs when there is back bleeding from a collateral artery, such as a lumbar artery. A type III endoleak occurs when there is a leak between the stent grafts. A type IV endoleak occurs when the material of the stent graft has high porosity. A type V endoleak occurs when there is endotension of unknown origin. Of all the endoleaks, type I and III should be repaired upon diagnosis to prevent continued transmission of systemic pressure into a confined sac. Last but certainly not least, there are several organ systems that can fail postoperatively. Renal failure is not uncommon secondary to contrast nephropathy from the large amounts of contrast used during the procedure. Renal failure may also result from atheroemboli, acute renal artery obstruction, and cephalad graft migration. Meanwhile, mesenteric ischemia is a known and feared consequence when the inferior mesenteric artery is covered and there is otherwise poor blood supply to the bowels. Pelvic ischemia may result when there is coverage of both internal iliac arteries. Furthermore, spinal cord ischemia is another potential consequence when an extensive length of descending aorta is covered.

Conclusion

In conclusion, EVAR has revolutionized the treatment of AAA by allowing for decreased mortality and morbidity. Proper imaging and sizing of stent graft are crucial for its success. The durability of EVAR is dependent on long-term surveillance and being mindful of potential postoperative complications.

References

1. Gillum RF. Epidemiology of aortic aneurysm in the United States. J Clin Epidemiol. 1995;48(11):1289–98.
2. Melton LJ III, Bickerstaff LK, Hollier LH, Peenen JHV, Lie J, Pairolero PC, et al. Changing incidence of abdominal aortic aneurysms: a population-based study. Am J Epidemiol. 1984;120(3):379–86.

3. Svensjö S, Björck M, Wanhainen A. Update on screening for abdominal aortic aneurysm: a topical review. Eur J Vasc Endovasc Surg. 2014;48(6):659–67.
4. Kostun ZW, Malik RK. Screening for abdominal aortic aneurysms. Clin Imaging. 2016;40(2):321–4.
5. Ulug P, Powell J, Sweeting M, Bown M, Thompson S, SWAN Collaborative Group. Meta-analysis of the current prevalence of screen-detected abdominal aortic aneurysm in women. Br J Surg. 2016;103(9):1097.
6. Hoornweg LL, Storm-Versloot MN, Ubbink DT, Koelemay MJW, Legemate DA, Balm R. Meta analysis on mortality of ruptured abdominal aortic aneurysms. Eur J Vasc Endovasc Surg. 2008;35(5):558–70.
7. Kontopodis N, Tavlas E, Ioannou CV, Giannoukas AD, Geroulakos G, Antoniou GA. Systematic review and meta-analysis of outcomes of open and endovascular repair of ruptured abdominal aortic aneurysm in patients with hostile vs. friendly aortic anatomy. Eur J Vasc Endovasc Surg. 2020;59(5):717–28.
8. Bown MJ, Sutton AJ, Bell PRF, Sayers RD. A meta-analysis of 50 years of ruptured abdominal aortic aneurysm repair. Br J Surg. 2002;89(6):714–30.
9. Robinson WP, Schanzer A, Li Y, Goodney PP, Nolan BW, Eslami MH, et al. Derivation and validation of a practical risk score for prediction of mortality after open repair of ruptured abdominal aortic aneurysms in a U.S. regional cohort and comparison to existing scoring systems. J Vasc Surg. 2013;57(2):354–61.
10. Salata K, Hussain MA, de Mestral C, Greco E, Awartani H, Aljabri BA, et al. Population-based long-term outcomes of open versus endovascular aortic repair of ruptured abdominal aortic aneurysms. J Vasc Surg. 2020;71(6):1867–78.e8.
11. Heller JA, Weinberg A, Arons R, Krishnasastry K, Lyon RT, Deitch JS, et al. Two decades of abdominal aortic aneurysm repair: have we made any progress? J Vasc Surg. 2000;32(6):1091–100.
12. Patel R, Sweeting MJ, Powell JT, Greenhalgh RM, EVAR Trial Investigators. Endovascular versus open repair of abdominal aortic aneurysm in 15-years' follow-up of the UK endovascular aneurysm repair trial 1 (EVAR trial 1): a randomised controlled trial. Lancet. 2016;388(10058):2366–74.
13. Parodi JC, Palmaz JC, Barone HD. Transfemoral intraluminal graft implantation for abdominal aortic aneurysms. Ann Vasc Surg. 1991;5:491–9.
14. Suckow BD, Goodney PP, Columbo JA, Kang R, Stone DH, Sedrakyan A, et al. National trends in open surgical, endovascular, and branched-fenestrated endovascular aortic aneurysm repair in Medicare patients. J Vasc Surg. 2018;67(6):1690–7.e1.
15. Varkevisser RRB, O'Donnell TFX, Swerdlow NJ, Liang P, Li C, Ultee KHJ, et al. Fenestrated endovascular aneurysm repair is associated with lower perioperative morbidity and mortality compared with open repair for complex abdominal aortic aneurysms. J Vasc Surg. 2019;69(6):1670–8.
16. Pitoulias GA, Torsello G, Austermann M, Pitoulias AG, Pipitone MD, Fazzini S, et al. Outcomes of elective use of the chimney endovascular technique in pararenal aortic pathologic processes. J Vasc Surg. 2021;73(2):433–42.
17. De Bruin JL, Baas AF, Buth J, Prinssen M, Verhoeven EL, Cuypers PW, van Sambeek MR, Balm R, Grobbee DE, Blankensteijn JD, DREAM Study Group. Long-term outcome of open or endovascular repair of abdominal aortic aneurysm. N Engl J Med. 2010;362(20):1881–9.
18. Lal BK, Zhou W, Li Z, Kyriakides T, Matsumura J, Lederle FA, Freischlag J, OVER Veterans Affairs Cooperative Study Group. Predictors and outcomes of endoleaks in the veterans affairs open versus endovascular repair (OVER) Trial of abdominal aortic aneurysms. J Vasc Surg. 2015;62(6):1394–404.
19. IMPROVE Trial Investigators, Powell JT, Sweeting MJ, Thompson MM, Ashleigh R, Bell R, Gomes M, Greenhalgh RM, Grieve R, Heatley F, Hinchliffe RJ, Thompson SG, Ulug P. Endovascular or open repair strategy for ruptured abdominal aortic aneurysm: 30 day out-

comes from IMPROVE randomised trial. BMJ. 2014;348:f7661. https://doi.org/10.1136/bmj.f7661.

20. Malkawi AH, Hinchcliffe RJ, Hold PJ, et al. Percutaneous access for endovascular aneurysm repair: a systematic review. Eur J Vasc Endovasc Surg. 2010;39:676–82.
21. Talor PR, Reidy J, Scoble JE. Endovascular abdominal aneurysm repair and renal function. Nephrol Dial Transplant. 2006;21:2362–5.
22. White GW, Yu W, May J, et al. Endoleak as a complication of endoluminal grafting of abdominal aortic aneurysms: classification, incidence, diagnosis and management. J Endovasc Surg. 1997;4:152–68.

Chapter 19
Putting It All Together: An Algorithmic Approach to Treat Patients with Peripheral Arterial Disease

Nicolas W. Shammas

Approaching the peripheral arterial disease (PAD), patient starts with understanding the severity of the disease on presentation and the patients' cardiovascular risk factors. A comprehensive history and exam are imperative to gather the information needed to optimally treat each patient. Furthermore, an understanding of the patient's quality of life on presentation and the goals of treatment can help the vascular specialist tailor therapeutic interventions uniquely to each individual. A shared decision between the provider and the patient is critical to achieve excellent patient's satisfaction and the intended goals of interventions.

The first target of therapy is to reduce cardiovascular mortality and morbidity in the PAD patient who is at an exceptionally high risk for cardiac death, amputation, and strokes. An intense preventative program that consists of quitting smoking, structured exercise, tailored cardiovascular diet, high-dose statins, baby aspirin, and low-dose rivaroxaban should be implemented as soon as possible and when feasible [1–12]. In diabetics with established cardiovascular disease including PAD, the addition of SGLT2 inhibitors or GLP agonists has also been shown to reduce major adverse cardiovascular events [13–17]. This first-line approach applies to nearly all PAD patients whether they present with symptomatic or asymptomatic PAD.

When the initial presentation is chronic limb-threatening ischemia (CLTI) with rest pain or ulcerations, the consensus is to proceed with revascularization with a straight in-line flow to the foot in the majority of patients to prevent amputation and possibly death [8, 18]. The only exception will be a patient with severe leg contracture or overall multiple medical comorbidities where revascularization does not change the overall prognosis or outcomes of the patient. Amputation in this case may be considered.

Claudicants, on the other hand, are not at immediate risk of losing their legs, and therefore a period of structured exercise (supervised or home-based) along with

N. W. Shammas (✉)
Midwest Cardiovascular Research Foundation, Davenport, IA, USA

N. W. Shammas (ed.), *Peripheral Arterial Interventions*, Contemporary Cardiology, https://doi.org/10.1007/978-3-031-09741-6_19

cilostazol should be considered for several months before revascularization [19–21]. This approach however needs to be tailored to the individual patient as some patients have severe symptoms that are disabling and are unable to adhere to a structured exercise program. Also, patients with large inflow severe disease such as the iliac arteries are likely to benefit from revascularization as a first approach. The failure of medical therapy and exercise to relieve symptoms warrants a revascularization approach. In order to reduce the recurrence of symptoms and additional future treatments, a structured exercise program is recommended following revascularization.

The endovascular approach to revascularization varies with the target segments. Stenting of the iliac arteries is generally preferred and has excellent long-term outcomes [22–25]. In severely calcified iliac arteries, Shockwave Lithoplasty can be considered as an adjunctive treatment before stenting to help achieve full-stent expansion [26, 27]. In contrast, in the common femoral artery and infrainguinal arteries, we have adopted the strategy of leaving the least metal behind. With this strategy, the use of the Tack Endovascular System or spot stenting is reserved for vessels with flow-limiting dissections or suboptimal results on angiography. Although data from the TOBA observational trials also included repairing a good proportion of type A and B dissections with promising long-term outcomes, there are no randomized data to confirm the superiority of this approach versus no treatment [28, 29]. When more precise imaging is used such as intravascular ultrasound (IVUS), more dissections are noted when compared to angiography [30–33]. We generally reserve repairing these dissections that appear to involve the adventitia and those with a wider arc (≥180°) although data on this approach are needed (Fig. 19.1). Drug-coated balloons may partially mitigate the negative effect of dissections on restenosis, but the full interaction with dissection severity, drug-coated balloons, and dissection repair remains poorly understood [34]. Despite the overall short and intermediate low target lesion revascularization, particularly with drug-eluting stents in the femoropopliteal segments, stents may carry several problems on longer follow-up including fracture and restenosis and can potentially limit future therapies. In our opinion, technologies that can leave the vessel with no or least metal and result in successful acute and long-term outcomes would be preferred. This latter strategy has gained significant momentum and is now a preferred approach by many endovascular specialists.

In order to optimize acute procedural results, there are several approaches that can be taken. Vessel prepping prior to definitive therapy is a key step to obtain maximal luminal gain while limiting dissections and bailout stenting. Angioplasty alone can lead to high rate of dissections and bailout stenting and has been shown to have a high patency loss and TLR. Vessel prepping consists of different approaches to prepare the vessel for a more definitive treatment to gain the maximum luminal diameter while limiting the extent of damage to the vessel wall. Vessel prepping can be achieved by three primary modalities:

(a) Remove part of the plaque, a concept of debulking that is accomplished by atherectomy.

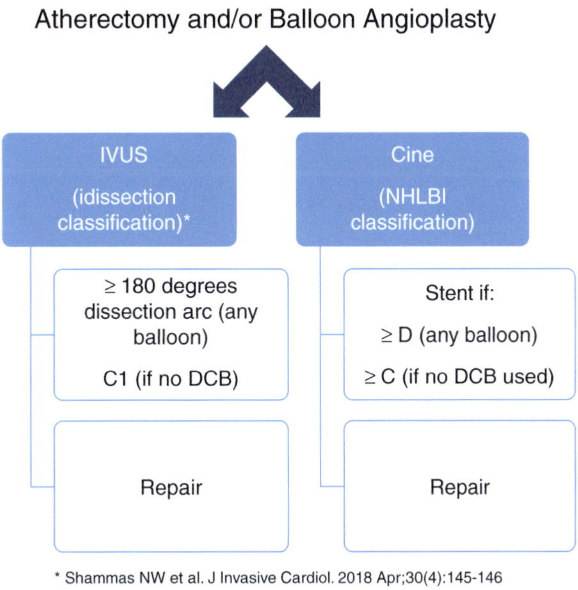

Fig. 19.1 Dissection repair based on the presence of angiographic (NHLBI) and intravascular ultrasound-based dissections (iDissection classification)

(b) Modify the plaque itself by various methods based on morphology. A severely calcified plaque can be modified by lithoplasty, while other softer plaques can be modified my microincision such as with the Flex VP longitudinal microincisional catheter.

(c) Redistribute the force of the balloon in focal areas such as with the use of specialty balloon including the chocolate balloon and other focal force balloons [35–39].

There are no data to compare the differences between these vessel prepping devices. Also, the degree of debulking with atherectomy devices remains unknown (soft vs aggressive). Vessel prepping has been shown to mostly impact the short-term acute procedural results reducing the need for bailout stenting and maximizing the overall success of the procedure. Also, vessel prepping can increase antiproliferative drug uptake (paclitaxel), and this may in return improve long-term patency and reduce TLR. Randomized, well-powered data are needed however to prove this concept.

Vessel prepping is part of a broader strategy of optimizing the outcome of endovascular treatment of peripheral arterial disease (Fig. 19.2) [40, 41]. Protecting the distal vascular bed and applying antiproliferative therapy are important steps to maximize short- and long-term outcomes. Protecting the distal vessels can be done by using atherectomy devices with aspiration capabilities (Auryon laser or Jetstream atherectomy and others) and the use of embolic protection filters [42–45]. These filters are shown to be highly effective in capturing debris. Although no randomized trials are available with and without filters, data suggest that filters reduce radiation exposure, amount of contrast use, and procedure time. Also, some nonrandomized

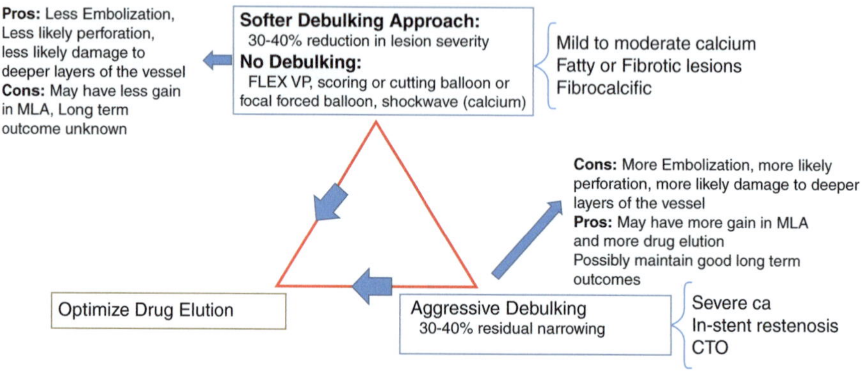

Fig. 19.2 Approach to vessel prepping with debulking or non-debulking strategies

data suggest a positive impact on overall long-term outcome [46–48]. Antiproliferative therapies (drug-coated balloons and stents) can be very effective in reducing TLR and improve patency when compared to treatments that do not include antiproliferative therapies [49–52]. Recently, there has been a concern about an increase in mortality with paclitaxel-based antiproliferative therapies [53], but most recent data could not confirm these findings [54]. Of interest, data from the AcoArt I trial suggest that when dissections are not visualized angiographically post-endovascular treatment, the overall primary patency is similar to those patients who received DCB [55]. This emphasizes the importance of vessel prepping to reduce dissections which may reduce the need for additional paclitaxel therapy. This concept needs to be proven with randomized prospective data and with the use of precise imaging such as IVUS which is more accurate in identifying dissections.

There is no one algorithm to treat infrainguinal symptomatic PAD. Our approach (Fig. 19.3) has been to define lesion morphology and complexity. Complex disease warrants vessel prepping typically with some debulking or non-debulking methods to minimize vessel barotrauma and limit dissections and bailout stenting. Complex disease includes CTO, calcified disease, and long lesions. ISR, particularly in the setting of an occluded stent, will respond well to debulking followed by angioplasty and drug-coated balloons [56–60]. Angioplasty alone is not an optimal treatment and should be avoided in ISR. Noncomplex disease can be treated with angioplasty (with or without vessel prepping) followed by angioplasty and DCB (if no flow-limiting dissection) or DES (if flow-limiting dissection or significant residual narrowing). Stenting remains a class I indication in the guidelines because of randomized trials that show its superiority to angioplasty. The Zilver PTX stent was superior to angioplasty, but there is conflicting data to its superiority versus bare-metal stents [61, 62]. The Eluvia stent was superior to the Zilver PTX stent in the IMPERIAL randomized trial [63]. Bare-metal stents such as the Supera stent and more recently the BioMimics 3D stent seem to have very good long-term results

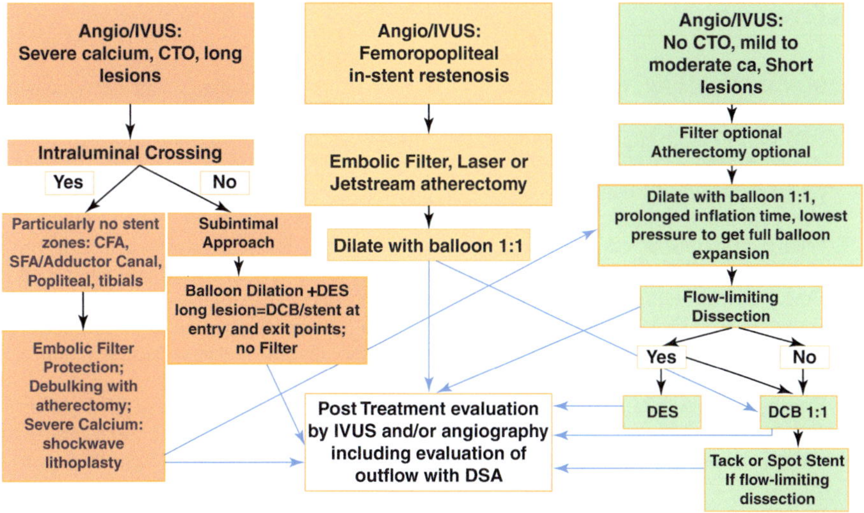

Fig. 19.3 Proposed algorithm in treating infrainguinal arterial disease based on lesion complexity and morphology

[64]. On the other hand, well-powered, large randomized trials with atherectomy versus angioplasty and/or stenting are not available, and therefore atherectomy remains a class III indication in the guidelines except for ISR. Observational data however support the role of atherectomy in improving acute procedural results although it is unclear if long-term outcomes are improved. The combination of atherectomy and DCBs however seems to have promising good long-term results, but also larger randomized trials are needed to conclusively demonstrate its effectiveness.

In conclusion, PAD patient should receive aggressive preventative therapies to reduce their morbidity and mortality. Modifying risk factors and exercise are important therapies for all PAD patients. Low-dose rivaroxaban with baby aspirin needs to be considered to reduce major adverse limb and cardiovascular events. Revascularization is reserved for those with severe limiting symptoms including severe claudication and advanced limb ischemia. A strategy of leaving the least behind has gained momentum in treating infrainguinal arterial disease (with vessel prepping and DCB). Bailout stenting or focal Tack Endovascular repair is considered with flow-limiting dissections. Primary stenting needs to be avoided when possible in no-stent zones such as the common femoral artery, distal superficial femoral artery, and popliteal artery. Stents are superior to balloon angioplasty, but well-powered randomized data comparing vessel prepping and DCB versus stenting (DES or BMS) are not available.

References

1. Biswas MP, Capell WH, McDermott MM, et al. Exercise training and revascularization in the management of symptomatic peripheral artery disease. JACC Basic Transl Sci. 2021;6(2):174–88. https://doi.org/10.1016/j.jacbts.2020.08.012. eCollection 2021 Feb.
2. Vogel J, Niederer D, Jung G, Troidl K. Exercise-induced vascular adaptations under artificially versus pathologically reduced blood flow: a focus review with special emphasis on arteriogenesis. Cell. 2020;9(2):333. https://doi.org/10.3390/cells9020333.
3. Fakhry F, Spronk S, van der Laan L, et al. Endovascular revascularization and supervised exercise for peripheral artery disease and intermittent claudication: a randomized clinical trial. JAMA. 2015;314(18):1936–44. https://doi.org/10.1001/jama.2015.14851.
4. Treat-Jacobson D, McDermott MM, Beckman J, et al. Implementation of supervised exercise therapy for patients with symptomatic peripheral artery disease: a science advisory from the American Heart Association. Circulation. 2019;140:e700–10.
5. Hirsch AT, Haskal ZJ, Hertzer NR, et al. ACC/AHA 2005 practice guidelines for the management of patients with peripheral arterial disease (lower extremity, renal, mesenteric, and abdominal aortic): a collaborative report from the American Association for Vascular Surgery/ Society for Vascular Surgery, Society for Cardiovascular Angiography and Interventions, Society for Vascular Medicine and Biology, Society of Interventional Radiology, and the ACC/AHA task force on practice guidelines (writing committee to develop guidelines for the Management of Patients with Peripheral Arterial Disease). Circulation. 2006;113:e463–654. https://doi.org/10.1161/CIRCULATIONAHA.106.174526.
6. Kumbhani DJ, Steg PG, Cannon CP, et al. Statin therapy and long-term adverse limb outcomes in patients with peripheral artery disease: insights from the REACH registry. Eur Heart J. 2014;35:2864–72.
7. Fowkes FG, Price JF, Stewart MC, Butcher I, Leng GC, Pell AC, Sandercock PA, Fox KA, Lowe GD, Murray GD, Aspirin for Asymptomatic Atherosclerosis Trialists. Aspirin for prevention of cardiovascular events in a general population screened for a low ankle brachial index: a randomized controlled trial. JAMA. 2010;303:841–8. https://doi.org/10.1001/jama.2010.221.
8. Gerhard-Herman MD, Gornik HL, Barrett C, et al. 2016 AHA/ACC guideline on the management of patients with lower extremity peripheral artery disease: a report of the American College of Cardiology/American Heart Association task force on clinical practice guidelines. J Am Coll Cardiol. 2017;69(11):e71–e126.
9. Bonaca MP, Bhatt DL, Storey RF, Steg PG, Cohen M, Kuder J, Goodrich E, Nicolau JC, Parkhomenko A, López-Sendón J, et al. Ticagrelor for prevention of ischemic events after myocardial infarction in patients with peripheral artery disease. J Am Coll Cardiol. 2016;67:2719–28. https://doi.org/10.1016/j.jacc.2016.03.524.
10. Eikelboom JW, Connolly SJ, Bosch J, Dagenais GR, Hart RG, Shestakovska O, Diaz R, Alings M, Lonn EM, Anand SS, et al. Rivaroxaban with or without aspirin in stable cardiovascular disease. N Engl J Med. 2017;377:1319–30. https://doi.org/10.1056/NEJMoa1709118.
11. Anand SS, Bosch J, Eikelboom JW, Connolly SJ, Diaz R, Widimsky P, Aboyans V, Alings M, Kakkar AK, Keltai K, et al. Rivaroxaban with or without aspirin in patients with stable peripheral or carotid artery disease: an international, randomised, double-blind, placebo-controlled trial. Lancet. 2018;391(10117):219–29. https://doi.org/10.1016/S0140-6736(17)32409-1. Epub 2017 Nov 10.
12. Bonaca MP, Bauersachs RM, Anand SS, Debus ES, Nehler MR, Patel MR, et al. Rivaroxaban in peripheral artery disease after revascularization. N Engl J Med. 2020;382(21):1994–2004.
13. Verma S, Rasmussen S, Saevereid HA, Ripa MS. Abstract 11456: Liraglutide and Semaglutide reduce cardiovascular events in patients with type 2 diabetes and peripheral arterial disease. Circulation. 2019;140:A11456.
14. Verma S, Mazer CD, Al-Omran M, Inzucchi SE, Fitchett D, Hehnke U, George JT, Zinman B. Cardiovascular outcomes and safety of Empagliflozin in patients with type 2 diabetes mellitus and peripheral artery disease. Circulation. 2018;137:405–7.

15. Bonaca MP, Wiviott SD, Zelniker TA, et al. Dapagliflozin and cardiac, kidney, and limb outcomes in patients with and without peripheral artery disease in DECLARE-TIMI 58. Circulation. 2020;142:734–47.
16. Neal B, Perkovic V, Mahaffey KW, et al. Canagliflozin and cardiovascular and renal events in type 2 diabetes. N Engl J Med. 2017;377:644–57.
17. Matthews DR, Li Q, Perkovic V, et al. Effects of canagliflozin on amputation risk in type 2 diabetes: the CANVAS program. Diabetologia. 2019;62:926–38.
18. Levin SR, Arinze N, Siracuse JJ. Lower extremity critical limb ischemia: a review of clinical features and management. Trends Cardiovasc Med. 2020;30(3):125–30. https://doi.org/10.1016/j.tcm.2019.04.002. Epub 2019 Apr 15.
19. Thompson PD, Zimet R, Forbes WP, Zhang P. Metaanalysis of results from eight randomized, placebo-controlled trials on the effect of cilostazol on patients with intermittent claudication. Am J Cardiol. 2002;90:1314–9.
20. Dawson DL, Cutler BS, Hiatt WR, et al. A comparison of cilostazol and pentoxifylline for treating intermittent claudication. Am J Med. 2000;109:523–30.
21. Iida O, Nanto S, Uematsu M, Morozumi T, Kitakaze M, Nagata S. Cilostazol reduces restenosis after endovascular therapy in patients with femoropopliteal lesions. J Vasc Surg. 2008;48:144–9.
22. de Donato G, Bosiers M, Setacci F, Deloose K, Galzerano G, Verbist J, et al. 24-month data from the BRAVISSIMO: a large-scale prospective registry on iliac stenting for TASC a & B and TASC C & D Lesions. Ann Vasc Surg. 2015;29(4):738–50.
23. Gabel JA, Kiang SC, Abou-Zamzam AM Jr, Oyoyo UE, Teruya TH, Tomihama RT. Trans-atlantic inter-society consensus class D aortoiliac lesions: a comparison of endovascular and open surgical outcomes. AJR Am J Roentgenol. 2019;213(3):696–701.
24. Suzuki K, Mizutani Y, Soga Y, Iida O, Kawasaki D, Yamauchi Y, et al. Efficacy and safety of endovascular therapy for aortoiliac TASC D lesions. Angiology. 2017;68(1):67–73.
25. Ichihashi S, Higashiura W, Itoh H, Sakaguchi S, Nishimine K, Kichikawa K. Long-term outcomes for systematic primary stent placement in complex iliac artery occlusive disease classified according to trans-atlantic inter-society consensus (TASC)-II. J Vasc Surg. 2011;53(4):992–9.
26. Radaideh Q, Shammas NW, Shammas WJ, Shammas GA. Shockwave™ lithoplasty in combination with atherectomy in treating severe calcified femoropopliteal and iliac artery disease: a single-center experience. Cardiovasc Revasc Med. 2021;22:66–70.
27. Armstrong EJ, Soukas PA, Shammas N, et al. Intravascular lithotripsy for treatment of calcified, stenotic iliac arteries: a cohort analysis from the disrupt PAD III study. Cardiovasc Revasc Med. 2020;21:1262–8.
28. Brodmann M, Wissgott C, Brechtel K, et al. Optimized drug-coated balloon angioplasty of the superficial femoral and proximal popliteal arteries using the Tack endovascular system: TOBA III 12-month results. J Vasc Surg. 2020;72:1636–1647.e1.
29. Gray W, Cardenas JA, Brodmann M, et al. Treating post-angioplasty dissection in the femoropopliteal arteries using the tack endovascular system: 12-month results from the TOBA II study. JACC Cardiovasc Interv. 2019;12:2375–84.
30. Shammas NW, Torey JT, Shammas WJ. Dissections in peripheral vascular interventions: a proposed classification using intravascular ultrasound. J Invasive Cardiol. 2018; 30:145–6.
31. Shammas NW, Torey JT, Shammas WJ, Jones-Miller S, Shammas GA. Intravascular ultrasound assessment and correlation with angiographic findings demonstrating femoropopliteal arterial dissections post atherectomy: results from the iDissection study. J Invasive Cardiol. 2018;30:240–4.
32. Shammas NW, Shammas WJ, Jones-Miller S, et al. Optimal vessel sizing and understanding dissections in infrapopliteal interventions: data from the iDissection below the knee study. J Endovasc Ther. 2020;27:575–80.
33. Shammas NW, Torey JT, Shammas WJ, et al. Intravascular ultrasound assessment and correlation with angiographic findings of arterial dissections following Auryon laser atherectomy

and adjunctive balloon angioplasty: results of the iDissection Auryon laser study. J Endovasc Ther. 2022;29(1):23–31. https://doi.org/10.1177/15266028211028200; 15266028211028200. Online ahead of print.
34. Tepe G, Zeller T, Schnorr B, et al. High-grade, non-flow-limiting dissections do not negatively impact long-term outcome after paclitaxel-coated balloon angioplasty: an additional analysis from the THUNDER study. J Endovasc Ther. 2013;20:792–800. https://doi.org/10.1583/13-4392R.1.
35. Shammas NW, Coiner D, Shammas GA, et al. Percutaneous lower-extremity arterial interventions with primary balloon angioplasty versus Silverhawk atherectomy and adjunctive balloon angioplasty: randomized trial. J Vasc Interv Radiol. 2011;22:1223–8.
36. Dattilo R, Himmelstein SI, Cuff RF. The COMPLI-ANCE 360° trial: a randomized, prospective, multi-center, pilot study comparing acute and long-term results of orbital atherectomy to balloon angioplasty for calcified femoropopliteal disease. J Invasive Cardiol. 2014;26:355–60.
37. Shammas NW, Lam R, Mustapha J, et al. Comparison of orbital atherectomy plus balloon angioplasty vs. balloon angioplasty alone in patients with critical limb ischemia: results of the CALCIUM 360 randomized pilot trial. J Endovasc Ther. 2012;19:480–8.
38. Shammas NW, Shammas WJ, Jones-Miller S, Radaideh Q, Shammas GA. Femoropopliteal arterial dissections post flex vessel prep and adjunctive angioplasty: results of the flex iDissection study. J Invasive Cardiol. 2019;31(5):121–6.
39. Tepe G, Brodmann M, Werner M, et al.; Disrupt PAD III Investigators. Intravascular lithotripsy for peripheral artery calcification: 30-day outcomes from the randomized disrupt PAD III trial. JACC Cardiovasc Interv. 2021;14(12):1352–1361.
40. Shammas NW. Optimal strategy in lower extremity peripheral percutaneous interventions: an interventionalist perspective. Vasc Dis Manag. 2009. https://www.hmpgloballearningnetwork.com/site/vdm/content/optimal-strategy-lower-extremity-peripheral-percutaneous-interventions-interventionalistaos. Accessed 3 July 2021.
41. Shammas NW. An overview of optimal endovascular strategy in treating the femoropopliteal artery: mechanical, biological, and procedural factors. Int J Angiol. 2013;22:1–8.
42. Roberts D, Niazi K, Miller W, et al. Effective endovascular treatment of calcified femoropopliteal disease with directional atherectomy and distal embolic protection: final results of the DEFINITIVE Ca++ trial. Catheter Cardiovasc Interv. 2014;84:236–44.
43. Shammas NW, Dippel EJ, Coiner D, et al. Preventing lower extremity distal embolization using embolic filter protection: results of the PROTECT registry. J Endovasc Ther. 2008;15:270–6. https://doi.org/10.1583/08-2397.1.
44. Shammas NW, Chandra P, Brodmann M, et al.; EX-PAD-03 Investigators. Acute and 30-day safety and effectiveness evaluation of Eximo Medical's B-laser™, a novel atherectomy device, in subjects affected with infrainguinal peripheral arterial disease: results of the EX-PAD-03 trial. Cardiovasc Revasc Med. 2020;21(1):86–92.
45. Shammas NW, Pucillo P, Jenkins JS, et al. WIRION embolic protection system in lower extremity arterial interventions: results of the pivotal WISE LE trial. JACC Cardiovasc Interv. 2018;11(19):1995–2003. https://doi.org/10.1016/j.jcin.2018.05.025.
46. Armstrong E, Brilakis E, Banerjee S, Shammas N, Radaideh Q. Events in femoropopliteal arterial interventions in a matched cohort of patients with critical limb ischemia: results from the XLPAD registry. J Am Coll Cardiol. 2020;76(17 Supplement S):B157–8.
47. Dippel E, Parikh N, Egeland R, Wallace K. TCT-162 distal embolization and protective devices: mortality, operating room time, length of stay, and costs. J Am Coll Cardiol. 2012;60(17_Supplement):B47.
48. Shammas NW, Shammas GA, Dippel EJ, Jerin M. Intraprocedural outcomes following distal lower extremity embolization in patients undergoing peripheral percutaneous interventions. Vasc Dis Manag. 2009;6:58–61.
49. Tepe G, Laird J, Schneider P, et al. Drug-coated balloon versus standard percutaneous transluminal angioplasty for the treatment of superficial femoral and popliteal peripheral artery disease: 12-month results from the IN.PACT SFA randomized trial. Circulation. 2015;131:495–502.

50. Rosenfield K, Jaff MR, White CJ, et al. Trial of a paclitaxel-coated balloon for femoropopliteal artery disease. N Engl J Med. 2015;373:145–53.
51. Ouriel K, Adelman MA, Rosenfield K, et al. Safety of paclitaxel-coated balloon angioplasty for femoropopliteal peripheral artery disease. JACC Cardiovasc Interv. 2019;12:2515–24.
52. Schneider PA, Laird JR, Tepe G, et al. Treatment effect of drug-coated balloons is durable to 3 years in the femoropopliteal arteries: long-term results of the IN.PACT SFA randomized trial. Circ Cardiovasc Interv. 2018;11:e005891.
53. Katsanos K, Spiliopoulos S, Kitrou P, Krokidis M, Karnabatidis D. Risk of death following application of paclitaxel-coated balloons and stents in the femoropopliteal artery of the leg: a systematic review and meta-analysis of randomized controlled trials. J Am Heart Assoc. 2018;7:e011245.
54. Dinh K, Limmer AM, Chen AZL, et al. Mortality rates after paclitaxel-coated device use in patients with occlusive femoropopliteal disease: an updated systematic review and meta-analysis of randomized controlled trials. J Endovasc Ther. 2021;28:755–77. https://doi.org/10.1177/15266028211023505. Online ahead of print.
55. Ren H, Liu J, Zhang J, et al. Association between postballoon angioplasty dissection and primary patency in complex femoropopliteal artery disease: 2-year clinical outcomes of the AcoArt I trial. J Int Med Res. 2021;49:1–12.
56. Zeller T, Langhoff R, Rocha-Singh KJ, et al. Directional atherectomy followed by a paclitaxel-coated balloon to inhibit restenosis and maintain vessel patency: twelve-month results of the DEFINITIVE AR study. Circ Cardiovasc Interv. 2017;10:e004848.
57. Cioppa A, Stabile E, Popusoi G, et al. Combined treatment of heavy calcified femoro-popliteal lesions using directional atherectomy and a paclitaxel coated balloon: one-year single centre clinical results. Cardiovasc Revasc Med. 2012;13:219–23.
58. Dippel EJ, Makam P, Kovach R, et al. Randomized controlled study of Excimer laser atherectomy for treatment of femoropopliteal in-stent restenosis: initial results from the EXCITE ISR trial (excimer laser randomized controlled study for treatment of femoropopliteal in-stent restenosis). JACC Cardiovasc Interv. 2015;8(1 Part A):92–101.
59. Gandini R, Del Giudice C, Merolla S, et al. Treatment of chronic SFA in-stent occlusion with combined laser atherectomy and drug-eluting balloon angioplasty in patients with critical limb ischemia: a single center, prospective, randomized study. J Endovasc Ther. 2013;20:805–14.
60. Shammas NW, Shammas GA, Jones-Miller S, et al. Long-term outcomes with Jetstream atherectomy with or without drug coated balloons in treating femoropopliteal arteries: a single center experience (JET-SCE). Cardiovasc Revasc Med. 2018;19(7 Pt A):771–7.
61. Gouëffic Y, Sauguet S, Desgranges P, et al. A polymer-free paclitaxel-eluting stent versus a bare-metal stent for De novo femoropopliteal lesions: the BATTLE trial. JACC Cardiovasc Interv. 2020;13(4):447–57. https://doi.org/10.1016/j.jcin.2019.12.028.
62. Dake MD, Ansel GM, Jaff MR, et al. Paclitaxel-eluting stents show superiority to balloon angioplasty and bare metal stents in femoropopliteal disease: twelve-month Zilver PTX randomized study results. Circ Cardiovasc Interv. 2011;4:495–504.
63. Gray WA, Keirse K, Soga Y, et al. A polymer-coated, paclitaxel-eluting stent (eluvia) versus a polymer-free, paclitaxel-coated stent (Zilver PTX) for endovascular femoropopliteal intervention (IMPERIAL): a randomised, non-inferiority trial. Lancet. 2018;392(10157):1541–51.
64. Garcia LA, Rosenfield KR, Metzger CD, et al. SUPERB final 3-year outcomes using interwoven nitinol biomimetic supera stent. Catheter Cardiovasc Interv. 2017;89(7):1259–67.

Index

N. W. Shammas (ed.), *Peripheral Arterial Interventions*, Contemporary Cardiology, https://doi.org/10.1007/978-3-031-09741-6

MIX
Papier aus verantwortungsvollen Quellen
Paper from responsible sources
FSC® C105338

If you have any concerns about our products, you can contact us on
ProductSafety@springernature.com

In case Publisher is established outside the EU, the EU authorized representative is:
Springer Nature Customer Service Center GmbH
Europaplatz 3, 69115 Heidelberg, Germany

Printed by Libri Plureos GmbH
in Hamburg, Germany